A Guide to
Practical Toxicology

A Guide to Practical Toxicology

Evaluation, prediction and risk

Adam Woolley

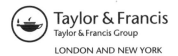

Taylor & Francis
Taylor & Francis Group

LONDON AND NEW YORK

First published 2003
by Taylor & Francis
11 New Fetter Lane, London EC4P 4EE

Simultaneously published in the USA and Canada
by Taylor & Francis Inc,
29 West 35th Street, New York, NY 10001

Taylor & Francis is an imprint of the Taylor & Francis Group

© 2003 Adam Woolley

Typeset in Goudy by Exe Valley Dataset Ltd, Exeter
Printed and bound in Great Britain by MPG Books Ltd, Bodmin

Every effort has been made to ensure that the advice and information in this
book is true and accurate at the time of going to press. However, neither the
publisher nor the author can accept any legal responsibility or liability for
any errors or omissions that may be made. In the case of drug
administration, any medical procedure or the use of technical equipment
mentioned within this book, you are strongly advised to consult the
manufacturer's guidelines.

British Library Cataloguing in Publication Data
A catalogue record for this book is available from the British Library

Library of Congress Cataloging in Publication Data
A catalog record for this book has been requested

ISBN 0-748-40923-8

For Sandy, David, Stewart and Kate

Contents

List of illustrations   xi
Preface   xiii
Acknowledgements   xv

1 Introduction to toxicology: the necessity of measurement   1

Introduction 1
The beginnings of toxicological measurement 2
Strong toxins and weak toxins 3
Toxicity defined 5
It is natural so it must be safe 8
General objectives of toxicological study 13
Nature and outcome of toxic reactions 14
Expression of toxicity 20
The necessity for toxicological assessment 27
The three Rs – reduce, refine and replace 31

2 Normality: definition and maintenance   34

Introduction 34
What is normality? 35
Experimental normality 37
Protocol design and procedure as sources of abnormality 41
Control groups as normality 41
Establishing and maintaining normality in experimental groups 43
The normality of baseline data 45

3 Determination of toxicity: basic principles   54

Introduction 54
Effects sought in toxicity studies 55
Regulatory framework and influences 56
Basic principles of toxicological investigation 59

4   Determination of toxicity *in vitro*   72

Introduction 72
Rationale for in vitro *toxicology; strengths and weaknesses 72*
Validation of in vitro *methods 73*
Test types and test systems 74
Toxicity in silico *74*
'Traditional' in vitro *toxicology 77*
Future utility 78
Pitfalls 78
Overview 79

5   Determination: general and reproductive toxicology   80

General toxicology 80
Test systems for general toxicology 80
Study designs in general toxicology 82
Examinations for specific toxicities 90
Pitfalls in general toxicology 93
Reproductive toxicology 95
Test systems for reproductive toxicology 97
Study designs for reproductive toxicology 100
Pitfalls in reproductive toxicology 105

6   Determination: genotoxicity and carcinogenicity   107

Genotoxicity 107
Test battery and study design 109
Test systems and tests 112
Pitfalls in genotoxicity 118
Carcinogenicity 119
Test systems for carcinogenicity 121
Study design and methods of assessment 123
Other systems for carcinogenicity assessment 126
Pitfalls in carcinogenicity studies 129
Overview of the future of carcinogenicity assessment 131

7   Determination: irritation and sensitisation   135

General principles 135
Factors in dermal toxicity 136
Test systems 137
Study design and parameters measured 137
Pitfalls in irritation and sensitisation 139

8   Determination: environmental toxicology and epidemiology   140

Environmental toxicology and ecotoxicology 140
Pollution, routes of entry and environmental ADME 141
Factors in testing for environmental effect 142
Test systems and study types for ecotoxicology 144
Pitfalls in environmental toxicology 147
Epidemiology – a brief review 148

9   Interpretation   151

Introduction 151
Steps in interpretation 153
Use of background data in interpretation 155
Statistics and significance in toxicology 156
Assessing exposure 161
The reality of difference – the interpretation of small differences 166
The reproducibility of difference 168
Interpretation of different data types 168
Case studies – ciprofibrate and genetically modified potatoes 189
The fundamentals of interpretation 194

10   Prediction of hazard   195

Introduction 195
Principles of prediction 197
Steps in the prediction process 199
Factors for consideration in prediction 203
Prediction from minimal databases 207
Computer models for toxicity prediction 209
Prediction for individuals 217
Prediction summary 218

11   Background to risk due to toxicity   219

Introduction 219
Overview of risk assessment 219
Levels of risk and factors that affect risk 220
Risk perception 223
Comparative risk 227
Risk expression and quantification 231
Summary 232

12   Risk assessment in practice and setting exposure limits   234

Introduction 234
Single effect versus general risk assessment 234

Tools and models in risk assessment 235
Target population, dose and exposure 239
Process and factors in risk assessment 243
Setting safety factors and margins 250
Exposure limits 252
Summary 258

13　Risk assessment and management in the workplace　260

Introduction 260
The historical and regulatory background 260
Factors in workplace risk assessment 261
Workplace risk assessment 262
Risk management in the workplace 264
Overview 268

**14　Risk assessment: carcinogenicity; the environment;
evolution and overview of risk assessment　270**

Introduction 270
Notes on risk assessment and carcinogenicity 270
Notes on risk assessment and the environment 280
The evolution of risk assessment 285
Overview of risk assessment 286

15　The future of toxicity testing　290

Introduction 290
Current practice 290
Current dynamics and pressures 291
Utility of animal experiments in risk assessment 292
Development of new test methods 293
In vitro toxicology and the future 294
Toxicology in silico 296
The future of safety evaluation 296

Appendix: useful websites　298
Select glossary　300
Notes　304
Bibliography　311
Index　313

Illustrations

Figures

1.1	Mechanism of paraquat toxicity	19
1.2	Ipomeanol	20
2.1	Characteristics of the normal distribution	36
5.1	The river of reproduction	95
5.2	The stages of human embryogenesis	96
9.1	Statistical process for continuous data	160
10.1	Structure of 4-hydrazinobenzoic acid	209
12.1	A simple physiologically based pharmacokinetic model	237

Tables

1.1	Comparative toxicity – approximate lethal doses (mg/kg) for various compounds according to chemical class, route of administration and species	4
1.2	Acute toxicity of TCDD in different species	4
1.3	Factors in target organ toxicity	23
2.1	Probability of a given sample of animals containing at least one case for different background incidence levels	49
2.2	Maximum background incidence that would yield a zero result in a sample	49
4.1	In vitro test systems	75
5.1	Test systems for general toxicology	81
5.2	Summary of basic designs for general toxicology	83
5.3	Organs and tissues that may be retained after post-mortem	88
5.4	Stage of reproductive cycle and preferred test systems	97
5.5	Reproductive parameters	103
6.1	Genetic associations with cancers	107
6.2	Direct-acting positive controls used in the Ames test	110
6.3	Principal genotoxicity test systems	113
6.4	Comparative data from transgenic models	128
6.5	Processes or mechanisms in carcinogenicity and markers of effect	132
9.1	The effect of variability in data on summary statistics	159
9.2	Selected ADME factors and their impact on toxicity	164
9.3	Classic associations in toxicology	170

9.4   Troubleshooting in general toxicology   171
9.5   Troubleshooting in reproductive toxicology   176
9.6   Guide to genotoxicity interpretation   177
9.7   Troubleshooting in genotoxicity   178
9.8   Carcinogen classification   179
9.9   Guide to carcinogenicity interpretation   181
9.10   Factors to consider in environmental toxicology   182
9.11   Factors in epidemiology and occupational toxicity   186
10.1   Endpoints predicted by expert systems   210
12.1   Models for risk assessment   238
12.2   Definitions of exposure limits   253
12.3   Calculating an OEL for thalidomide using different methods   256
12.4   OEL calculation for ethinyl oestradiol, a synthetic oestrogen   256
13.1   A basic system of compound categorisation   265

Boxes

1.1   Toxicities associated with natural remedies   10
1.2   Studies with the constituents of mushrooms   30
3.1   Factors in test system selection   65
3.2   Troubleshooting dose range-finding results   70
5.1   Characteristics of test systems for general toxicology   81–2
5.2   In-life observations and measurements in general toxicology   85
5.3   Characteristics of test systems for reproductive toxicology   98–9
5.4   Outline designs for example reproductive studies   101
6.1   Additional means of assessing carcinogenic potential   126–7
6.2   Transgenic animals in carcinogenicity assessment   127–8
9.1   Confirmation of the validity of the control data   154
9.2   Questions in assessment of exposure   162
10.1   Desirable database for prediction of human relevant hazard   202
10.2   Prediction from minimal databases   208
10.3   Prediction of toxicity in paracetamol overdose   218
11.1   Cholinesterase inhibition: factors in risk determination   221–2
11.2   Genetically modified foods   225–6
11.3   Elements of comparative risk   228
11.4   Risk and chemicals naturally present in food   230
12.1   Assessment of exposure – basic principles   241
12.2   Factors to be considered in risk assessment   244
12.3   Choosing safety factors   250–1
12.4   Setting exposure limits   257–8
13.1   Risk management in the workplace   267
14.1   DNA vulnerability – endogenous damage and repair   272
14.2   Thresholds in carcinogenicity   275–6
14.3   Methylene chloride and cancer   278
14.4   Environmental risk assessment of MTBE use in Europe   282–3
14.5   Notes on international management of toxic risks   285
14.6   Methylene chloride and evolution in risk assessment   287

Preface

This book arose out of my perception that there is a large amount of toxicology lore which is widely accepted as fact and used in toxicological reports but is not supported by easily accessible references. I also felt that there was a need for a practical, user friendly introductory text for those coming to toxicology from related fields or professions and who need some insight into how toxicity studies and investigations are carried out. This was seen as including new graduates starting careers in toxicology as well as specialists in particular areas of toxicology who need some background on the other areas. I felt that the book should be informative but readable and should also act as a gateway to the subject, indicating where further information can be found, including the use of websites for literature searches and other areas such as regulations and guidelines.

Throughout the book words like 'may', 'could' and 'however' appear frequently; this is tacit recognition that there are few certainties in life beyond the single gold standard that wherever a statement is made there will be someone to disagree with it. This is particularly true for any aspect or judgement or interpretation; differing opinions between toxicologists, especially toxicological pathologists, can be extremely frustrating for anyone needing a definite answer to a question of safety. Getting a decision wrong in toxicology can be associated with far reaching adverse effects and with consequent litigation or (politically far worse) loss of votes. For this reason toxicologists (especially those in regulatory agencies) tend to be conservative in their opinions; this is not necessarily a bad thing.

In view of the vastness of the subject, this book cannot hope to be detailed or complete; for reasons of brevity and time, there is no section on safety pharmacology and treatment of epidemiology is kept short. In view of this the intention is to provide a basis of knowledge – a series of pointers – which can be expanded through use of the bibliography and references given. There are many different ways of achieving an objective in toxicological study and evaluation and this book cannot pretend to address them all or to be absolutely definitive in any one area. Toxicologists are known for their differences in opinions and I am just another opinionated toxicologist.

Acknowledgements

It is unlikely that such a wide ranging text could be prepared in isolation and I have sought people to review individual sections for sense. Having said that, all the opinions expressed are my own, as is responsibility for any errors that may still lurk in the text. I would particularly like to acknowledge and thank the following for their assistance with the indicated sections: Genotoxicity – Patricia Collins (Sequani) and Mike Kelly (Oxford Glycosciences); Reproductive toxicity – Mandy Irvine (Quintiles); Environmental toxicity – Reinhard Laenge (Schering); Risk assessment and management in the workplace – Neil Bradshaw (Pharmaceutical Consultant). Advice on pathology was received from Moira Jones at Quintiles. I also wish to register my thanks for significant input and encouragement from Guy Healing, John Fowler and Sandy Woolley in making comments which helped form the book. Finally I want to thank Dilys Alam and Grant Soanes at Taylor & Francis for their patience in tolerating the painfully slow gestation of this project.

Chapter 1

Introduction to toxicology

The necessity of measurement

Introduction

Toxicology is the science of poisons and the definition of a poison can be as wide or as narrow as considered appropriate by the author or speaker. Toxicology is a science which has a direct impact on, and responsibility to, the public in a way that other subjects, for instance astronomy or particle physics, do not. This responsibility arises from the role that toxicology has in assessing the safety of chemicals that have been or will be, in daily use or to which the public are exposed. If the assessment is wrong there is a distinct probability that adverse effects will be seen in exposed populations or that the benefits of a new chemical will be denied to people who would be advantaged by its use.

The public perception of toxicity is very important to people who conduct or interpret toxicological investigations. A change may be perceived as adverse through incomplete access to all information and this will provoke questions. When is a cluster of disease patients significant? How do you investigate? Who should we believe? Why? What is the true, unprejudiced significance of this finding for the exposed population? Major concerns of the public are cancer, loss of 'special senses' (especially sight), general debilitation, reproductive effects, disease or shortened lifespan. Much emphasis is placed on exposure to pesticides in food, without concern about the natural chemicals that occur in the same plants (e.g. mushrooms), or on exposure to low-level radiation but not on sunbathing and consequent increased risk of skin cancer, including melanoma.

The science of toxicology progresses by default. Accidents and emergencies, whether involving human, animal or plant life, often provide salutary lessons. After the discharge of dioxins at Seveso in 1976, prolonged investigations told us that dioxin is very toxic to animals in various ways; it is clear that humans suffer chloracne but other effects in humans are unproven or unknown. The discharge of inorganic mercury waste at Minimata bay in Japan taught us that nature does not always make things safer – it can increase hazard – in that case by methylation and increasing lipophilicity of the mercury such that the human food-chain was affected. It is automatically assumed by many that synthetic chemicals are harmful, but this assumption may ignore significant benefits.

In the developed world, pharmaceutical standards and purity are assumed and are regulated; not so the quality of 'designer drugs' or the diluent of pharmaceutical cocaine. The expanding market for herbal extracts and remedies provides real cause for concern; are the sources correctly identified, processed, stored and labelled?

Treatment of some foods, such as peanuts in store, with mould-preventing chemicals carries some risk from the chemical but markedly reduces risk of liver cancer due to aflatoxin, which is produced by the mould *Aspergillus flavus* growing on damp-stored peanuts. Aflatoxin is a particularly potent hepatotoxin and carcinogen which may induce cancer at levels as low as 1 ppb; it has been found in trace amounts in peanut butter prepared from untreated peanuts. This could be sold as 'organic' peanut butter; does this support the campaign for organic production?

The beginnings of toxicological measurement

Although not always known as toxicology, this fascinating amalgam of different disciplines has had a long history, stemming from the Eberus papyrus of the ancient Egyptians and progressing steadily through ancient Greece and Rome. In Greece and Rome the knowledge of poisons was crucial in eliminating unwanted politicians, rivals or relatives; this was particularly noted in some Roman wives who used contract poisoners to do away with rich husbands so that they could inherit the wealth and move on to the next hapless, but temptingly rich, victim. This cheerful habit was revived in Rennaisance Italy, a society in which dwarves were created by feeding known growth inhibitors to children; in *A Midsummer Night's Dream* Shakespeare writes 'Get you gone, you dwarf . . . of hindering knotgrass made'.

It was clear to the practitioners of the day that the dose was the critical factor determining success or failure. However, it was Paracelsius, born in 1541, who linked dose with effect by stating that the dose differentiates between a poison and a remedy. To put this in a modern context, a daily glass of red wine is considered to be therapeutically beneficial; increase that to a bottle or more a day and cirrhosis of the liver beckons.

It is usually fairly easy to say what dose of a chemical is toxic or harmful but much more difficult to predict safety. While the concept of 'poisonous' was understood, for instance in the seventeenth century, as the effect of poisons or of an excess of something, the concept of safety was of little concern. The work of people like Percival Potts, who linked scrotal cancer in former chimney sweeps with prior exposure to soot, led to gradual recognition of safety as a concept. However, in line with modern practice, it took many years to do anything about it.

With the enormous increase in the use of chemicals that has taken place during the late nineteenth century and in the twentieth century, it has become apparent that there should be an increasing emphasis on demonstration of safety. This concern for safety is applied in many areas, including novel or genetically modified foods. In some cases, where a traditional or long-used chemical is known to be unsafe, efforts are made to find a substitute. When the search is successful it is sometimes the case that the substitute removes the old problems while introducing new ones. However, it is generally accepted that to predict safety – given that there is no such thing as a 'safe' chemical or a risk-free existence – it is necessary first to demonstrate what dose of the study chemical is toxic and how that toxicity develops as dose increases.

In the modern context there is public recognition that there are chemicals to which people are exposed voluntarily (cigarette smoke, medicines and alcohol, for example) and those in which exposure is involuntary (pesticides in vegetables, other people's cigarette smoke, pollution, food preservatives, antibiotics in food animals and so on). There is a lively public debate on many of these substances, which often takes extreme views due to lack of knowledge or wilful misinformation or misinterpretation by interested parties. It is a fact that promotion of tobacco was discontinued in UK in 1965 – so what are the advertisements for? To cause smokers to switch brands? Such fine lines are drawn by politicians but it is the responsibility of the toxicological community to define safe doses or inclusion limits for these various chemicals. Above all, this must be done in a credible manner, within the existing framework of regulation and ethical behaviour.

In addition, there is a growing body of scientific work investigating the effects of chemicals that occur naturally in our food. For instance, it has been shown in several papers that some constituents of mushrooms can cause cancer in mice when given at high dosages. It should be borne in mind that, in the correct circumstances, administration of water might be capable of inducing cancer, although it is more often a cause of drowning. If a study was conducted that demonstrated that water was a carcinogen, would this mean that we should give up drinking water or convert it to beer? The relationship between dosage and harmful effects is crucial in the assessment of chemicals, including those that occur in a natural diet. Given that much of the exposure of people to individual chemicals is at low levels, the fact that many may cause cancer at high levels is probably not significant for everyday life. Furthermore, it is important to remember that the majority of testing is performed on single substances, whereas the majority of exposure is to many substances simultaneously, for example in a normal diet. Life is about mixtures.

Strong toxins and weak toxins

A reasonably clear ranking of potency among chemicals can be established when appropriate compounds are selected for comparison (Table 1.1). Thus TCDD (tetrachlorodibenzo-p-dioxin) is one of the most potent chemicals known, and can be lethal to guinea pigs at 1 μg/kg of bodyweight, while the lethal dose of an everyday substance such as paracetamol (acetaminophen) is very much higher. However, this type of ranking is, in some ways, distorting as the potency of any chemical can change markedly depending on the species under consideration, TCDD being 20–50 times less toxic in rats (Table 1.2). Organophosphate insecticides are much more toxic, by design, in insects than in mammals. Table 1.1 also shows the differing toxicities according to species and route of administration.

Table 1.1 Comparative toxicity – approximate lethal doses (mg/kg) for various compounds according to chemical class, route of administration and species

Compound (class)	Species	Route of administration		
		Oral	Parenteral[a]	Dermal
Botulin toxin	Mice		0.000002 (ip)	
Ethanol	Man (est.)	7000		
	Mice	10,000		
Digitoxin (cardiac glycoside)	Cat	0.18		
	Guinea pig	60		
DDT (OC insecticide)	Rats	113		
Methoxychlor (OC insecticide)	Rats	6,000		
Nicotine	Rat	50		
	Rabbit			50
Paracetamol (analgesic)	Man (est.)	250		
	Mice	340	500 (ip)	
Pentobarbital (barbiturate)	Mice	280	80 iv.: 130 (im, ip)	
Phenytoin (anticonvulsant)	Mice	490	92 (iv)	110
Malathion (OP insecticide)	Rat	1000		>4000
Parathion (OP insecticide)	Male rat	4		
	Female rat	13		
Soman/VX (OP nerve gas)	Man (est.)	0.007 (iv)		0.142
	Rat	0.012 (sc)		
	Guinea pig	0.008 (sc)		

Notes: [a]Parenteral routes: iv, intravenous; im, intramuscular; ip, intraperitoneal; sc, subcutaneous.
OC, organochlorine; OP, organophosphorus.
Compiled from the various reference texts listed in the Bibliography.

Table 1.2 Acute toxicity of TCDD in different species

Species	LD50 (µg/kg)
Guinea pig	1
Male rat	22
Female rat	45
Mouse	114
Rabbit	115
Hamster	5000
Monkey	70

Source: Compiled from Poland, A and Knutson, JC. '2,3,7,8-Tetrachlorodibenzo-p-dioxin and related halogenated aromatic hydrocarbons: examination of the mechanism of toxicity'. Annual Review of Pharmacology and Toxicology 1982 22: 517–54.

The toxicity of a substance is determined by the following factors:

- Dose
- The individual exposed
- Species
- Presence or absence of receptors
- Frequency of dosing – single or repeated
- Duration of exposure or administration
- Route of exposure
- Absorption/metabolism
- Protein binding and disturbance due to competitive binding or deficiency of sites
- Physical form
     Liquid – viscous or free flowing, volatile or inert; aqueous or organic
     Solution – concentrated or not
     Solid – dust, inert mass, crystalline or amorphous
- Presence of other chemicals – synergistic, additive or inhibitory effects

When a substance is a strong or potent toxin it is usually readily apparent from its effects on humans or other animals. The majority of debate comes at the lower end of the potency spectrum, particularly with synthetic chemicals such as pesticides, to which people are exposed at homeopathic low levels in everyday life. The bottom line is that we are exposed daily to thousands of chemicals, the majority of which occur naturally in our food and environment and about which very little is known in terms of toxicity. As far as food is concerned, as a result of culture and tradition, foods that are harmful are avoided or are treated specially before consumption. Thus, red kidney beans and cassava root are harmful if they are not properly prepared before eating due to the presence of toxins in the raw food. Fugu fish, a delicacy in Japan, requires careful removal of the skin, liver and ovaries, which contain a potent nerve poison, tetrodotoxin, to which there is no antidote. Equally, there are ancient remedies, such as some herbal teas, which were given to people who were ill; the tendency to use these teas daily can result in unwanted side effects. Thus, a traditional remedy may be safe when used as tradition indicates but becomes harmful if used incorrectly or in combination. Ginseng and gingko is a newly popular combination that was not used in history and that has not been fully evaluated by modern techniques.

Toxicity defined

The *Dictionary of Toxicology* (2nd edition, Macmillan Reference Ltd, 1998) defines toxicity as 'the ability of a chemical to cause a deleterious effect when the organism is exposed to the chemical'. The *Oxford English Dictionary* indicates that toxicity is a 'toxic or poisonous quality, especially in relation to its degree or strength'. These definitions contain a number of important concepts, such as deleterious effect, exposure of an organism and that of degree or strength. However, in many ways they throw up more questions than they answer. What is a deleterious effect or a toxic or poisonous quality? A simpler definition might be that it is an adverse change from normality, which may be irreversible; but this requires definition of adverse change and, crucially, of normality.

An adverse change is one that affects the well-being of the organism, either temporarily or permanently, while normality is probably best considered in statistical terms of the normal distribution with a mean plus or minus two standard deviations. Towards the upper and lower limits of such a population the decision as to whether a value is normal or abnormal may become more complex and open to debate. In the absence of quantitative or semi-quantitative data the decision as to what constitutes normality becomes subjective and dependent on the judgement or prejudices of the decision-maker. In crude terms it is easy to define some changes as adverse; for instance cirrhosis of the liver is an irreversible change which is often associated with early death. In cases where this is brought on by drinking excessive amounts of alcohol it is easy to conclude that alcohol is toxic. However, at low doses alcohol is considered to be beneficial.

How, then, to separate toxicity from the norm or from effects that are potentially beneficial? This question is valid for all substances to which we are exposed, whether these are natural constituents of our diet or synthetic chemicals such as pharmaceuticals or pesticides. At what point does alcohol cease to be beneficial and to have an adverse effect? The advice given by doctors tends to conflict with that given by fitness instructors; should you abstain completely, take a daily dose of your preferred drink, leave one day per week alcohol-free or what? With medicines the question becomes much more complex because beneficial effects, such as treatment to kill a tumour, may be associated with unpleasant side effects that, in a normal person, would be clearly adverse. Nausea and vomiting would be unacceptable as routine side effects of an analgesic for headaches but are accepted in cancer treatment where the 'cost' of side effects is offset by the benefit of a potential cure.

Much of the effort that is put into the determination of toxicity has the ultimate motive of assessing or predicting safety in terms of daily exposure levels that can be expected to have no long-term adverse effect. Some toxicity investigations are undertaken to elucidate the mechanism by which a substance is toxic, when effects have been shown in toxicity studies or through epidemiological investigation or clinical experience. The discovery of the mechanism by which paracetamol (acetaminophen) is toxic has greatly contributed to the successful treatment of overdose.

For synthetic chemicals, whether they are intended to be pharmaceuticals, pesticides, industrial chemicals or intermediates used in the synthetic pathways for these substances, there is a clear need to define toxicity so that any adverse effects can be understood and their effects in humans can be predicted. This need is relevant as much to the people producing the chemical as to the eventual consumers. The definition of toxicity is important for natural chemicals as well, although the usual reaction to the toxicity of such substances – for instance vitamin A – is one of surprise and disbelief. If a small amount is good for you, essential even, then getting a large dose must be particularly beneficial. Vitamin A is, perhaps, a special example in that it occurs at the correct levels in a normal, balanced diet, but is taken widely as a supplement to the extent that there have been incidences where it has been taken to excess and caused toxicity, such as birth defects. Early Arctic explorers recorded that polar bear liver made them ill, which is due to its very high content of vitamin A.

The necessity for the study of toxicity becomes less clear when the chemical in question is a natural constituent of a normal diet. For example, much effort has been invested in the various chemical constituents of mushrooms. At high doses, it has been shown that it is possible to induce cancer in Swiss mice when they are fed unrealistically high concentrations of the individual chemicals found in mushrooms or of whole or processed mushrooms. Once again it is necessary to invoke Paracelsius and point out that response is dependent on dose. We should question the conclusion of research that implies that we should be careful about or give up eating a vegetable because a constituent can cause cancer at high levels of ingestion in rodents. There is also the paradox that fruit and vegetables are known to be 'good' for you but there is also the realisation that they contain many chemicals that may be toxic if enormous doses are taken. This is especially true when they are taken or administered in isolation from their natural source or context.

In assessing safety, one of the prime concerns is whether the test chemical is capable of causing or promoting cancer. However, one of the basic problems here is that cancer is expected to develop in between 25 and 40 per cent of the population, depending on source of estimate, and that it is very diverse in form and causation. Its origins are multifactorial and often cannot readily be ascribed individually to a particular cause, with some exceptions such as lung cancer due to smoking. Thus, if someone regularly consumed 100 g of mushrooms each day, as part of an otherwise balanced diet, it would probably not be possible to ascribe a stomach cancer diagnosed in old age to the ingestion of unusually large amounts of mushrooms. In addition, many cancers have latency periods that may last many years and a tumour such as mesothelioma, due to asbestos, may occur 30–40 years after the causative exposure. Many dietary constituents are potentially carcinogenic at high doses but that does not mean that we should give up eating the normal foods in which they occur. Some toxicities that are related to diet are ascribable to chemicals that result from deterioration of the food during storage. For instance, Balkan endemic nephropathy has been linked to ochratoxin resulting from fungal growth on grain that has been badly stored. Clearly, it is important that we should understand such effects and attempt to reduce the risk as far as possible.

It is natural so it must be safe – everyday toxicity conundrums

At the end of 1999, the website of the American Council on Science and Health (ACSH) published a Christmas dinner menu listing the chemicals that are found naturally in an everyday diet. The listing included hydrazines in mushroom soup, allyl isothiocyanate in broccoli spears, aniline and caffeic acid in carrots, psoralens in celery and, finally, a long (and incomplete) list of chemicals found in coffee. No one is suggesting that consumption of normal quantities of a Christmas dinner is going to be associated with unacceptable toxicity but the list gives some perspective on the relevance of chemical intake and the fact that many toxins cannot be avoided. Bruce Ames and Lois Swirsky Gold have pointed out that over 99 per cent of the chemicals that people ingest occur naturally in a normal diet. However, the chemicals listed in this article, although safe when eaten in a normal diet, are variously mutagenic, carcinogenic in rodents, associated with contact hypersensitivity and phototoxicity or are simply toxic when given in their pure form at high concentrations to rodents. It is not sensible to assume that natural chemicals are safe, just as it is not sensible to assume that a synthetic chemical is inevitably toxic.

For the majority of chemicals it is possible to plot increasing toxic effect against increasing dose to produce a dose–response curve which is sigmoid in shape. For some chemicals, the response curve is U-shaped. For chemicals that are essential for the well-being of an organism, such as vitamin A, there is an optimum range of dose over which normality is found. Below this dose, increasing evidence of deficiency is seen and above it there is evidence of toxicity that increases with dose. This type of finding is common to many vitamins or other essential naturally occurring chemicals. Another type of response curve is shown by aspirin, which inhibits platelet aggregation at low dose (reducing the incidence of heart attacks), is active at normal doses for inflammation or pain, but becomes toxic at high doses. The difference with aspirin is that it is not essential and absence from a normal diet will not be associated with adverse effect.

At what point should findings in toxicological experiments alert us to hazards arising from routine exposure to individual chemicals? To answer this requires that the toxicological hazard is actually due to the chemical under study and confirmation that the mechanism of toxicity is relevant to humans. For some rodent carcinogens, this question is easy to answer. Where there is a direct effect on DNA that can lead to cancer, often at low doses as for aflatoxin, there is a clear human-relevant hazard. Where the mechanism of carcinogenicity is not related to direct DNA damage but to a non-genotoxic effect the answer is less clear. Many rodent carcinogens achieve their effects through non-genotoxic mechanisms that are not relevant in humans. d-Limonene is carcinogenic in the kidney of male rats through formation of slowly degraded complexes with α-2u globulin, a protein found at high concentrations in the urine only of male rats.

This protein is normally degraded in lysosomes in the kidney, but when it is complexed with d-limonene, this degradation is slowed, resulting in overload of the lysosomes and necrosis in the proximal tubule cells and regenerative cell division. The resulting hyperplasia can lead to the formation of cancers. Because α-2u globulin is specific to male rats, this effect is of no relevance to human health.

A further example of non-genotoxic carcinogenicity in animals that is not relevant to human health is peroxisome proliferation and the subsequent induction of liver tumours in rats and mice. Other species have been shown not to respond to these agents in this way, notably in a seven-year study with a peroxisome-proliferating hypolipidaemic compound in marmosets (see the ciprofibrate case study in chapter 9). This same study indicated that stomach tumours seen in rats were also specific to that species. The risks of peroxisome proliferation and the relevance of this to humans are looked at in greater detail in the chapters on risk assessment (chapters 12–14).

This should not be taken to imply, however, that non-genotoxic carcino-genicity is irrelevant to humans, as a large number of human cancers, such as colon or breast cancer, are attributable to such mechanisms. However, in general if a chemical is carcinogenic by a non-genotoxic mechanism in one species of rodent (perhaps in one sex), at doses that are very much higher than those found in routine human exposure, it is probable that this effect is not relevant to humans.

It is relatively easy to identify chemicals that damage DNA and are muta-genic by *in vitro* tests. Detection of human-relevant non-genotoxic effect is more complicated as there are many more endpoints, but this would seem to be the route of the future for investigations of carcinogenic potential.

The fear of cancer is very real as it is a widespread condition that very often has unpleasant side effects and is frequently fatal. However, this fear is usually reserved for new untried factors or for occupational exposures that become associated over a period of years with cancer. Furthermore, cancer is not the only hazard of which people should be aware; there are many toxic properties contained in apparently innocuous preparations and foods which are used routinely and without concern.

Natural medicines and poisons

A wide range of herbs has been used in traditional medicines, often in teas and infusions that were taken as indicated by a physician or herbalist. There has been an unfortunate tendency to drink these teas regularly as a tonic and this over-frequent use can result in serious unwanted effects. Herbs often contain pharmacologically active compounds of great potency and, apart from toxicity arising from excessive pharmacological action, can have carcinogenic and teratogenic properties.

Box 1.1 Toxicities associated with natural remedies[1]

Traditional remedies, often taken as herbal teas, sometimes have highly pharmacologically active constituents and innocent overuse can have significant adverse effects.

- Ginseng is used in Chinese medicine for impotence, fatigue, ulcers and stress. It contains active compounds that produce CNS stimulation and increase gastrointestinal motility. Chronic or excessive use can be associated with diarrhoea, nervousness, cardiac effects and nervous system disturbances and imbalance of fluids and electrolytes.
- Comfrey (*Symphytum* sp.), which has been used as a wound healer, anti-irritative, anti-rheumatic, anti-inflammatory, contains pyrrolizidine alkaloids, which are highly hepatotoxic and potentially carcinogenic through damage to DNA. Daily consumption of comfrey over several years in salads or teas can lead to liver toxicity, teas derived from the roots being particularly hazardous; in addition the preparations may be fetotoxic.
- Fresh garlic has wide antimicrobial activity, fibrinolytic activity, reduces blood cholesterol and lipid concentrations and reduces formation of atherosclerotic plaque. However, taken to excess it can induce nausea, vomiting, diarhoea and bronchospasm; it is also associated with contact dermatitis attributed to the presence of antibacterial sulphides.

There are many instances of interactions between herbal remedies and prescribed drugs, either through increased or decreased effect. Even simple dietary components can have unexpected effects; grapefruit juice consumption is known to be associated with inhibition of cytochrome P450 (CYP3A4), which is responsible for the metabolism of a wide range of drugs. This has been associated with increased plasma concentrations of cisapride, a drug given for irritable bowel syndrome, leading to cardiac arrythmias in some patients. Inhibition of cisapride metabolism, which probably takes place in the small intestine, can increase the likelihood of these life-threatening effects. A similar effect has been reported with carbamazapine, a drug given in epilepsy. Equally, administration of metabolism inhibitors can have useful effects, for instance in reducing the doses of some drugs needed to achieve therapeutic effect.

With the commonplace example of grapefruit juice, it becomes clear that there are unsuspected risk factors in everyday existence; equally, given the multitude of such risks, attempts to account for all of them and lead a risk-free existence are probably doomed to failure. Another unsuspected source of risk is honey. There would normally be no reason to suspect honey as potentially harmful, but when it is produced from rhododendron flowers it is very toxic, two teaspoons being enough for adverse effect in some subjects.

Many natural substances or mixtures have been associated with abuse and resultant toxicity, prime examples being tobacco, cannabis and opium.

Natural versus synthetic

Digitalis from the foxglove has been known for hundreds of years and was commonly used in cases of oedema (dropsy), essentially as a diuretic with cardiac side effects that gradually came to be appreciated as a primary action of the drug. The foxglove contains a number of pharmacologically potent cardiac glycosides, which have a complex range of actions on the cardiovascular system, seen at low doses. They are used in congestive heart failure and sometimes to decrease the ventricular rate in atrial fibrillation. The initial mixture of numerous active constituents has been refined to the extent that single compounds are now used, for example digoxin. However, absorption tends to be variable and this, together with a steep dose–response curve, makes therapy more hazardous than is desirable. With the advent of modern pharmaceutical research, new cardioactive agents were discovered that are safer than digitalis, especially the calcium channel blockers, such as verapamil, diltiazem or nifedipine. These have dose–response curves that are less steep than digitalis drugs and so are easier to use because the toxic dose is appreciably higher than the therapeutic dose. In this instance the synthetic drug is safer to use than the naturally derived agent, having a more targeted action and a much smaller range of adverse side effects. The original problem with digitalis extract, that of administering an imprecisely defined mixture of highly potent alkaloids with wide-ranging effects, has been gradually circumvented by purification and finally by synthesis of carefully targeted molecules.

The effects of endogenous chemicals are, in some cases, mimicked by those of foreign compounds. Compounds such as opium and morphine have well-known addictive properties and share some properties with neuropeptides that are present naturally in mammals. Opium is a mixture of alkaloids that includes morphine, of which codeine is a methyl derivative; as with digitalis, use of opium, which was known to the ancient Greeks, gave way to the use of the individual compounds. The complex range of actions of opioids is explained by the presence of several receptor types for which endogenous peptides have been discovered. These peptides – the endogenous opiates – of which endorphins are one example, are produced in reaction to stress, such as exercise, and there is increasing evidence that, like their natural plant-derived counterparts, they have addictive properties. Exercise-induced euphoria – runner's high – is a relatively frequent term in the literature and endorphin release is associated with alterations in pain perception, feelings of well-being and lowered appetite. It has been suggested that the euphoria leads to altered perception of risk and may be associated with some accidents where joggers are hit by cars. Another possible side effect of excessive exercise is that addiction to the endogenous opioids may be associated with eating disorders, including anorexia.[2–4]

The natural versus synthetic debate should not be left without consideration of the issue of transgenic materials. Transgenic indicates the transfer of genetic material from one species to another, often from another taxonomic phylum. One example is transgenic maize produced by inclusion of a gene from *Bacillus thuringensis* that expresses an insecticidal protein which kills maize borers, a significant source of damage to crops. Other insertions delay deterioration of fruit and vegetables or seek to improve flavour. There is concern that the novel foods thus produced may not be 'safe' either in terms of human use or in terms of their environmental safety. One of the cited environmental advantages of the modified maize is the reduced use of pesticides, although this has to be confirmed in practice. Where a novel gene is inserted with the intention of expressing a protein or peptide, this type of inclusion is highly unlikely to be of any danger to consumers of the products, due to the normal process of digestion and consequent low absorption of intact peptides from the gastrointestinal tract. Although the individual nucleotides of the inserted genes and the resulting amino acids from their protein products will be absorbed, they will be biochemically equivalent to the natural nucleotides and amino acids and will, as such, be indistinguishable from them. Where insertion is intended to express a small molecule that can be absorbed intact or have local effects in the gastrointestinal tract, there may be greater risks to consumers.

Much debate was caused by reports of the effects of genetically modified potatoes that expressed a lectin from snowdrops as a countermeasure to attack by insects and nematodes. Lectins, which are glycoproteins, include natural chemicals such as abrin, which attacks the gastrointestinal tract and ricin from the castor bean; they are known toxins. The study of the potatoes by dietary administration to rats concluded that there was significant hazard for consumers in the genetic modification and extended this conclusion to other genetically altered foods. However, the study was of short duration, used small numbers of animals and unrealistically high inclusion levels of the potatoes, which was probably a confounding factor in this study. In short it was considered that the experiment was poorly designed, executed and interpreted and not a suitable basis for drawing conclusions. At most it was adequate as a basis for the design of more definitive studies (see case study in chapter 9).[5]

It is clear from this that toxicological research in this area has to be conducted to very high standards. The risks of getting it wrong – either in overstating the risk with attendant effects on future food production levels or in understating risk which might result in unacceptable toxicity in consumers – are clearly high. Either way, the toxicologists concerned will be at the forefront of the debate, and their independence and scientific standing must be unimpeachable.

Environmental risks are another matter and genetic transfer between herbicide-resistant crops and weeds has been shown, requiring the use of more toxic chemicals, which the original insertions were supposed to make redundant. This is the type of situation where indirect toxicity could result. If pesticide use increases, there could well be environmental detriments that affect the public indirectly, for instance through increased concentrations in drinking water or through less easily measured changes in the ecosystem.

General objectives of toxicological study

Toxicology is a wide-ranging subject with many applications and, as a result, there are many reasons for starting a toxicological investigation. Among these are:

- To establish a dose–response curve: the quantitative relationship between dose and response. It is important to define the steepness of the response; for some drugs such as phenytoin, digitalis or warfarin, a small increase in dose can produce very large increases in adverse side effects that can be life threatening. The safety margin for these compounds is very small; for other classes of drug it can be much greater and a doubling of dose will have little extra effect.
- To assure safety of new chemicals for use as pesticides, drugs or food additives before they are registered for general use in industry or doctors' clinics. This type of toxicity study is regulated by government and international guidelines which describe minimal study designs and the types of study that must be conducted and the test systems which may be used. Toxicologists in regulatory authorities tend to be conservative in their approach as they have a responsibility to the public to ensure as far as possible that the safety of new chemicals or the relevance of new methods is thoroughly investigated before significant human exposure is allowed.
- To establish the mechanism for a toxic effect that may have been seen in other studies.
- To produce epidemiological studies to explain observations in the population, for instance the long investigation into the association of smoking with lung cancer and other diseases. This type of study may also be used to seek explanations for toxicities seen in patients or workers in particular industries.
- To investigate or validate new methods of testing or investigation, particularly those conducted *in vitro* rather than in animals.

The last point is particularly important as the extensive use of animals in toxicological experiments is becoming increasingly questioned. There is a considerable dilemma here; animals offer a whole multi-organ system in which to conduct experiments and the interrelationships of the various organs can be investigated in a way that they cannot (at present) in a single cell or tissue system in a static vessel. A patient who takes a diuretic orally does not give it directly to the kidney where it is expected to have its effect. In order to get to the site of action in the kidney, the drug has to pass through the gastrointestinal tract and then the liver and the bloodstream. In the blood, on the way to the kidney, the drug passes through every other organ in the body where there are opportunities for unwanted effects; for instance certain classes of antibiotic (e.g. gentamycin) and diuretic (e.g. furosemide) have been associated with effects on the hair cells in the inner ear leading to hearing impairment. Any programme of work that seeks to investigate the effects of a novel compound intended for extensive, regulated use in man must, at some point, include experiments in animals that will examine these interrelationships.

The down side is that animal research is expensive and may not give a wholly reliable result when related to humans. The best test system for humans is, undoubtedly, other humans but even this is complicated by differences between ethnic groups and individuals and by ethical questions as to whether human volunteers should be asked to take potentially toxic pesticides and/or new drugs for which the toxicity is completely unknown. Knowledge of the differences in human populations also indicates that one group of humans may not be a good model for another, as a result of genetic diversity. For instance, Eskimos tend to be able to metabolise the anti-tuberculosis drug isoniazid faster than Egyptians and would therefore give erroneous results were they to be used as a test system to investigate safety of use in Egyptians. Finally there is no doubt that giving even small doses of an unknown chemical to humans is not ethically acceptable. For these reasons experiments that attempt to find new methods of investigation and to validate them for use in safety evaluation comprise one of the more important avenues of toxicological exploration.

Nature and outcome of toxic reactions

Chemicals interact with animal cells in numerous ways; these can be broadly categorised as having effects at the level of the cell organelle, the cell, the tissue or organ (or part of an organ) or the whole organism. Interactions at the cellular level are often associated with a precise molecular target, such as a pharmacologically important receptor, an enzyme or other molecular component. Such interactions may result simply in changes in the biochemistry of the cell, which may or may not be visible microscopically, or in effects so severe that they result in cell death. Cell organelles, such as the endoplasmic reticulum, which carries many enzymes responsible for metabolism of foreign chemicals, can be disrupted by lipid peroxidation brought about by free radicals generated by metabolism of the chemical. This autodestructive process can be so extensive that the whole cell is affected and dies through necrosis. Equally the endoplasmic reticulum may become more extensive as a result of increased amounts of enzymes produced to metabolise a particular chemical. This process of enzyme induction is classically associated with hepatocytic hypertrophy around the central vein in the liver, which produces a characteristic appearance in histological sections and is often associated with an increase in liver size.

When many cells in a tissue are affected, the whole organ may be changed in functional terms or have a different appearance under the microscope when compared with controls or expectation. The kidney is a good example of an organ in which particular parts may be affected while leaving the rest of the tissue apparently untouched. Damage to the glomerulus or the proximal convoluted tubule may not be reflected by changes in other parts of the organ. However, the function of the kidney as a whole may be affected by influences such as blood pressure or hormonal diuresis, which may result in unwanted side effects in the rest of the organism.

All toxic reactions have a biochemical basis, which may be more or less precise. Cyanide specifically inhibits cytochrome oxidase in the mitochondria, preventing oxidative phosphorylation through inhibition of mitochondrial electron transport. Fluorocitrate, a metabolite of the rodenticide fluoroacetate, is bound by aconitase, an enzyme in the tricarboxylic acid cycle. Thus the central cycle of carbohydrate metabolism is inhibited by blocking the conversion of citrate to isocitrate, leading to the death of the recipient.

Many chemicals are not toxic themselves, but become so when metabolised. This toxicity-inducing metabolism may be a normal fate for the molecule; fluoroacetate is always metabolised to fluorocitrate. Paracetamol, however, is normally eliminated from the body by conjugation with sulphate or glucuronide, while a small proportion (about 4 per cent) is metabolised via cytochrome P450 to a metabolite that is normally conjugated with glutathione (GSH). Although GSH is present in the liver at high concentrations relative to other peptides, in paracetamol overdose it becomes depleted, so freeing the toxic metabolite to bind covalently to liver proteins, leading to liver necrosis. Paracetamol overdose is often fatal, but, in survivors the effects may be transient; liver biopsies taken a few months after overdose may reveal no evidence of previous damage due to the liver's enormous powers of self-repair.

The toxic reactions discussed above are examples of effects that are immediately obvious and which usually follow a high, or relatively high, dose. Other toxic reactions may be expressed slowly, through gradual reduction of functional reserve. The kidney of a young adult has a large excess of functional capacity, which declines with age. If high doses of non-steroidal anti-inflammatory drugs are taken, through prescription or abuse, this normal age-related decline can be accelerated to a point where renal failure occurs. The same situation can exist in the nervous system, where normal age-related decline may be accelerated by constant exposure to doses of chemical that are not individually toxic but have a disastrous additive effect. This has been seen following daily work-related exposure over long periods to n-hexane or methyl n-butyl ketone. The long-term result is a neuropathy and muscular weakness, which begins in the extremities and progresses toward the centre with continued exposure.

Another type of reaction to toxins is one characterised by a biochemical and then a morphological response to a chemically induced imbalance in the organism, often hormonal. Drugs such as some hypolipidaemic fibrates, which inhibit secretion of gastric acid in rats, can be associated with carcinoid tumours of the rodent stomach. This is due to an increase in the plasma concentration of gastrin, which stimulates the neuroendocrine cells, resulting in their hyperplasia. This hyperplastic response is translated, in a proportion of the animals, to malignant tumours. Similarly, hormonal imbalance can result in an increased incidence of breast cancer or prostate cancer. In this respect the recent increase in testicular cancer amongst younger men is of interest; studies have been set up to see if there is a relationship with low levels of environmental pollutants.

Through effects in the reproductive tract or on the reproductive cycle, which may not be apparent at the time of exposure to the responsible chemical, toxicity can also be expressed in succeeding generations. Thalidomide is the classic example of this and is interesting from several standpoints. A sedative given to pregnant women to reduce nausea in early pregnancy, thalidomide was associated with a range of defects in the offspring, the most apparent being shortening of the long bones of the limbs (phocomelia). The defects seen were closely dependent on the day the drug was taken, usually in the fourth or fifth week of pregnancy; furthermore it is a chiral molecule and the $S(-)$ form is more embryotoxic than the $R(+)$ form. Thalidomide illustrates the precision of effects on the developing fetus and the importance of time of exposure relative to the stage of embryonic development. A further example of unsuspected reproductive effect is diethyl stilboestrol which was given to pregnant women as an anti-abortion agent but was associated with the appearance of clear cell adenocarcinomas in the vagina and testicular defects in their offspring, effects that did not become evident until puberty.

Toxic reactions, severe or trivial, may be reversible or irreversible according to which tissue is affected. As indicated above for paracetamol, the liver has a large capacity for repair of extensive lesions; other tissues associated with easy repair are those that can divide and replicate themselves quickly, such as the skin and gastrointestinal tract. The kidney falls into both the reparative and the next, non-reparative category. The epithelium of the proximal tubule is a common target for toxic attack but, as long as the basement membrane on which these cells rest is not breached, repair can be very rapid if exposure is stopped. Other parts of the kidney, notably the glomerulus and the pelvis, do not repair so readily, in part due to differences in embryonic origin. As suggested by the example of the kidney, tissues which do not divide readily do not repair easily or, in some cases, at all. Of these the usual example is the central nervous system, another tissue with a large functional reserve that can be overwhelmed by insidious toxic actions over a period of years.

Cellular basis and consequences of toxic change

With the exception of a few substances that are corrosive, direct effects of toxic substances are expressed in individual cells. According to the extent of exposure (dose) the number of cells affected increases to the point where the whole organ or tissue is changed, biochemically or morphologically. There are relatively few substances that have direct effects in cells without first being metabolised. Those that are active without prior metabolism are often intrinsically reactive or have activity at specific receptors on the cell membrane or in the cell itself. Corrosive substances tend to act from outside the cell and have widespread effects that result in the deaths of many cells but in a different manner to toxins that work from the cell membrane or inside. In other words, in corrosion, there is no initial molecular event that could be said to be the initiating reaction in starting toxicity. With something like an acid, the corrosive effect is equal on all molecules in the cell and the effects devastating for the exposed tissue, which is often the skin. Although the corrosive effects may be local initially, depending on the substance involved, the toxicity expressed may become systemic as the protective barrier of the skin is broken down and absorption takes place.

In individual cells, toxicity may be classified in broad terms as either reversible or irreversible and there may be a change in functional competence or morphological or biochemical lesions that impair the well-being of the cell. Irreversibility may not be associated with immediate expression of effect, as with the development of adenocarcinoma in young women following maternal exposure to diethyl stilboestrol or with mesothelioma years after exposure to asbestos. In the case of minor functional changes, which might be associated with the activity of cellular pumps or signal transmission capabilities, the changes may be repairable and so prove to be reversible. Where repair is not possible due to extent of the lesions, the cell may die through two possible routes – necrosis or apoptosis. Necrosis is a process over which the organism's biochemistry has no control and consequently is accompanied by characteristic morphological changes indicating an almost violent death. It is often associated with the presence of inflammation, typified by the presence of leucocytes that have migrated into the tissue to the site of damage. Apoptosis, or programmed cell death, on the other hand, involves a series of defined biochemical events that result in the removal of the cell contents and membranes in a manner that, in comparison with necrosis, leaves little morphological evidence. Correct regulation of apoptosis is essential in normal embryonic development.

Where a cell is damaged in some way that does not result in immediate necrosis or later apoptosis, the effects may persist for years without causing any further damage. In cases where there is an unrepaired change in the DNA this may lie dormant until the cell is stimulated to divide and, if this division is repeated and the process not controlled, the result may be a tumour – benign or malignant. In this way an apparently benign or invisible change may have devastating effects years after the relevant exposure has been forgotten.

Receptors – as distinct from the active sites of enzymes – play an important role in many toxicities. Binding of a foreign chemical at a receptor instead of, or in competition with, the natural ligand can be expected to result in adverse effects if the receptor is inappropriately activated or inactivated. As with other mechanisms of toxicity, the effects of receptor binding may be acute, as with tetrodotoxin to sodium channels in the neuronal axons, or delayed, as in tumour promotion by phorbol esters. In the latter case, the phorbol ester binds to protein kinase C which triggers a cascade response, ultimately resulting in cell division in which existing DNA damage can be fixed, leading to tumour growth from previously initiated cells.

For toxicities that are expressed through non-covalent binding to pharmacological receptors, it is probable that when the stimulus or ligand for the receptor is removed, the undesirable effect will cease. Receptor effects can be induced indirectly by toxicants reacting at the active sites of enzymes. The reversibility of effect, driven by strength of binding to the site of action, is illustrated by the difference in toxicity between organophosphate and carbamate insecticides. Both these classes of insecticide bind to the active site of acetylcholinesterase, which hydrolyses the neurotransmitter acetylcholine. Whereas carbamate binding to the active site is relatively transient, the binding of organophosphates lasts much longer, to the extent that it is, in some cases, considered irreversible. Where the target cholinesterase is the neuropathy target esterase, 'ageing' of the enzyme takes place, resulting in a permanent change. This is the basic mechanism behind organophosphate-induced delayed neuropathy, a persistent effect of exposure to some organophosphates. The role of organophosphate-based sheep dips in the occupational health of farm workers will be considered in the chapter on risk assessment (Box 11.1).

Where cellular homeostasis is affected, there can be severe consequences for the cell and, where there is widespread effect, for the whole organism. A classic example of this is the effects of ricin, from the castor bean plant, which is a mixture of enzymatic proteins that fragment ribosomes, inhibiting protein synthesis. Although ricin is known as a parenteral toxin, ingestion of castor beans can be associated with severe toxicity, particularly in the gastrointestinal tract, with large ingestions producing haemorrhagic gastritis, diarrhoea and dehydration. The effects are exacerbated by the presence of ricinoleic acid in the oil of the seed, which increases the peristalsis in the intestine; beyond the intestine, target organs are the kidney and liver. Thus, action at a vital cellular target produces adverse effects in the whole organism.

The interaction of one cell with another is another aspect of the cellular basis of toxicity. In normal tissue, adjacent cells have channels between them through which small molecules can pass; cells in which these gap junctions are still patent are less prone to proliferation than when they are closed. Several tumour promoters, for example phorbol esters and phenobarbital, reduce intercellular communication through gap junctions and this is thought to lead to transformation of the cells and so to neoplasia.

The axons of neurons can be extremely long and are dependent on the transport of nutritional components from the neuron cell body. When this transport is disrupted, the axon dies back in the type of reaction that is seen in response to chronic exposure to n-hexane. In this case, metabolism of the hexane to 2,5-hexanedione is associated with cross-linking of neurofilaments in the axon and subsequent blockage of transport at the nodes of Ranvier. In this case, effects on one type of cell are associated with adverse change (progressive peripheral paralysis) in the rest of the organism.

Toxic attack on specific cell types is characteristic of many chemicals, for instance the effects of paraquat and 4-ipomeanol in the lung. Paraquat is a widely available herbicide, which has two nitrogen atoms that are the same distance apart as in two endogenous polyamines, putrescine and spermine. This similarity allows it to be taken into the type I and II pneumocytes in the lung, where it accumulates and, with the high local concentration of oxygen, undergoes redox cycling (Figure 1.1). This process involves reduction of paraquat by an electron donor (e.g. NADPH) and its reoxidation by transfer of an electron to oxygen. This results in the generation of superoxide radicals, which go on to form hydrogen peroxide through the action of the protective enzyme superoxide dismutase (SOD). Where this enzyme activity is too low to remove all the available superoxide, reactive hydoxyl radicals are produced, with subsequent attack on the cellular lipid membranes through lipid peroxidation. The ability of these cells to concentrate paraquat and the locally high concentration of oxygen work together to cause severe local toxicity, affecting the whole animal. The fact that the molecule is not metabolised to a less toxic form but is regenerated, leaving it free to repeat the cycle many times, leads to depletion of NADPH with significant effects on cellular homeostasis. Paraquat also has effects in the kidney and other organs but it is the lesion in the lung that is

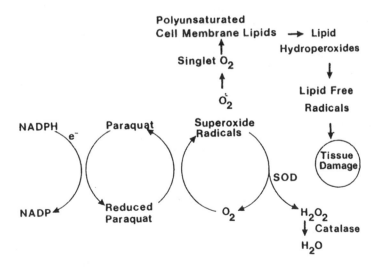

Figure 1.1 Mechanism of paraquat toxicity.
Source: Timbrel, JA. *Introduction to Toxicology*. London: Taylor & Francis, 1999: 99.

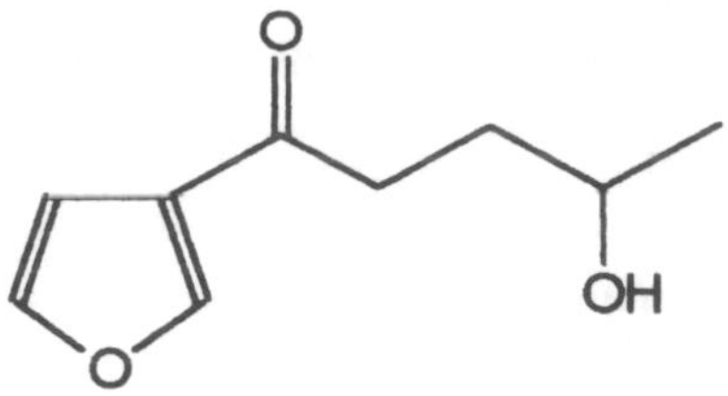

Figure 1.2 Ipomeanol.
Source: Timbrel, JA. *Introduction to Toxicology*. London: Taylor & Francis, 1999: 290.

responsible for the death of the patient. The effect of the kidney change is to reduce renal function, slowing excretion and thus exacerbating the toxicity.

The mould *Fusarium solani*, found on sweet potatoes, produces 4-ipomeanol (Figure 1.2) which attacks the Clara cells of the lung specifically, through production by cytochrome P450 of an epoxide on its furan ring. This enzyme is also present in the liver but, although it is present there in larger amounts than in the Clara cells, it is less active. In addition, the liver has large concentrations of glutathione, a tripeptide that is crucial in protection against oxidative attack. Consequently the Clara cells are at a disadvantage in comparison with the hepatocytes and show the effects caused by binding of the reactive intermediates to cellular macromolecules, leading to necrosis and pulmonary oedema.

The most significant target in the cell is the DNA. This is subject to a wide range of direct attacks, such as covalent binding and formation of adducts, intercalation of planar molecules and radiation damage. Indirect effects result from the up- or downregulation of gene expression, which can be detected through the burgeoning sciences of genomics and proteomics. The ability to relate changes in gene expression or protein levels to specific toxicities will be a powerful tool in the earlier detection of toxicity.

Expression of toxicity

The following is a brief review of ways in which toxicity can be expressed, or its expression influenced, in individuals exposed to unusual concentrations of any chemical, natural or synthetic; it is not intended to be exhaustive. The expression of toxicity is influenced by factors inherent in the exposed subject, in addition to the factors listed on p. 5, including age, disease, pregnancy, genetics, nutrition, lifestyle, sex and occupation.

The ability to metabolise and eliminate chemicals at the two extremes of age is notably different to that seen during the majority of a lifespan. Neonates and geriatric people show different sensitivities to drugs due to differences in liver and kidney function; this can be extrapolated to other chemicals with which they may come in contact. Benoxaprofen was introduced as a new drug for use in arthritis but, due to the normal age related decline in kidney function and metabolising capability, was associated with serious toxicity in some geriatric patients. Neonates also show lower drug metabolising capabilities; in some cases this deficiency is protective, in others it is not.

Disease is also a factor to be considered. This may be pre-existing or induced by the exposure to the toxicant. The two major organs of concern are the kidney and the liver, in an analogous way to the effects of age. Where there is pre-existing cirrhosis of the liver, hepatic function will differ significantly from normal. Damage in the liver inflicted by paracetamol has the effect of prolonging exposure to the drug. Where liver disease is associated with bilirubinaemia, drugs bound to plasma proteins may be displaced by bilirubin, markedly increasing the plasma concentration of free drug. For drugs such as phenytoin or warfarin, which are highly protein-bound and have steep dose-response curves, a small decrease in protein binding can more than double the amount of free drug available for pharmacological effect. Protein binding can also be affected in kidney disease, where reduced filtration rates lead to slower elimination, and vital blood flows can be affected by other factors such as cardiac disease.

Pregnancy is associated with an increase in plasma volume and consequent borderline anaemia and with changes in protein binding. The extracellular space is increased with an associated increase in the amount of fluid available for dissolution of drugs (increased volume of distribution). There is increased cardiac output and changes in respiratory parameters, seen as increased tidal volume, increased distribution and faster gaseous equilibrium. Retention of contents in the upper gastrointestinal tract is prolonged.

Genetics may affect the response to a chemical through differences in the way in which it is handled – absorption, distribution, metabolism and elimination (ADME). The most common factor is variation or deficiency in enzyme activity. Early discoveries of this were made with isoniazid and debrisoquine, both of which were associated with genetic polymorphisms – slower acetylation of isoniazid and deficient hydroxylation of debrisoquine. There is great variation in paracetamol metabolism between individuals by a factor of up to ten, the highest rate being comparable to that in the most sensitive animal species (hamsters) and the lowest to that in the least sensitive (rats). These differences have been exploited in the development of animal models with deficiencies in particular enzyme systems. For instance, the Gunn rat has a deficiency in glucuronosyl transferase, which is responsible for conjugation (phase 2 metabolism) of initial metabolites of chemicals (phase 1 metabolism). Ethnic differences are important, for instance Canadian Indians have a lower capacity for ethanol metabolism than Caucasians. Sex is another factor, especially in hormonal terms; sensitivity to chloroform's renal toxicity is much greater in male mice than in females. This difference is removed by castrating the males and restored by administration of male hormones. There are significant differences between male and female rats in drug metabolism and physiology, which can result in different toxicological responses.

Diet and nutrition are also significant. The importance of diet is illustrated by the tumour profile for Japanese people in Japan, which is different to that found in west coast Americans. However, Japanese people living in California show a profile of tumours similar to that of their American neighbours. Food restriction in rats and use of a low-protein diet produces an increase in lifespan and a reduction in the incidence of several tumours. Lipid content of diet may be important in affecting absorption of lipophilic chemicals and the fibre content of diet affects the bioavailability of toxicants by binding and thus reducing absorption. Nutrition, as distinct from diet, is also important; anorexia or a diet low in protein can result in lower synthesis of enzymes responsible for metabolism and elimination of chemicals. Related to diet are lifestyle factors such as smoking and alcohol consumption, which can also influence expression of toxicity.

Occupation can determine the likelihood of toxic expression, either directly or indirectly. Exposure to vinyl chloride was associated with a rare liver cancer, haemangiosarcoma, its rarity and presence in a clearly defined segment of the population leading to epidemiological identification of the cause. In uranium miners there was a greatly increased probability of lung cancer in those who smoked. Occupational toxicity can be found in more mundane forms. People harvesting parsnips or celery may show phytophotodermatitis which results from the transfer of psoralens from the plants to the skin and exposure to sunlight, a relationship that may not be readily identified clinically.

Toxicity is manifested in an enormous number of different ways and can be seen as changed organ function, reproductive effects (sterility, impotence, terato-genicity, loss of libido, transplacental cancer), changes in normal biochemistry, excess pharmacological action, phototoxicity, or as cancer. There are indirect effects, for instance due to stress, or non-specific changes, for which no direct cause can be identified, such as lowered appetite and associated loss of body-weight. The end result, however, is that toxicity is usually expressed through specific organs, known as target organs. The problem with this approach is that many of the more potent, often less biochemically specific, chemicals affect a wide range of organs or tissues.

Target organ expression of toxicity

As suggested, the disadvantage of the classic approach to target organ toxicity is that, too often, the organ is considered in isolation from other organs or from the rest of the organism. It is convenient to teach toxicology in this way but it means that it can be difficult to cross-link information so that interrelationships are evident. In considering the toxicity of a compound it is important to keep the general view in mind; equally in looking at the effects in one organ or tissue it is important to remember the rest of the organism. Paracetamol is one of the classic hepatotoxins but it also affects the kidney. Phenytoin, used in the control of epilepsy, can result in convulsions in overdose (it has a low therapeutic index or safety margin), chronic use is associated with gingival hyperplasia, it is a teratogen and can cause hypersensitivity with extensive dermal reactions. Lead has effects on learning ability, in the nervous system, in the blood and in the kidney and is associated with reproductive changes and may be carcinogenic. The susceptibility of organs to the effects of chemicals is influenced by a number of factors, some of which are discussed below.

Determinants of target organ toxicity

There are a number of factors that influence the extent to which the effects of a chemical are expressed in particular tissues and these are summarised in Table 1.3 and expanded in the following text.

Blood supply

The blood is the main vehicle for distributing chemicals of all kinds around the body and it is logical that the blood supply is important in defining the degree of exposure of individual tissues to the chemicals in the blood, endogenous as well

Table 1.3 Factors in target organ toxicity

Factor	Examples
Blood supply	Liver, kidney and lung have greater blood supplies than adipose or muscle tissue
Oxidative exposure	Lung and paraquat toxicity
Cell turnover	Gastrointestinal mucosa, bone marrow and toxicity of cytotoxic chemotherapies
Repair and reversibility	Hepatic change may be easily repaired while change in the CNS is not
Physiology	Concentration effects in the distal renal tubule
Morphology	Length and diameter of axons in the peripheral nervous system
Processing ability or metabolic activity	Liver and xenobiotic metabolism. Renal proximal tubule versus the Loop of Henle. Oxygen concentrations
Hormonal control	Reproductive tract and endocrine organs. Induction of hepatic metabolism and increased clearance of thyroid hormones
Accumulation	Lung and paraquat; adipose tissue and TCDD; cadmium in kidney; lead in bone. Environmental accumulation of pesticides such as DDT
Protection mechanisms	High concentrations of antioxidant glutathione in the liver. DNA repair differences or deficiencies

as foreign. The liver receives all the blood supply from the gastrointestinal tract via the inferior vena cava, from where it goes to the heart and thence to the lungs. Thus chemicals absorbed in the gut go to the liver, the main site of xenobiotic metabolism, and are distributed, with any persistent metabolites, to the heart and then on to the lungs and kidneys, which receive 25 per cent of the cardiac output via the aorta.

Oxidative exposure

Much toxicity is due to oxidative attack on macromolecules and this is affected by blood supply and, of course, in the lung where the locally high concentration of oxygen is partly responsible for the high toxicities seen with compounds like paraquat.

Cell turnover

Tissues that have an intrinsically high turnover of cells are at risk from chemicals that inhibit cell division. These include the mucosa of the gastro-intestinal tract, the skin, the bone marrow and the testes. Inhibition of the division in the bone marrow can affect the whole organism through induction of anaemia and/or reductions in the numbers of circulating leucocytes, in turn leading to reduced immunocompetence. Where there is a high level of apoptosis, for instance in developing embryos, disturbances in cell turnover have the potential to result in malformations in the fetus. Where cell turnover is increased, for instance through necrosis with replacement through increased cell division, there are inherent risks of DNA replication errors which can lead in the long term to tumour formation.

Repair ability and reversibility

An important aspect of assessing the significance of toxic effect is whether it is reversible, either on removal of the stimulus or through repair of tissue damage. The extent to which tissues can repair themselves differs markedly according to tissue type and, to an extent, embryonic origin. Some tissues are able to repair themselves readily, especially the liver. In rats given toxic doses of carbon tetrachloride, early evidence of liver damage seen in the plasma a few days after administration is frequently not reflected in histopathological evidence of damage after 14 days. This considerable capacity for self-repair means that it is possible to miss toxicologically significant hepatotoxicity in standard acute toxicity tests, which require single administration followed by 14 days observation before autopsy. This repair capability is seen in humans following overdose with paracetamol (acetaminophen) where there is often severe liver toxicity; in survivors biopsy of the liver three months after the overdose sometimes shows no evidence of persisting liver damage. Equally some tissues do not readily repair themselves, especially the nervous system. In these tissues regeneration does not take place or is very slow. Whereas a necrotic hepatocyte can be quickly replaced, a necrotic neuron is lost completely and the function of that part of the nervous system reduced proportionately. In some organs, particularly the kidney, different parts have different capabilities for repair. Thus damage to the glomerulus and the renal pelvis is not readily repaired but the proximal tubule epithelium shows considerable repair capability, providing the basement membrane (on which the cells lie) is not breached.

Physiology

Cells or tissues with specific characteristics are susceptible to toxicants which disrupt or take advantage of those characteristics. Paraquat is an example of this, through its accumulation in the lung, via the uptake mechanism for the endogenous polyamines. In the kidney, the passage of the urine through the distal tubule can lead to toxicity as the toxins increase in concentration as water is reabsorbed.

Morphology

The length and small diameter of axons in the peripheral nervous system contribute to the axonopathy induced by n-hexane due to cross-linking of the microfilaments and subsequent poor nutrition of the distal parts of the cell. This is an instance where physiology is also important, as the axon depends on transport of nutrients from the neuronal body and appears to be unable to acquire them from elsewhere. With the passage of nutrients blocked the axon dies distally from the blockage.

Processing ability

Tissues that have high processing or metabolic activity are also frequent targets of toxicity. The liver has high activities of enzymes responsible for chemical metabolism and, therefore, if toxic metabolites are produced they are likely to be produced in higher concentrations than in other tissues, increasing the risk of local effect. The difference between the liver and the lung in terms of enzymic activity is one of the determining factors in the toxicity of 4-ipomeanol. The proximal tubule of the kidney is another site of high metabolic activity and is a frequent target. High metabolic activity may also mean greater potential for oxidative attack through oxygen radicals, which can be produced as a result of normal metabolic processes. The kidney is also at risk through its normal physiological function of producing concentrated urine; this can increase the exposure of cells in the nephron to a point at which toxicity is elicited.

Hormonal control

Tissues that are subject to hormonal control will be affected when the concentrations of the relevant hormones are increased or decreased. When hepatic enzymes are induced in rats, there is often an increase in follicular hypertrophy or hyperplasia in the thyroid due to increased removal of thryoid hormones from the plasma as a result of the increased hepatic metabolism. The plasma levels of thyroid stimulating hormone (TSH) are controlled by circulating thyroid hormone concentrations by negative feedback; where this feedback is reduced, the pituitary is stimulated to produce more TSH, which acts on the thyroid. The endocrine system is extremely complex and effects in one part can have a number of knockon changes in other tissues.

Accumulation

Tissues that are able to accumulate specific toxins are also frequent targets for toxicity. Paraquat features here again in lung toxicity. Cadmium is widespread in the environment and accumulates in shellfish and plants. In mammals, cadmium is complexed with a metal-binding protein, metallothionein, which accumulates in the kidney. When a critical level of cadmium content in the kidney is reached – generally quoted as being approximately 200 μg/g of kidney tissue in humans – nephrotoxicity becomes evident and renal failure follows. Constant low intake at slightly raised levels can produce gradual accumulation over many years, which ultimately results in renal failure.

Accumulation in bone is a feature of toxicity of lead and strontium, which is a cause for concern if the strontium is the radioactive isotope. Bisphosphonates, used in the treatment of osteoporosis, also bind tightly to bone and this is a source of some of their toxicity.

Environmental accumulation is also a factor to consider because it can have dire consequences, as illustrated by increasing concentrations of fat-soluble compounds such as DDT in bird of prey populations. DDT, and similar compounds such as TCDD, tend to accumulate in lipid tissue from which they are released very slowly. At one time Americans were, by their own regulatory standards, inedible due to the amounts of DDT they had accumulated in their adipose tissue. For such compounds, toxicity can be expressed if there is a sudden loss of weight, reducing adipose tissue and releasing large amounts of toxin into the plasma where it can pass to the target organs, as in migration or pregnancy in malnourished people. In the development of brown-field sites care must be taken that the residues of any industrial waste are considered in licensing use of the land, especially for growing food crops. This was a major source of toxicity at Love Canal in New York State, where a housing estate was built on a toxic waste dump.

Protection mechanisms

Some tissues, particularly the liver, have high concentrations of endogenous compounds that have protective functions – normally against active oxygen species. Glutathione, which may be present in the liver at a concentration up to

5 mM, is a good example of this. Enzymes such as superoxide dismutase, which catalyses the conversion of superoxide to hydrogen peroxide, are also important in protection of the cell. There are also differences between tissues in the activity of DNA-repair mechanisms. For example the brain is less able than the liver to excise the DNA base guanine methylated at the O^6 position, making it more susceptible to tumour formation following administration of dimethyl-nitrosamine. Defective DNA repair is also seen in patients with xeroderma pigmentosum, which gives a high incidence of skin cancer in response to exposure to UV light.

The problem in drawing such distinctions is the same as with describing toxicity in terms of target organs. A single chemical may be associated with effects in several organs and have a different mechanism of toxicity in each due to the differences in tissue susceptibility. This breadth of possible effects makes testing for toxicity extremely complex until a mechanism is suspected. The enormous range of potencies of the chemicals to which we are exposed is an additional complication.

The necessity for toxicological assessment

It is a moral requirement that new drugs, pesticides or food additives should be as safe as is reasonably possible when they are made available to the doctors, farmers or consumers. The degree to which a product must be safe is determined by its intended use. Pesticides or food additives should be entirely safe at the levels to which consumers are exposed. Pesticides, by their nature, are toxic to the target species but should be safe for non-target species. Food additives, whether added for processing reasons or flavour or as preservatives have a lower margin of tolerance for safety than pesticides, for which an interval between treatment and harvest can be set, together with an acceptable daily intake. With drugs the acceptable margin of safety – the difference between therapeutic and toxic doses – is dependent to a large extent on the indication for which they are intended. Toxicity, seen as side effects, is more tolerable in an anti-cancer drug than in an analgesic sold over the counter.

To ensure that the required margin of safety is demonstrated, for instance for a new drug, it is essential to conduct a programme of experiments to assess the toxicity of the new molecule, specifically to describe a dose–response curve. From these data it should be possible, with appropriate interpretation and experimental support, to extrapolate the effects seen to humans. For chemicals that are already marketed, toxicological assessment becomes necessary when effects are seen in consumers that have not been seen or noticed before. In this case, the intent is to establish a mechanism for the toxicity observed and to recommend appropriate changes in the way the chemical is sold or in the way in which it is used. It is a fact of life that it is not considered ethical to administer new drugs to humans without some assessment of their effects in other test systems. With chemicals that are not intended primarily to be administered to people (e.g. pesticides), the restraints on giving them to humans are even greater. As a consequence of this it is routine, at the current development of the science, to use animals in toxicological safety evaluation programmes or in experiments that investigate mechanisms of toxicity seen in humans.

In using animals it is increasingly understood that their use should be regulated to high ethical standards. A plethora of evidence indicates that animals can be good models for the behaviour of chemicals in humans and that they are the only ethical and valid test system. Evidence also suggests that they are not good models and that their use should be discontinued completely. Both positions are extremes and inevitably the truth probably lies between them. In other words, an ideal situation is where the use of animals is reduced to an extent where there is sufficient scientific 'comfort' to make a sensible, secure assessment of the risks. For some chemicals, one species will be a better model for humans than another and, for this reason, it has become normal practice to study toxicity of new drugs or pesticides in two mammalian species. Considerable savings could arise from validating one or other species, or at least not requiring work in 'invalid species'.

Ethics of toxicological assessment

The use of animals instead of humans in toxicity testing has been considered briefly above. In a sense humans are used, at lower doses than in animals, in safety studies with new drugs. These early studies are to assess the pharmaco-kinetics and any adverse effects in healthy volunteers (phase I clinical studies) and then to study safety, together with some aspects of efficacy, in greater detail in patients (phase II studies). However, no administration to volunteers is allowed until an initial battery of toxicity tests has been conducted to assess the new molecule and to provide data from which to calculate a safe starting dose in humans. The costs of such clinical trials bear out the contention that using humans as test models for humans is hugely expensive and, as patients can be scattered across centres around the globe, inconvenient and slow. There is the additional concern, as with animal models, that experiments in some groups of humans may not be relevant to other groups, as indicated above for isoniazid in Eskimos and Egyptians. In fact the inherent variability of humans is being exploited in pharmacogenetics, which studies the genetic basis for variations in drug metabolism and toxicity and should eventually give data that allow design of specific treatment regimens for patients with specific phenotypes. If a valid cross section of the human global population were used, the variability present would be so great as to obscure subtle but important changes from normality.

The traditional view is that there is no escape from the premise that for effective toxicity testing the variability in the test system must be controlled to allow a satisfactory definition of normality. Change from a carefully defined and understood baseline can be more readily detected than in a diverse population of unmatched individuals. The test system must also be inexpensive and easy to look after as the volume of toxicity testing is so great that the expense would become prohibitive otherwise. The volume of toxicological research and experiment is partly due to the numbers of new chemicals under development and partly due to regulatory guidelines imposed by governments. Mostly it is a compromise, balancing cost against failure; some might say that science has lost out, but science and politics are uneasy bedfellows.

The cost benefit of the chemical has to be assessed in deciding the necessity or ethical acceptability of undertaking toxicity studies in animals. In the case of cosmetics it has been decided that the use of animals to test cosmetic ingredients or products is now unacceptable, meaning that cosmetic toxicity has to be assessed in other ways. However, although such methods of safety assessment may be acceptable in testing of voluntarily used cosmetics, they are not applicable to food additives, pharmaceuticals or pesticides to which human exposure may be involuntary or indicated by illness. Furthermore, cosmetics are nearly all for use on the skin or in the mouth and the risks of using them are very different to those encountered with a pharmacologically active drug given by mouth or injection. Some of the most aggressive chemicals used in our personal lives are fragrances.

There are, at present, no ethical concerns about using long-lived cell cultures in toxicity testing. Some cells for use as test systems can be obtained by taking a blood sample from a healthy volunteer, for example leucocytes, or from tissues obtained at operations from patients; these also pose no ethical problem, unless the tissues are obtained without patient consent.

Primary cell cultures and preparations of cell organelles such as microsomes, however, require fresh cells derived from a freshly killed animal. Is an experiment that uses an animal in this way more ethical than one that uses a complete and conscious animal? In assessing the relevance of the data for humans, the process of extrapolation from an isolated culture of rodent hepatocytes to humans is much more precarious than making the same leap from a complete animal having all the organ interrelationships intact.

It is fundamental that if some toxicity studies are ethically essential, there are some that should not be conducted. The ban on the use of animals to investigate cosmetics and their ingredients has been discussed above. Other examples are more complex; is it necessary to investigate the acute toxicity of a household cleaner if it is thought that it may be ingested accidentally by children or purposefully by adults? In the case of natural constituents of a traditional food, for example mushrooms, is it ethical to investigate the toxicity of individual components? Possibly, especially if there has been evidence gathered from humans that there is a problem for which it is considered that the food or its constituent is responsible. Is it ethical to undertake an experiment on such a constituent that exposes a single group of mice to an unrealistically high dose in the drinking water for two years? The inescapable conclusion from the published data for the mouse study by McManus and co-workers (see note 7 in Box 1.2) is that the experimental design was deficient (at the very least), the study was not reported adequately and that it served no useful purpose; consequently, in my opinion, the animals were needlessly used. In the absence of dose response information, no risk assessment for humans was possible, yet one of the conclusions was that humans should not eat mushrooms

---

Box 1.2 Studies with the constituents of mushrooms

The natural constituents of mushrooms have been widely investigated for their carcinogenic potential and the results published in a number of papers.

- One study[6] looked at the carcinogenicity of a constituent of *Agaricus xanthodermus*, an inedible species, albeit related to the common field mushroom; this experiment used subcutaneous administration and, as a result, is of dubious relevance to people who ingest their food. Production of tumours at the site of administration could have been expected.
- In another study[7] 4-hydrazinobenzoic acid, a constituent of the common mushroom, was given in drinking water at 0.125 per cent to a single group of Swiss mice, equivalent to approximately 5 mg/day/mouse or about 125 mg/kg/day for a 40 g mouse. There was 'substantial' early mortality due to rupture of the aorta. In survivors, a proportion of the mice developed unusual tumours in the aorta – the site of the initial toxicity – diagnosed as leiomyomas or leiomyosarcomas.
- No dose-response information could be gained from this experiment (there was only one group); the formulation of the chemical in the drinking water did not mimic the natural occurrence of the chemical.
- The only conclusion that could be drawn directly was that hydrazinobenzoic acid given in the drinking water caused tumours in Swiss mice *in this study*. In the absence of dose–response information – especially a no effect level – no risk assessment for human use is possible from these data and conclusions about human use cannot sensibly be drawn.
- Other studies have failed to show carcinogenic potential for the common mushroom or its constituents.[8,9] The study by Toth and co-workers in 1997 suggested that the negative finding was due to insufficient mushroom intake, acknowledging the fact that if you are sufficiently dedicated you can induce cancer in mice eventually, so long as the strain, dose levels and design are chosen appropriately.

– despite the many years of human consumption without any serious suggestion from epidemiological studies of any hazard when eaten at normal amounts. If this flawed reasoning were rigorously applied to the whole human diet, we would soon die of starvation or boredom. Hopefully, this type of ill-conceived experiment would not be considered ethical in the current or, indeed, in any climate.

In assessing the ethical need for a toxicological experiment using animals, it is important to question the objective of the study and to assess the design in the light of that objective. If the experiment is not being undertaken to answer a specific question of human concern or the design will not allow the generation of meaningful data, the need for that experiment should be carefully questioned.

The three Rs – reduce, refine and replace

One of the cornerstones of toxicological investigation is the concept of the three Rs – reduce, refine, replace – put forward by Russell and Burch.[10] The intention is to reduce the numbers of animals used in toxicological experiment, to refine the methods by which they are used and to replace the use of animals as appropriate alternative methods become available. A successful example of this approach is the increasing replacement of rabbits in pyrogen testing. Pyrogens, sterilisation-resistant components of bacteria which may be of importance especially in parenteral solutions, may be detected in batches of finished product by injection into the ear veins of rabbits and monitoring the temperature response. This test is costly in terms of labour and animals and is also subject to interference by the presence of pharmaceuticals in some preparations; in addition it does not give a measure of the amount (only the potency) of pyrogenic substances present. The rabbit has popularly been replaced to a large extent by an *in vitro* system using a lysate of amoebocytes from the horseshoe crab *Limulus*; this test is considerably more sensitive than the rabbit test and is one of the best examples of a fully validated alternative assay in use in toxicology. Even so, the output from the two tests is not identical. A high endotoxin level does not necessarily lead to pyrexia. The use of rabbits or mice in bioassays for potency of various biological pharmaceutical preparations, such as insulin, has been greatly reduced by the use of more precisely targeted pharmacological or analytical tests. This is exemplified by the large reduction in numbers of biological tests described in the *British Pharmacopoiea* for 1993 in comparison with that for 1988. Replacement of animals in toxicological testing is inherently simpler if a specific endpoint is being investigated, whether pyrogen content or DNA damage. The more complex or uncertain the endpoint, the more difficult it is to devise a simple test that will answer the question. Refinement of testing methods and protocols is also a long-term goal; the use of guinea pigs in allergenicity testing is being superseded by the local lymph node assay in mice. Animal experimentation has also been refined by careful application of statistics in the design of experiment protocols.

The pursuit of the three Rs is an ongoing process but it can be expected to be long and, in all probability, ultimately incomplete. The achievement of the first 10–20 per cent has been relatively easy; the next 20 per cent will be much more difficult as the endpoints to be studied become less amenable to simplification. It follows that the next 20 per cent beyond that will be harder and slower still but this should not be taken as a reason for not investigating further. Much is made of the minimal study design which results from use of the three Rs; this approach is fraught with risk as, like a net with a wider mesh, more errors can creep through. Much better would be an optimised study design.

If it is accepted that the development of new chemicals is necessary or inevitable (or the use is proposed of naturally occurring chemicals in an unnatural context or quantity) it should be accepted that their safety, or otherwise, should be investigated up to state of the art. Such investigation is essential in the development of new drugs, food additives or pesticides or veterinary medicines. While the two first categories are expected only to be in contact with humans, pesticides and veterinary products are not intended for human exposure. Pesticides are subject to a wide range of other tests to examine their effects on beneficial species such as bees and fish in an assessment of their likely environmental effects. Toxicity testing is also useful in investigating the effects of chemicals or dietary components that are believed to be associated with, or which exacerbate human disease. The necessity of such testing is decided in part by regulatory guidelines (for the three major categories of registered chemicals) and partly by scientific need judged from the expected properties of the chemical. Where animals are used there should be local ethical review committees that monitor numbers and procedures and ensure that the highest possible standards of ethical research are maintained.

Toxicity testing therefore has to assess the probability of an enormously wide range of reactions – covalent, non-covalent, hormonal and metabolic, the basis for which is at the cellular level, although this extends in many instances to the whole organism and is dependent on interrelationships between organs or tissues. The simplest way to do this for unknown or unpredicted mechanisms is to examine the response of a whole organism to the test chemical and to screen for as many endpoints as possible in a set of general tests. Where an unexpected reaction is seen, mechanistic studies can be undertaken to investigate precise endpoints and it is in these precisely targeted experiments that *in vitro* systems become powerful and effective.

In the final analysis, toxicological data cannot be interpreted unless the significance and meaning of detected change is thoroughly understood. When the meaning of the test results is known, it should be possible to take the relationships shown and the targets identified and related these to expected effects in humans. For chemicals which are coming to market and significant public exposure for the first time, the process of evaluation continues after sales begin, to monitor for unexpected effects, which can then be investigated in appropriate mechanistic or epidemiological studies. It should be borne in mind that correct interpretation of data is often lacking in the immediate aftermath of a crisis.

The rest of this book looks at how toxicity tests are conducted, how the results are interpreted and then at the process of how these conclusions are used in risk assessment. However, the first step in all this is to define normality so that change from expectation can be detected in the first place. This is the subject of chapter 2.

Normality

Definition and maintenance

Introduction

The whole basis of toxicological investigation is to detect differences from experimental normality that are attributable, with reasonable certainty, to the influence of the substance under investigation. This simplistic overview, however, then begs the question as to what is normal or, by association, natural. Dictionary definitions of normal use words such as usual, typical or expected; the normal state or condition or being in conformity with a standard, for instance as shown by body temperature. Natural is defined as existing in or derived from nature; not artificial; in accordance with nature; normal. In terms of public perception, normality is seen so routinely that it may be more useful to think of abnormality, which can provoke a reaction that is not seen in response to the normal. Equally there are degrees of abnormality. Someone in a wheelchair, with shortened limbs due to exposure to thalidomide, may be seen as more abnormal than a person in a wheelchair because of an accident; the former will always be disabled while the latter may be 'normal' again. Such simple judgement is based on perception, which may not be readily supportable in scientific terms. In toxicological terms normality can usually be defined by numerical data, means or incidence data or, less verifiably, experience. For characteristics that are defined by presence or absence or narrow ranges of values, definition of normality is relatively simple in comparison with those that are present on a graduated scale or have a wide range of value.

Deviation from normality may be determined through the circumstances of the observation and according to experience or expectation; left-hand-drive cars are not normal in the UK but are clearly normal in France. Similarly a tumour may be expected routinely in old age (when it could be said to be 'normal') but unexpected at the age of 21. It was this characteristic that indicated diethylstilbestrol (DES) as a carcinogen; vaginal adenocarcinoma is unusual in young women but was seen in the young daughters of women who had taken DES in pregnancy to prevent abortion.

What is normality?

Normality, or abnormality, may also be indicated by the presence or absence of an observation. The thalidomide tragedy was shown by the presence of severely shortened limbs, phocomelia, in babies born to mothers who had taken thalidomide in the first 40 days of pregnancy, although other abnormalities became apparent as investigations continued. This was a demonstration of an increase in a rare observation in a specific population, associated with exposure that was definable in terms of dose and day or week of pregnancy. Abnormality may be defined in biochemical terms usually by the absence of enzymes responsible for some aspect of basal metabolism. Phenylketonuria is associated with a recessive deficiency for phenylalanine hydroxylase. This leads to increased excretion of metabolites of phenylalanine that are responsible for neurological effects, including mental retardation and low IQ; many mutations have been reported for this gene.

Deviation from normality is also definable through changes in the incidences of observations, which may then be associated with exposure (in epidemiological studies) or with treatment (in toxicity studies). Phocomelia and haemangiosarcoma (due to occupational exposure to vinyl chloride) are both seen in a normal population but at incidences that are so low as to make them abnormal. In contrast to this, lung cancer may be seen in people who do not smoke; however, there is a clear association of lung cancer with cigarette smoking, marking this as a deviation from normality that is attributable to a toxic exposure. In a similar way, excessive consumption of alcohol during pregnancy is associated with fetal alcohol syndrome seen in the babies born to these mothers.

The above are examples where the incidences of presence or absence data have changed in response to exposure or treatment. Where toxicological, as opposed to epidemiological, investigation is concerned, the most usual way of demonstrating deviation from normality is through statistical analysis of continuous data from the tests conducted. Continuous data, as opposed to positive or negative, presence or absence can be readily exemplified by height in people. It is relatively easy to say if someone is abnormally short or tall – for example 1.2 m or 2.2 m. However, this judgement becomes much more difficult if the subject is between 1.5 m and 1.8 m. The average male height in a population may be around 1.70 m but that population would probably encompass the very short and very tall, grouped in a classic bell-shaped or normal distribution (Figure 2.1). This distribution is characterised by a mean that falls at the centre of the distribution but which does not reflect its width or range of values in the population. The range of values present is defined by the standard deviation of the mean, which tends to be large when there is a wide range of values and smaller with a narrow range. The standard deviation will also tend to get smaller with increasing sample size (n). In a group of 500 men taken from different sports, the mean heights of two samples of 100 randomly

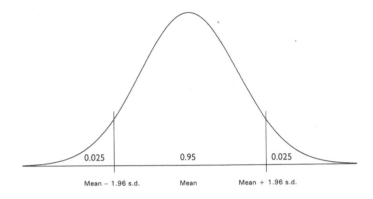

Figure 2.1 Characteristics of the normal distribution.
Source: Modified from Heath, David. *An Introduction to Experimental Design and Statistics for Biologists.* London: Taylor & Francis, 2000.

chosen individuals are unlikely to be significantly different. Equally, the mean height of a sample of 50 football goalkeepers is likely to be fairly uniform and so have a small standard deviation. In fact, in comparison with the mean height of 50 jockeys, the goalkeepers might be seen as unusually tall and the two samples would probably be significantly different when compared statistically. If the two samples of 50 were combined, the mean would fall somewhere in the middle and the standard deviation would increase to reflect the wider range of values in the more diverse sample. In this instance, two samples of defined individuals have been extracted from a relatively undefined population. In toxicology the definition of the two samples is provided by treatment of a test system in comparison with untreated controls.

The characteristics of the normal distribution mean that 95 per cent of values lie within 1.96 standard deviations of the mean; these are the 95 per cent confidence limits. However, this does not necessarily mean that the values falling outside these limits are abnormal; can abnormality be assigned arbitrarily to obvious outliers? The normal distribution plays a central role in assessment of numerical data in toxicology because it forms a basis from which to make comparisons of treated groups against controls. Effect is demonstrated by showing the null hypothesis (that there is no difference between controls and treated groups) to be false (i.e. that there is a difference between the two populations, treated and control). However, demonstrating such a difference does not necessarily imply abnormality; two samples of 21-year-old males may have mean heights that are significantly different but this does not mean that one group is abnormal.

Although it is useful to consider normality within populations, it is also applicable to individuals and is affected by factors that influence normal function, including disease. In pregnancy there are a number of important changes from individual normality that affect the composition of the blood and how chemicals are cleared from the body. Paradoxically, pregnancy is a normal condition with its own limits of normality. Age is also an important consideration and normality for an individual, defined by an assortment of parameters, drifts with increasing age. Factors that change with age include protein binding, clearance, metabolism, renal and CNS function. There is a general tendency for normal function to decline with age, for example in the kidneys or central nervous system. Normal age-related decline in clearance may result in abnormal reaction to drugs, such as that seen in adverse reactions to benoxaprofen. These affected a number of elderly patients and eventually led to the drug's withdrawal from the market. Such decline is normal but it may be accelerated in some cases by chronic exposure to chemicals; this acceleration clearly results in abnormality at an earlier stage than expected. Normality in the very young is also different from that in adults. Neonatal absorption for different chemicals can be more or less extensive than that seen in adults – young or old – and this clearly has an effect on the way babies handle drugs or other chemicals.

Abnormality may be singular, in that an individual may be normal in every respect except one – deformity of one arm for instance – or multiple. However, a single genetic defect can have multiple effects as in trisomy 21 or cystic fibrosis, the abnormalities of which are interconnected.

At some point a judgement becomes necessary as to what is normal and what is not; ideally this is based on numerical data or a scientific appreciation of qualitative data. Frequently, however, a subjective judgement is made and the perceived abnormal is treated with suspicion. This tendency has a huge influence on the public perception of the effects of chemicals of all kinds – food additives, pesticides, components of genetically modified crops, new drugs, etc. Normality may be judged against difference from expectation; this is simple for presence or absence phenomena but more complex for a sliding scale such as height. A distinction may be made between an objective, mathematical definition and the subjective perception of normality. At what point is a tall man abnormally tall and is this perception the same for everyone? A very tall person might consider people of average height to be short, when in fact they are mathematically normal in height. Clarity of difference makes these judgements much simpler; however such clarity is a luxury that is not often available in toxicology. Some treatment-related effects may not render the treated test system abnormal, but could significantly affect life expectancy if allowed to continue. It is this subtlety of effect that makes definition of normality in toxicology so important.

Experimental normality

In any toxicological experiment it is vital that the test system should be as defined as possible, always bearing in mind that it is a biological organism. For the most part this means the exclusion of any factor that might impede the experimental objective being achieved. In animal experiments it is important to ensure that the animals are free from the effects that may be induced by disease or parasitic infection or poor husbandry practices – amongst numerous sources of abnormality. It should also be realised, however, that normality in a test system may not equate to normality in the wild-type organism, particularly in the case of bacteria. The Ames test is conducted with strains of *Salmonella typhimurium* that have had specific characteristics designed into them; deviation from these characteristics invalidates the test results. Equally, the laboratory rat may be said to be normal in laboratory terms but is clearly not so in comparison with the wild rat from which it is derived. In an analogous manner to bacterial strains, there are strains of rat bred with specific abnormalities for purposes of metabolism investigation, for example the Gunn rat or transgenic mice for investigation of specific toxicological mechanisms or for accelerated assessment of carcinogenicity. From this it is clear that a distinction should be drawn between wild-type normality and experimental normality.

There are many factors that can affect the test system and so have direct or indirect effects on the responses to treatment with chemicals. This can be reflected in lack of reproducibility of data between laboratories or in data which mislead interpretation, particularly if an abnormality conceals a response to treatment that is present in a 'normal' test system.

Of these factors one of the most difficult to assess is stress. Although this refers particularly to animals, it should be noted that incorrect storage or preparation of *in vitro* test systems will also compromise the experiments undertaken. In animals a degree of stress is normal in everyday life but this leaves the question as to what is a normal level of stress. Assessment of excessive stress is relatively easy, as the changes seen in comparison with an unstressed control are usually plain. Low-grade chronic stress and its effects are much more difficult to distinguish and, as a result, it may be impossible to separate subtle effects of treatment from the effects of stress.

Aside from treatment itself, one of the most important sources of stress in animal studies is inappropriate husbandry. In general, the animals used in toxicological experiments are social and benefit from housing in groups, which reduces stress and so produces a more normal animal. Studies of animals implanted with telemetry devices that relay data on heart rate, blood pressure or body temperature have shown that heart rate and blood pressure increase when cage mates are separated, when a new cage is provided or when an unfamiliar person enters the room. Recently, the increasing practice of housing primates in groups, instead of in individual 1 m^3 steel cages has shown the benefits of attention to good husbandry technique. Individually housed primates are likely to show atypical behaviour, including self-mutilation and repetitive movements that can in no way be said to be normal. In gang-housed experiments the animals are housed together in single-sex treatment groups and have the opportunity to socialise and interact with each other; they are visibly more relaxed and outwardly normal. In a similar way it is generally accepted that rats housed together are better models for toxicity experiments than singly housed animals.

One argument for single housing is that food consumption data are more precise; also if an animal dies unexpectedly there is no chance of cannibalisation by cage mates. However, food consumption measurement may be hampered by bedding, preventing measurement of spillage, and better husbandry should reduce the numbers of unexpected deaths. In other species also, the benefits of individual food consumption data of dubious accuracy or utility are outweighed by the advantages of group housing in providing a less stressed animal. For rodents, individual housing has the downside that the animals are subject to low-grade chronic stress which has the potential to produce hypertrophy in the adrenal cortex with increased adrenal weight. In studies of up to 13 weeks, the adrenal changes are often accompanied by reductions in thymus weight, which may mask immunotoxic change, although stress itself can lead to immuno-suppression. In longer studies with individually housed rats, the lifespan of the animals is somewhat shorter than with group housing and the animals tend to be more difficult to handle and have a different tumour profile. Group housing alleviates much of this stress, although dominant animals may have some counter-effect on this in the case of individual cage mates. However, some animals are better housed individually, usually due to fighting, male mice and hamsters being two good examples of this. New studies are indicating, however, that male mice can be housed together if they are kept together from a very early age; this means allocating them to cages at delivery and then randomising cages rather than animals.

Another factor increasingly used in animal experiments is environmental enrichment, where toys are provided or activities, such as foraging, encouraged. Although group or pair housing is good environmental enrichment in itself, provision of cage furniture for dogs and primates or cardboard cage inserts for rodents are also used increasingly. For primates the use of small bits of food hidden in the bedding or a honey and seed mixture smeared on wooden perches is a very good way of promoting behavioural patterns that are closer to normality.

While husbandry is a potential source of continuous low-grade stress, other causes of stress may be transient. These include handling, treatment (or the prospect of treatment), irregular examinations such as recording of electro-cardiograms, blood or urine collection, or simply removal from the home cage for examination. While stress is generally accepted as being an important factor to avoid in toxicological experiments, its effects are inherently difficult to quantify, as the investigation is itself often stressful and reaction to stress, especially hormonal, can be very rapid. Experimental design and conduct should be optimised to reduce stress as far as possible. Stress reduction can start with the choice of study personnel. In studies with animals, the choice of people who will carry out the majority of the handling and procedures is very important because their attitude and approach will affect the behaviour of the animals. A relaxed, caring technician will have animals that are themselves relaxed and easy to handle, while the opposite is true of those who are impatient or bad tempered.

In routine toxicity studies with dogs or primates it is usual to record electro-cardiograms from unanaesthetised animals. Unless the animals are thoroughly acclimatised to the procedure, heart rate will be significantly increased above normal values, along with blood pressure; careful handling of the animals is vital to minimise stress. Procedure-related effects can conceal reductions in blood pressure and smaller increases in heart rate that can result in histo-pathological lesions in the heart, an effect to which the papillary muscle of the laboratory beagle dog is known to be sensitive. Although it is possible to perform these measurements on anaesthetised animals, the choice of anaesthetic is important as it too can affect blood pressure or heart rate. To avoid such experimentally induced abnormality and to track real changes in this type of parameter, it is advisable to use telemetric equipment which gives a remote reading of these data in an unrestrained animal and indication of change from 'true' normality.

It may also be useful to draw a distinction between psychological and bio-chemical or physiological stress, the latter two being more likely to be treatment induced in a well-designed experiment. Poor protocol design can be a source of unwarranted stress, especially when an excessive blood sampling regimen is pursued, producing a marginal anaemia that may itself make the animal more susceptible to the toxicity of the test substance.

The distribution of animals in the treatment room is also worth considering to avoid minor environmental differences that may become significant in longer studies. In this respect, rodents on the top row of cage racking can show ocular abnormalities, due to greater levels of light in that position, relative to the lower rows which are inevitably more shaded. Incautious distribution of controls or treated groups can produce an uneven distribution of ocular changes, which may be misinterpreted as treatment-related.

The source from which animals are obtained is also important. In terms of continuity and comparability of historical control ranges, a consistent supplier for each species should be used wherever possible. Significant differences were apparent between wild-caught primates and those bred in captivity in special facilities. The wild-caught animals were of unknown age, except in general terms, and were of unknown medical history – especially with respect to parasitic infections. The results of this included behavioural abnormalities and pre-existing histopathological lesions, which could confound the study findings. These problems have been largely circumvented by use of captive breeding, which produces an animal that is notably more relaxed and which, with group housing, is much easier to work with. Husbandry practices at dog breeders have also improved, with people employed to familiarise the animals with handling and interaction with technicians; this also produces a more relaxed animal that is easier to work with and, possibly, also safer.

Protocol design and procedure as sources of abnormality

Much of the above refers to abnormalities that may be present in the test system before the study starts. However, it is also possible to introduce abnormality into the study by poor protocol design. Taking samples, for toxicokinetic determinations, from dogs and primates is often performed only on treated animals or to a much lesser extent in the controls. For this reason it is vital that samples for clinical pathology are collected before the toxicokinetic (TK) samples. The extensive sampling normally associated with collection of samples for TK may induce a marginal anaemia, which will be more apparent in treated animals than in the controls which were sampled less extensively than treated animals. This can give a false impression of a treatment-related effect. The order and time of day at which investigations are undertaken must be consistent in order to ensure that diurnal variations are discounted. It may be useful to consider large studies as a number of replicates, with equal numbers from each treatment group in each replicate; this helps to ensure that the investigations are evenly spaced across the groups and that the variation between replicates is accounted for.

Control groups as normality

The contemporary control or untreated test system is always assumed to represent the experimental standard of normality from which treatment-related deviation may be assessed. However, the group sizes in toxicity experiments are usually quite small, and in a typical rat study a control group of 10 males would typically be randomly allocated from a group of about 45 males, allowing five animals as replacements, the remaining animals going to the treatment groups. Within the four groups it is quite possible to have differences in various parameters, that are statistically significant before the effects of treatment are added; this level of difference tends to increase as the diversity or heterogeneity of the original population increases. To assess the 'normality' of the control group their data may be compared with those from similar groups from other studies conducted in the same facility. This gives a valuable check that the controls have behaved in a similar manner to those on previous studies (i.e. that the controls of the current study are producing data that are in line with expectation). This type of check is routine for *in vitro* studies, particularly for positive control groups and in reproductive studies where the incidences of rare variants or malformations is a critical factor in determining the relevance of any differences seen from the contemporary control. These checks involve the maintenance and use of historical control data, which are discussed in detail below.

A protocol or experimental plan defines the endpoints or parameters to be examined and therefore defines the areas in which the controls must be normal. However, it should be appreciated that normality in scheduled parameters does not necessarily imply normality in others. In other words the test system should be normal in all respects in order to be valid for that experiment.

For the majority of experiments it is necessary to have a control group because of the relatively small differences that may be seen and also to facilitate the evaluation of dose–response curves and the presence of a no-observed-effect level. However, it may not be necessary to have controls where the change from normality is expected to be large or clearly evident, as in dose-finding studies early in an experimental series. The control group becomes essential in longer studies where 'experimental normality' can drift as the study progresses. Longer may be a relative term, as this can apply *in vitro*, especially with primary cell cultures, as well as in animals. Such change with time is seen typically with the plasma activity of alkaline phosphatase (ALP), which decreases with age. Increases in ALP activity are seen with some compounds that affect the liver, and when these increases are small they can be countered by the normal decrease in ALP activity, leaving the enzyme activity essentially unchanged from the previous examination. This lack of change, seen in treated animals, is an effect of treatment even though the ALP activity in those animals has not risen; the controls should show the expected decrease in activity.

In studies in which there is a statistically viable group size, it is not normally necessary to collect data before treatment, with the exception of non-invasive data such as bodyweight or food consumption. This is because the number of animals in each group allows a sensible statistical comparison to be made with the controls. Where the group size is smaller, usually seen in studies with dogs, non-human primates or *in vitro* studies, the scope for statistical analysis is greatly reduced because statistical power is affected by the sample size. In studies *in vitro* it is normal to compare the contemporary control against expectation as contained in the historical control ranges for the testing laboratory. In animal studies using dogs or non-human primates it is usual to collect data before treatment begins to indicate the baseline data for individual animals; these also act as a health check and individuals with abnormal results can be excluded or treated as appropriate. These data provide a within-animal control that, when evaluating data collected during the treatment period, can be used with the contemporary control data in a dual comparison to indicated treatment-related changes. Equally, change in the control groups in some parameters from one examination to the next may be contrasted with the absence of change in treated groups, thereby allowing the difference from controls to be interpreted appropriately. Carcinogenicity bioassays frequently have two control groups, allowing separate comparisons with treated groups to be made. If the high-dose group shows a difference from one control group but not the other, the difference may be dismissed as unrelated to treatment.

Inevitably there will be occasions when individual control cultures or animals show results that are clearly abnormal – either high or low; such results that lie grossly outside normal ranges are also occasionally seen in treated individuals at any treatment level. Examples of such deviation from expectation might include high colony counts *in vitro* in untreated controls or lack of response in positive control groups in bacterial mutagenicity tests or markedly high activities for single enzymes in the plasma of individual rodents. Some strains of rat are prone to early kidney failure, which is seen in controls and may be exacerbated or accelerated by treatment in test groups. In untreated controls it is obvious that the result has arisen by chance; where the individual has been treated such dismissal is more difficult, but can be achieved by reference to other data from that individual and to other members of the group or by the absence of dose response.

In some animal experiments it is normal to use the animal as its own control. This is true of experiments where individual data are collected before treatment but is a much more significant factor in some short-term tests. In studies such as skin sensitisation in guinea pigs, the Mouse Ear Swelling Test or in irritation studies, an untreated area of skin or the untreated ear or eye is assessed. This use of within animal control data is based on the assumption that the chemical administered will not enter the systemic circulation and that all effects are therefore confined to the site of administration.

Establishing and maintaining normality in experimental groups

An experiment has been planned and the test system has been delivered, prepared or taken from the freezer. As a first step it may be assumed, initially at least, that the population of cells, bacteria or animals that has been provided for the experiment is itself normal. However, some degree of heterogeneity in this population must be assumed and a commensurate degree of heterogeneity of response expected from the individuals. Before the experimental variable of treatment can be applied, it is necessary to distribute any inherent variability in the individuals of the test system evenly amongst the groups, in order to avoid experimental bias that may be seen as spurious differences between treatment groups. With cellular systems the stock culture may be mixed and subsampled to provide the cultures for the different control and treated groups, a process made more valid by the huge numbers of cells that are involved. With animals it is slightly more difficult because of the smaller numbers and the greater extent of genetic diversity that is to be expected. There are several methods available for random allocation of animals to treatment groups, which will achieve this even distribution. Usually the animals are allocated to treatment group by using a stratified bodyweight approach where the animals are listed by bodyweight and divided into as many ranges as there are treatment groups. Animals are then assigned in sequence to groups according to a rotation that ensures that an even number of animals from each range is assigned to each group. This is appropriate for smaller numbers of animals, especially when they are large, and usually gives treatment groups with similar group mean bodyweights. An alternative is simply to allocate them randomly to treatment groups as they are removed from their travel boxes or from stock cages. In either case, it may be necessary to adjust the distribution subsequently to remove any variation that becomes obvious during the period before the start of treatment or exposure to the test chemical. In some studies, especially those with large animals or in reproductive studies, it is important to ensure that litter mates are not grouped together, to avoid any genetic bias that may be introduced to a single group. Where a specific para- meter is considered of importance, it is good practice to examine it before treatment starts and to randomly allocate the animals to the treatment groups using these data. Use of pre-treatment cholesterol or triglyceride values as the basis for allocation to groups would be appropriate for a drug expected to affect plasma lipid concentrations, for example. The intention and overall result is to produce the correct number of treatment groups that are as similar as possible before treatment begins, in particular that the control groups are comparable with the groups destined for treatment.

Having completed the process of random allocation to groups or treatment, it is now necessary to ensure that the various groups remain comparable to each other, at least until treatment is applied. The groups also have to be comparable to previous control groups from similar experiments to allow comparison when necessary. For most test systems, but particularly for animals, an acclimatisation period is necessary to acclimatise them to the laboratory environment. For cell cultures this may mean that they are allowed to go through a few cycles of divisions to check for viability. For animals, a period of between one and four or more weeks is allowed; the former for rodents, the latter for larger animals such as dogs. This allows them to settle after transport to the testing laboratory and to become accustomed to the new procedures or cage mates. It is during this period that health checks are performed and the distribution among the groups is confirmed.

The importance of husbandry for test systems has already been mentioned and it is important that standards of husbandry should not change during experi- ments, especially short ones. In some cases it is necessary to change housing but this should not be undertaken lightly as the animals will be subject to stress as a result and this may affect their responses to the test compound.

In animal studies one of the most important factors to consider is the diet offered. The aim is to provide a diet that is well balanced and nutritious without compromising health. Correct nutrition has a critical role in toxicology; low- protein diets are known to affect metabolic capability and may increase the toxicity of directly toxic chemicals and decrease the effects of chemicals that require metabolism. Diets have been formulated traditionally to maximise growth and reproductive performance. However, a high-protein diet is not suited to mature rats and gives a different tumour profile in comparison with low-protein diets. In fact the growth of tumours may be enhanced by high levels of fat and protein. Conversely, the presence of antioxidants and trace elements can decrease tumour growth. There has been gradual realisation that high- protein diets can be responsible for excessive weight gain and adverse tumour profiles and poor survival, which has resulted in the use of low-protein diets or dietary restriction. The problem here is that a low-protein diet may not be appropriate for a growing animal. The apparently logical choice of changing from a high-protein to low-protein diet at the end of the growth phase is fraught with difficulty because this might affect the absorption of the test chemical and lead to increased or decreased exposure levels. Equally, the use of dietary restriction to reduce weight gain, for instance by offering food for 2 hours per day, means that the animals soon learn to eat only at that time of day. As a result the food intake is not significantly reduced in comparison with studies where diet is freely available. Also the practical considerations of giving and removing food each day adds to the study workload and increases costs. These factors are of particular concern in rodent studies, especially long ones, but are less of a problem with dogs, which are generally given a set amount each day. In any study there is a general preference for using the same batch of diet throughout; in any case, the batches offered should be known. It should be understood, however, that changing the diet offered or the feeding regimen will have a knock-on effect on the historical control ranges which will take some time to become re-established.

When studies are performed by mixing the test material in the diet, care must be taken that the inclusion levels do not affect the nutritional value of the diet. This is particularly difficult to achieve when testing novel foods; recent studies with genetically modified potatoes used dietary inclusion levels of potato that have been associated with pathological findings in the intestine. The presence of these changes was wrongly attributed to the genetic modification of the potato.

These various comments may also apply to consistency of media used for *in vitro* work, although as these are largely synthetic the overall significance may not be so great. Changing media routinely used in a particular type of *in vitro* study may be expected to change the response of the test system and will require the establishment of new historical control ranges.

One of the aims of study conduct should be to maintain consistency of design from one study to the next in order to obtain control data that may be referenced to the historical control ranges of the laboratory. This allows the performance of the controls to be measured against expectation at the laboratory and facilitates an answer to the question 'Are the controls normal?' The establishment and use of these historical control ranges or background data is a critical part of laboratory management.

The normality of baseline data

In any scientific experiment as many variables as possible are controlled in order to assess the truth or otherwise of the test hypothesis. The use of concurrent controls gives a baseline against which change in treated groups can be measured; they become the experimental definition of normality *for that experiment*. Within this narrow definition it is possible for each experiment in a series to stand alone, providing that controls remain valid as comparators for their test group or groups. However, when it becomes necessary to compare results across a series of experiments, it is important that the control groups are comparable historically with each other, otherwise deviation from expected control values in one experiment cannot be assessed with any confidence.

In toxicology, as in most scientific disciplines, the presence of a suitable control group, or groups, allows a judgement to be made as to the presence or absence of a treatment-related effect. It is possible, however, for control groups to provide data that are not consistent with normal expectation in the testing laboratory and to give results that are not consistent with previous experience. Even with the large, randomly allocated, double control groups typically used in carcinogenicity bioassays, each of 50 animals of each sex, it is possible to see statistically significant differences between the two control groups – especially in bodyweight or food consumption. It is therefore important to have a database of historical control data that will allow an assessment of the 'normality' of the controls, particularly when group size is small.

Uses for historical control data

Historical control data can be used to answer questions on the control data or on the deviation of treated group data from expectation if the concurrent control is in some way inappropriate – for example if the data are unexpectedly low. Equally they can be used to show that the occasional outlying result in treated groups is within the expected range of values. They are particularly important in tests such as those for mutagenicity, when they are used to check that the controls have produced the expected number of colonies or that the positive controls have shown a significant increase over untreated control values. In reproductive studies they are used routinely to compare the incidences of rare malformations with normal incidences in previous control groups.

If part of a study is finished earlier than the concurrent controls it is possible (although tricky) to use historical control data to assess any treatment-related changes in the 'uncontrolled' test group. This type of assessment is best when gross change from expectation is sought, as subtle changes cannot be confidently assessed in these circumstances. Changes in these cases can be assessed against presence or absence of similar change in groups that complete the treatment or exposure period.

Types of historical control data

It is important to consider the data type before trying to set up historical control data bases, as some data are not appropriate for this treatment. Data that are suitable are objectively derived and are typically for continuously variable parameters or are incidence data for findings that are present or absent. The numeric type includes colony counts, mitotic index, clinical pathology parameters, bodyweight and similar measurements. Incidence data are typically for reproductive malformations or variants and tumours. Subjective data – those that require some judgement to grade – are not generally suitable for historical control data. Non-neoplastic pathology findings are a good example of this because of their presence in a number of severity grades, which are dependent on the judgement of the individual pathologist and because of the inconsistency of nomenclature between pathologists. In rats a limited degree of basophilic tubules may be normal in the kidney but, because of the probability of different interpretation and grading between pathologists, it is not generally possible to assign a numeric value that would be consistent from one study to the next. With tumour data it is much simpler because the animal either has a tumour or it does not (always allowing for pathological disputes about what constitutes a tumour, for instance with hepatic foci and adenomas). It is also impossible to have background data for clinical signs, especially those that are largely subjective such as hypoactivity or the extent of thinning of background lawn in the Ames test.

Defining a normal range

In defining normal values the most important characteristic to be determined is the mean of the control values for the parameter in question. However, this single figure does not indicate by itself the extent of the variability of the data about that mean. While a range – minimum and maximum – will give some indication of that variability, it is usual to apply 95 per cent confidence limits to the data and give the mean plus or minus 1.96 standard deviations, which excludes any outliers at the extremes. This gives reasonable confidence that 95 per cent of values will be inside the 'normal' range and also indicates the inherent variability of the parameter. However, this basic approach does not take account of the variable sample size for the different parameters, which is typical of historical control databases. Thus a commonly measured enzyme such as alanine aminotransferase activity may have 200 or more values, while a less common enzyme such as sorbitol dehydrogenase may only have 30. In this case the use of the simple mean plus or minus two standard deviations may give a false impression of security for the lower sample size. To take account of this it is possible to use a formula that takes account of the sample size by applying degrees of freedom. The range is calculated using the formula:

$$t_{n-1} \times \text{s.d. divided by } \sqrt{n}$$

where t is the tabulated value for t at $P>0.05$ for that number of values less 1 for the degrees of freedom. When such a range has been calculated the data reported for that parameter should include the number of samples (n), the mean and the calculated normal range and the actual range of values. All these values indicate the reliability of the figures generated; a normal range quoted from 30 values of an inherently variable parameter, for instance an enzyme activity, will be less reliable than from a similar population of a consistent parameter, such as plasma sodium concentration.

A vital aspect of normal range definition is the origin of the data contained in relation to what they are being compared with. For valid comparisons to be made, the control groups have to be as similar as possible and if the experiment is in any significant way atypical then its control data should not be included in the historical control ranges for the laboratory.

Drift in historical control ranges

With any biological organism some drift in normality is to be expected. With humans the normal height of the general population has increased significantly since medieval times and the health profile of the population has also changed as diet, medical knowledge, patient care and a host of other factors have improved. In toxicological test systems, reasons for drift or evolution in historical control values include change in genetics, storage or husbandry, culture media or diet, environmental factors and subtle variations in methodology. It is unusual to be able to pinpoint a precise cause for such drift, as various factors tend to interact to produce values that may be far from expectation, leading to historical control subsamples that may not be consistent with the rest of the data.

Suppliers have huge influence over historical control data through the pressure to select for particular characteristics in cell lines or animals that have large litters; these animals tend to be larger and to grow more quickly, which may be associated with earlier sexual maturity. In the late 1980s it was noted that some strains of rat were eating more and gaining more weight than previously. This had the effect of reducing survival in long-term studies below 50 per cent at two years – the magic cut-off figure produced by regulatory authorities to define an 'acceptable' carcinogenicity bioassay. This was due in part to unexplained deaths but also to increases in renal disease and increased incidences of mammary and pituitary tumours. The weights of some organs had also increased over previous historical controls.[1]

Drift, which may be due to supplier influences, has also been important in the historical control data seen with reproductive studies in fetuses of rats and rabbits. A good example of this is the reduction in the number of extra ribs seen in some rat strains from over 20 per cent of fetuses to fewer than 5 per cent in a five-year period at one laboratory. Litter size has tended to increase in line with breeder pressures and this may be expected to influence the historical background incidences of study findings, quite apart from the expected reductions in fetal weights.

Another source of drift can be in the diagnostic criteria and nomenclature used by pathologists in evaluating the study tissues – especially in carcinogenicity studies. To a large extent this is an artefact, and comparison of tumour rates between laboratories is also made more complex by differences in these factors.

The consequence of this variability is that it is necessary to update historical control ranges at regular intervals to ensure that they stay relevant to contemporary studies. The best way of achieving this is to use a data capture system which has the facility to take control values from suitable studies for recent historical control data and from which studies are excluded as needed. Selection of studies for inclusion needs some care to avoid data bias.

How many data points?

The number of data points needed to give a viable historical control database for any one parameter is dependent on the data type and the inherent variability of the parameter in question. For a continuously variable parameter with low variability a smaller number of points will be adequate than with a highly variable parameter. Although it may be feasible to define the number of values necessary for statistical security in the light of the variability in a parameter, it may not actually be sensible to do so. The reason for this is that all too frequently the smaller data sets relate to rarely examined parameters, particularly enzymes, and in these cases any historical control data may be a bonus and cannot be ignored. The weakness of the comparison has to be taken into account in the interpretation and it may become necessary to refer to similar data from dissimilar studies or from other laboratories.

For incidence data, Tables 2.1 and 2.2 give some indication of the sample sizes needed for a viable comparison. In this case, which is typical for tumour incidence data in carcinogenicity bioassays, the more data available the better the security of the conclusions drawn from them. The principal caveat is that they should be recent data as some drift in tumour incidence may be expected

Table 2.1 Probability of a given sample of animals containing at least one case for different background incidence levels

Sample size	True population incidence level (%)				
	2	5	10	20	40
10	0.183	0.402	0.652	0.893	0.994
20	0.333	0.642	0.879	0.989	1.0
30	0.455	0.786	0.958	0.999	1.0
50	0.636	0.923	0.995	1.0	1.0

Source: Glaister, John R. *Principles of Toxicological Pathology*. London: Taylor & Francis, 1986.

Table 2.2 Maximum background incidence that would yield a zero result in a sample ($P<0.05$)

Sample size (n)	5	10	15	20	50
Background incidence (%)	45	26	18	14	6

Source: Glaister, John R. *Principles of Toxicological Pathology*. London: Taylor & Francis, 1986.

with time. The minimum incidence of a tumour that is possible in a treated group in a standard carcinogenicity bioassay is 2 per cent or one animal in 50. However, although the control groups in modern carcinogenicity bioassays are typically of 100 animals (in two groups of 50) for each sex, this does not necessarily give enough statistical sensitivity to dismiss a single tumour as incidental. This is because a control group of this size is only likely to show a tumour with a minimum incidence of between 3 and 4 per cent. The implication of the data in the tables, especially Table 2.2, is that to assign a tumour found in one treated animal to incidental causes, a historical database of a minimum of 200 animals would be desirable. With tumours, the statistical device of combining males and females, which would give a control group of 200 animals, is only viable when there is no sex-related bias in incidence. This is clearly not the case for prostate, testicular, mammary or other sex-specific tumours and cannot even be applied to liver tumours due to sex-related differences in metabolism. For analysis of rare tumours, it may be necessary to resort to outside sources of historical control incidences which are likely to be larger, although more diverse in origin and derived from different study designs.

Reproductive toxicity studies provide similar problems and it is likely that a minimum of 50 litters would be needed to give a secure historical control database. The litter is the unit of evaluation in reproductive studies and the number of individual pups is less significant.

For numerical data, such as clinical pathology or colony counts, 100 data points may be acceptable for an evenly distributed parameter with limited variability between individuals. For parameters where the variance about the mean is lower, for instance electrolyte concentrations in plasma, a smaller number may be acceptable. Where the parameter is highly variable between individuals and, in some cases, between occasions of examination, it is desirable to have a much larger data set for comparison.

Transferability of normality – data from other laboratories

In the same way that the contemporary control data is the best estimate of normality for any particular experiment, control data generated in similar experiments at the same laboratory are the best source of historical control data. However, there are occasions when the in-house experience is insufficient for confident interpretation of the results. This is so for parameters that are not frequently measured, or when it becomes necessary to compare in-house data with those from outside in order to verify correct performance of the test.

There are a number of factors that work against this, however, including differing environmental factors such as diet or noise, differences in analytical technique or instrumentation and pathological nomenclature. Despite these challenges, data from other laboratories are frequently better than nothing at all. The criteria for deciding the relevance of data from other laboratories for purposes of historical control use are the same as for in-house data, as discussed below. The greater lack of comparability of such data with those produced in-house must not be forgotten in the process of interpretation. This is illustrated by data published for control groups from a number of studies using Charles River rats and mice.[2–4]

Note

There are sources in the literature for other parameters such as those of clinical chemistry or haematology, however, these are probably less useful than tumour incidences and may well be subject to undefined methodological differences, rendering them essentially useless. Animal suppliers should have background data on their web sites, especially for parameters such as growth and food consumption or specialist data such as glucose concentrations in diabetic models.

Criteria for comparison of historical controls

The following uses a fairly arbitrary order to indicate the importance of the individual factors that need to be considered in deciding how much one set of data is comparable with another. The comparability of the data sets will increase as the number of similarities from the listings below increases.

- *Species and strain or derivation of culture or test system*   Use of the same species is clearly essential but different strains of mouse or rat, as with strains of *S. typhimurium* or *E. coli*, have their own characteristics which significantly influence the values for their various parameters. This distinction extends to primary or secondary cell cultures derived from animals; for strict comparability they should be from the same strain, similarly treated or derived from the same original culture source. Hepatocytes from rats pretreated with Aroclor 1254 (now more rarely used) will probably not be the same as those from pentobarbitone-treated animals.
- *Experimental protocol*   The procedures used in producing the data must be as similar as possible, extending to culture methods, husbandry, treatment or exposure period and data collection methods. Where the protocol delineates the criteria for data collection, it is critical that data from similar protocols are compared as small shifts in definition can produce large differences in incidence. This is particularly relevant in epidemiological toxicology and may be an Achilles' heel for future evaluation of records collected under COSHH regulations. Data collected from restrained animals may well differ significantly from those collected by telemetry, for example heart rate and blood pressure.
- *Age of the test systems must be comparable*   There are a significant number of parameters that change with age. In primary cultures of hepatocytes, metabolic capability declines over a period of hours so that data from a fresh

culture may be radically different from those given by older cells. In animals the most obvious change with age is seen in bodyweight but other parameters move in concert with this. In the plasma, alkaline phosphatase activity reduces as the growth phase slows and the bone-derived isoenzyme becomes less important. Renal function in older animals is significantly lower than in the young and this may influence response to toxins through slower clearance and possible changes in the importance of metabolic pathways. In addition, greater variability between individuals is a characteristic of old age.

- *Dose route or method of exposure*   Although this is less important *in vitro* there is still scope for significant difference, as with exposure in the vapour phase or in a solvent such as DMSO. In animals, ADME and toxicity following the various routes of administration can be very different. There may also be effects on parameters due to the procedure itself; muscle damage at the site of injection can be associated with increased release of enzyme markers of muscle damage into the plasma; e.g. creatine kinase, lactate dehydrogenase and aspartate aminotransferase. Such damage may be due to the vehicle used in the formulation.

- *Vehicle or culture media*   As compounds seem to have become more difficult to formulate, there has been a trend towards more exotic vehicles in an attempt to enhance bioavailability. A significant number of excipients used in formulations, such as suspending agents and, particularly, solubilising or wetting agents such as Tween 80, have their own toxicity which complicates comparisons between them. In addition, formulation differences, in terms of percentage content of individual agents give an extra layer of uncertainty.

- *Same source or supplier of test system*   The importance of environmental factors and genetic differences between suppliers may have effects that are determined by the inherent stability of test systems. Data from test systems that are not genetically homogeneous will tend to vary least between suppliers, in part due to the inherent variation between individuals in such species.

- *Similar environmental and housing conditions*   These include factors such as stocking density, breeding or culture procedures, etc. Housing and stocking densities, which affect stress levels, can have wide-ranging effects, including effects on tumour profile. Changes in husbandry practices, for instance to exclude or reduce disease, have far reaching effects on animals; this has been seen with rabbits where changes in housing conditions greatly reduced the mortality seen in older facilities.

- *Similarity of data recording*   Occasionally, new procedures or personnel can lead to a new observation that has been present before but simply missed due to lack of observation at the critical time or because the personnel or method of observation changes. The overall quality of data is also a factor but is one that cannot be readily established from tables in isolation.

- *Laboratory instrumentation and analytical procedures*   This is an important factor to consider (but not always available) when comparing analytical data from different laboratories. It may be a factor in published differences in the plasma activity of alanine aminotransferase in marmosets from different laboratories. Change from manual or visual data collection, for example differential cell counts, to instrumental methods can produce large changes in incidences. Inception of new analytical kits or data treatments can likewise have significant effects that make it impossible to compare early data with new.

At some point the decision must be made as to whether the historical control database offers sufficient comparability with the experimental controls to make a meaningful contribution to the interpretation of the results. If a significant number of the factors given above is not matched, it would probably be better to rely on the experimental controls rather than to use historical control data of dubious similarity.

Chapter 3

Determination of toxicity

Basic principles

Introduction

The following chapters examine the various areas of toxicity investigation that are routinely undertaken in a development programme, starting with a review of basic principles. A short chapter on *in vitro* systems is followed by chapters covering the main areas of regulatory toxicology, namely general and reproductive toxicity, genotoxicity, carcinogenicity and so called 'special studies' for effects such as contact hypersensitivity. There are also brief reviews of ecotoxicology and epidemiology, the intention being to give a complete picture of toxicological investigation without going into detail in these specialist areas. However, due to space, I have not made any effort to cover safety pharmacology for pharmaceutical products; the ICH guidelines (website given in the appendix) are a good source of information on this area.

Circumstances of toxicity testing

Nothing in this world is without toxicity of some kind. Investigations to determine the extent or seriousness of toxicity are undertaken for a number of different reasons and with various objectives in mind, often with evaluation of risk for human use or extent of exposure as an ultimate goal. The endpoint of such investigation can be precise – as in attempting to clarify the relationship between an effect and exposure to the test substance or to elucidate mechanisms of toxicity. Very frequently there is no such readily definable endpoint, merely the broad question – how toxic is this material? The answers to this question may well be used to predict effects in humans and to assess safe dose levels (drugs) or amounts to which people may be exposed without adverse effect (pesticides, food additives or chemicals at work). In terms of studies needed before release of a substance intended for public use or leading to human exposure, the investigations of a chemical's safety fall into two phases and, broadly, two types. The first set of investigations addresses two objectives. The first objective is to identify intrinsic hazard in the test chemical and the second is to estimate where and when that hazard may be manifested. The purpose of the second type of investigation is to confirm the predictions arising out of the first set, in the real world. In other words, before release to the public, the first step is to predict and suggest ways of controlling or preventing effects or events that might require investigation. In the second step, epidemiological studies are undertaken after distribution of the chemical has started to ensure that hazards to human health or the environment have been correctly predicted and assessed. The first set of studies is undertaken in a laboratory environment and the second conducted in the 'field' in patients or consumers or in the environment.

Before a marketing authorisation for sale to the public is granted, the testing of a chemical falls into the category of safety evaluation. The extent of such testing and the type of study conducted are closely regulated by government guidelines. Compliance with these guidelines is not optional; it is also a general proviso that the studies be conducted according to the scientific needs of the particular chemical under evaluation.

Once sales of a pesticide or drug have started and significant public exposure – either of consumers or patients has occurred, it is possible for untoward and unpredicted effects to be detected that may be associated with the chemical. It is popular in this increasingly litigious society to suggest that any abnormality in a population is attributable to chemical exposure, for instance to local use of agrochemicals. These effects become the subject of epidemiological investigation that is intended to establish a link, or otherwise, between the chemical and the effect. With drugs for which the dose given and the patient history and co-medication are known and for which the exposed population is easily defined, such investigations are relatively simple. For low-level exposures to pesticides where the dose is unknown or only roughly estimated, and for which there are numerous other exposures to contend with, certain establishment of a relationship between effect and the chemical is much more difficult. In both cases, once a relationship has been proven, specific mechanistic studies can be undertaken to show exactly how the substance exerts its toxicity and, in some cases, under which circumstances it has its undesired effect.

In order to bring a new chemical to the market place it is necessary to design a programme of investigation according to complex sets of regulatory guidelines specific to the area of use of the chemical. Although the studies prescribed for each class of chemical may be different in type or duration they are all conducted to the same basic set of principles or protocol. In essence, these are to define an objective, choose a test system and design and conduct a study according to a predetermined protocol, having a set of investigations and endpoints that are chosen to meet the objective.

Effects sought in toxicity studies

It is an inherent handicap of toxicity measurement that programmes of evaluation are necessarily designed to detect historically known effects, especially where a particular change is expected due to prior knowledge of similar chemicals. Unexpected – and therefore generally unwanted – effects may be found during the course of routine toxicity investigations and are then subject to mechanistic investigation to assess their relevance to humans. Occasionally, unpredicted effects are found in patients or consumers after marketing has started, e.g. cardiac arrythmias seen with the gastrointestinal drug cisapride, which were due to prolongation of the heart rhythm – the QT interval – in some patients. This has induced a general examination of new drug candidates for effects on QT interval prolongation in safety evaluation programmes. Such triggers for additional investigations are relatively frequent, adding to the guidelines for the range of tests that must be conducted before marketing is authorised. The classic example of a new previously unconsidered effect was that of thalidomide, in which serious reproductive effects were found. The thalidomide disaster had an enormous influence on the practice of toxicity testing and safety evaluation, ultimately leading to a rigid framework of investigative studies but also encouraging a conservative response to toxicological innovation that is still with us.

One of the objectives of pre-marketing toxicity evaluation must be to search for mechanisms of possible epidemiological concern. It is relatively straightforward to identify severe effects such as acute renal toxicity but much more challenging to find or predict the minimal effect that may accumulate in human subjects over years or a lifetime and lead to insidiously progressive renal failure. The longest study routinely conducted in evaluation of medicines is the carcinogenicity bioassay in mice or rats over the majority of the lifespan of the chosen species. These studies are primarily designed to evaluate the potential for tumour formation and are not necessarily, therefore, very good for revealing subtle changes due to true long-term toxicity.

Regulatory framework and influences

Particularly in the second half of the twentieth century, the regulation of toxicity testing increased tremendously in terms of practice and the types and duration of study conducted. Frequently, slightly different study designs were required in the USA, in Japan or in Europe. This resulted in duplication of tests and greater use of animals, with associated increases in development costs, which were not associated with significantly better quality of safety evaluation. In pharmaceutical regulation, the progress of the ICH process (International Conference on Harmonisation) has contributed greatly to the streamlining of testing programmes. This has been driven by industry and the regulatory authorities from the three main pharmaceutical markets. The process is likely to continue for the foreseeable future as our knowledge base develops and as new testing paradigms are produced and debated.

As new or unexpected effects have been detected, especially in the patient or consumer population, new studies or investigative programmes have been added to the guidelines. The type of study conducted for a particular class of chemical has also been influenced by precedent, where scientifically irrelevant studies were conducted for regulatory advantage. Omission of the test from future programmes for similar chemicals triggered questions from the box-ticking fraternity. The detection of unexpected effects in the human population, particularly for new drugs, inevitably has a huge influence on the practice of toxicological safety evaluation. In particular, the thalidomide tragedy had far reaching effects on testing regimens and methods and the marked growth in regulatory toxicity, and greater regulation, can be charted from that point onwards.

Regulation of study conduct

Another set of regulations, Good Laboratory Practice, governs how the tests are conducted. These grew from the experience of the FDA (Food and Drug Administration in the USA) in the early 1970s when it was discovered that a number of irregularities had been perpetrated in undertaking studies for new medicines. The regulations were set up to increase accountability and prevent fraud in the safety evaluation of drugs and have now been adopted globally. They define the requirements that a testing facility must fulfil in order to produce studies that are acceptable to the various authorities, and the term GLP has become pervasive as an adjective attached to facilities or studies. Good Laboratory Practices have had offspring that have grown up as Good Clinical Practices, Good Agricultural Practices and Good Manufacturing Practices. Their use has undoubtedly given immensely greater confidence in the results of toxicity testing; nevertheless some scientists still maintain that they are generally incompatible with pure research due to their tendency to impose inflexibility of study conduct. It should be borne in mind, however, that unfettered flexibility does not necessarily lead to good toxicological investigation. Although GLPs may be seen as inflexible, they do impose discipline on the subject of toxicity testing and this can only be seen as a good influence.

Legislation, guidelines and animal use

Animal welfare legislation is also an important factor to consider in toxicity testing, in terms of attainment of ideal housing standards and in the prevention or curtailment of suffering. In order to minimise the number of animals needed, it is important that testing is undertaken in healthy, unstressed animals, factors that have been reviewed above in chapter 2. The restraints on excessive use of animals have become stronger over the last 25 years of the twentieth century. In the UK it is now necessary to seek special Home Office approval for the use of non-human primates and the use of great apes is forbidden. Testing is discouraged in cases where the work is a simple repeat of a study, although the testing of drugs which have come 'off-patent' is a case where tests may be repeated because the original data files are not available to the generic producer. However, in many cases the new studies are conducted to the higher standards of the most recent legislation. Throughout this the concept of the three Rs – reduction, refinement and replacement – is central, the overall aim being to reduce the use of animals through refinement of investigative programmes and, where possible, by introduction of methods that replace them altogether.

The move away from animal experiments for routine toxicological safety evaluation has been slow and will continue to be so while the science is still growing and, in particular, while regulatory acceptance of the methodology is minimal. However, progress is being made. Replacement may be exemplified by the use of *in vitro* screening tests for dermal or ocular irritancy and the replacement of the rabbit in pyrogen testing by use of the *Limulus* amoeboeyte lysate (LAL) test for endotoxins. Reduction has been achieved through regulatory acceptance of the local lymph node assay instead of the guinea pig maximisation tests in sensitisation. The use of sparse sampling regimens in rodent studies reduces the need for large numbers of satellite animals for toxicokinetic evaluation, an effect that can also be achieved by the use of smaller sample volumes and more sensitive analytical techniques. Refinement of technique includes reduction of suffering by offering environmental enrichment, particularly important in primates, careful selection of dose levels and the reduction of pain. In particular the evolution of acute toxicity testing towards evaluation of severe toxicity rather than death – as required by the classic LD_{50} test – has markedly reduced animal use and suffering. The LD_{50} is still a useful concept, however, and may be estimated from the results of early studies and from the single dose toxicity studies that are still required.

COSHH (Control of Substances Hazardous to Health) Regulations

Further regulation for the workplace is provided by the requirements of health, safety and environmental control, covered in the UK by the Health and Safety Executive and monitored through the provisions of COSHH (Control of Substances Hazardous to Health). These regulations are aimed at protecting the workers involved in the testing or production of new chemicals and are the object of occupational toxicology. With some new medicines having therapeutic activity in microgram amounts the protection of the workforce becomes of paramount importance, even if some of the purpose is slightly cynical and aimed at the avoidance of litigation. The records of worker health which are retained as a result of COSHH will become an important epidemiological source of data in the assessment of health effects in the future.

The way forward

The inherent conservatism of regulatory authorities with regard to test models or methods is also a factor to consider. The general requirement is to use test systems or models that have been thoroughly validated, so that the data will provide a secure and fully understood basis for interpretation of the data and their significance for humans. This process of validation is complex and is often tied to extensive ring experiments – a series of similar or replicates of the same protocol performed in different laboratories around the world. There is an understandable tendency to use methods that are understood and have been shown to be reliable in scientific literature. In this way the local lymph node assay has gradually become more accepted in prediction of sensitivity reactions as a replacement for guinea pigs. The use of *in vitro* models in regulatory toxicology is likewise made difficult; at this point they are clearly acceptable in genotoxicity testing and may become so in some safety pharmacology tests, which can be considered to be a branch of toxicity testing.

Public perceptions

A further, and important, influence is provided by public and political pressure. This is rarely influenced by complete appreciation of the scientific data relating to a set of circumstances and is often based on a part set of the data. Partial understanding of a complete data set or complete understanding of a partial data set are unlikely to lead to a satisfactory understanding of the mechanisms leading to a particular set of effects or variation from normal, however normality is defined. Politics and science are often poor bedfellows and the use of science in political judgements, or vice versa, has to be carefully assessed according to the circumstances of the situation. The results may be over reaction and production of a set of regulations that can have worse consequences than the status quo.

Basic principles of toxicological investigation

Objectives

Investigations of toxicity may be carried out in isolation as single studies or part of a programme for the safety evaluation of a new chemical. In the case of novel drugs the purpose of testing is to support initial entry to humans in volunteer studies and subsequent trials in patients. The amount of testing required increases as the intended duration of treatment in humans increases. Other objectives include assessment of environmental impact for pesticides or the toxicity evaluation of intermediate chemicals used in the production of others, usually for occupational purposes. Broadly, the objectives and philosophy of a programme of testing are driven by the intended use of the test chemical.

Whether part of a programme or as a stand-alone study there should be a robust, preferably simple, study plan with a clearly stated objective. In animal-based tests this objective is likely to be broadly stated without precise endpoints, usually 'to determine the toxicity of . . .' This is in recognition of the complexity of animals and the large number of endpoints that are addressed in these studies. With simpler test systems the objectives are more precise, for instance to determine chromosome damage. This objective should be strictly adhered to if the integrity and interpretability of the study is to be maintained. It is not sensible to incorporate an assessment of reproductive toxicity into a 13-week general toxicity study because an animal becomes pregnant unintentionally. Re allocation of animals from one purpose to another may produce unwanted bias in the data, making interpretation more complex.

In regulatory toxicology there is considerable emphasis on demonstrating toxicity rather than safety, as a negative outcome cannot be proved with confidence; safety therefore has to be inferred and demonstration of a toxic dose supports this inference. Consequently, for chemicals of low toxicity, there is only reluctant acceptance of limit tests or doses, which may be the maximum practicable due to the physical characteristics of the chemical, for example low solubility. However, there is little sense in giving excessively high doses as there is frequently a dose beyond which absorption is saturated and no further systemic exposure can be achieved. As a consequence, toxicity expressed at high dose may be due simply to local effects in the gastrointestinal tract, which will probably not be relevant to humans in whom significantly lower doses or exposures can be expected.

Test substance considerations

The quality and characteristics of the test substance are crucial to the successful conduct of a toxicity investigation or to a development programme. Impurities can have far reaching effects on the toxicity of substances, both for study programmes and, when marketed, for human consumers or users. Impurities in tryptophan, used as a nutritional supplement in fitness programmes, were responsible for muscle wasting in many consumers and for a number of deaths; this debacle occurred after production changes which introduced new impurities that had not been present in the early batches. Production processes or the pathway of synthesis often involve the use of solvents which can be difficult to remove. The use of dichloroethane is controversial because it is known to be carcinogenic in rodents at high doses. Although the levels present in the final material may be far below the level for carcinogenicity to be evident, it is better to be safe and to remove it from the synthesis. Genotoxicity studies for mutagenic potential are particularly at risk from low levels of contaminants that may give a false positive to a non-mutagenic substance. It is normal to use the purest possible material in definitive toxicological investigations to avoid false reactions due to impurities. Impurities may express greater toxicity than the test molecule; for instance TCDD was a significant contaminant in Agent Orange used as defoliant in Vietnam by the US armed forces. When effects are receptor mediated, impurities may compete with the parent molecule at binding sites, thereby affecting toxicity or pharmacological response. When a toxicological programme as a whole is considered, it is best to use the same batch of test substance or batches of similar or better purity that are consistent with the product to be sold.

The quality of the test substance should be defined by suitable certificates of analysis or by information from the supplier in the case of studies that are not part of a development programme. By the time that early studies in patients begin, new pharmaceuticals should be accompanied by analytical certificates to Good Manufacturing Practice standards and the supporting toxicity studies should be conducted in material of the same standard.

The physicochemical characteristics of the test substance should also be considered as these can have significant impact on the choice of vehicle or carrier for toxicity studies and may determine whether such studies can be conducted. For example volatile compounds may be tested by inhalation in animals but need special testing apparatus for *in vitro*, genotoxicity experiments such as the Ames test.

The presence of a chiral centre in a molecule can also affect toxicity or action, as the enantiomers may be associated with different effects, either in degree or type. For this reason it is sometimes advisable to develop only one of the enantiomers; in fact this may well be the preferred strategy of the regulatory authorities. Development of the racemic mixture may be acceptable if there is rapid conversion between the two forms *in vivo* making distinction between them impossible.

Carrying system and route of administration

In order to bring the test substance together with the test system it is usual to formulate it with a solvent or carrier that allows the concentration or dose of the substance to be varied in a controlled manner. The choice of carrying system or vehicle in which the test substance will be dissolved or suspended is closely interlinked with the choice of test system and with the characteristics of the test substance. In an ideal world such carriers are simple and aqueous for use with easily soluble compounds; reality is often sadly different and increasingly complex formulations are being devised to achieve adequate exposure of the test system.

The intended route of administration has a profound influence on the choice of vehicle and is chosen according to the purpose and objective of the intended study. To examine the potential toxicity of a drug or agrochemical for which the expected route of therapy or exposure is oral, the most appropriate route of administration is also oral. For studies aimed at occupational health, dermal administration or inhalation are also likely to be relevant routes of exposure. For drugs, clinical intentions will drive the choice of route in the toxicity studies, although almost all drugs are also given intravenously at some point in order to generate comparative pharmacokinetic and bioavailability data. For dermal preparations that are not absorbed significantly, greater systemic exposure can be achieved by parenteral or oral administration, allowing 'worst case' systemic exposure to be investigated. This is an important consideration if the barrier functions of the patient's skin have been compromised by abrasion or other breakdown, allowing greater absorption than normal.

The best vehicles or carrier systems are the simplest, usually aqueous or with suspending agents that are toxicologically inert. For test substances that are poorly soluble in aqueous media, corn oil or a similar oil may be used. However, this is not suitable for *in vitro* experiments and cannot be used orally in some animals such as rabbits where the physiology of the gut is not compatible with large amounts of lipid. Wetting agents such as Tween 80 can have their own effects in the gastrointestinal tract, leading to faecal abnormalities and possible effects on absorption of the test substance. Use of simple aqueous media is unlikely to be associated with long-term effects. Use of corn oil in rats or mice at up to 5 ml/kg is usually associated with a compensatory decrease in food consumption and slight functional change in plasma lipid levels, which is unlikely to be of toxicological significance.

Increasingly complex vehicle systems, devised for insoluble compounds with a view to increasing test system exposure, can be associated with their own toxicity, which can mask the effects of the test substance. For substances with low solubility in water, it is more difficult to design a sensible *in vitro* assay, as these are generally water based. In these cases water-miscible solvents such as dimethyl sulphoxide can be used, providing the concentration is kept low; even then there is the possibility that the test substance will precipitate when it hits the water of the experimental medium. In some *in vitro* tests it is possible to claim exposure of the test system if the test substance is present as a precipitate.

Preparations for intravenous administration pose a particular problem and often mean that, with limited solubility, studies are conducted at low doses that are nearly meaningless unless continuous infusion techniques are used. It is important to avoid intravenous use of solvents that have their own toxicity, for example histamine release may be triggered in dogs by injection of polysorbates.

For dermal administration the vehicle is usually chosen to be similar to the circumstances of exposure in the human target population. For drugs this means that the formulation tested in toxicology studies should be as close as possible, preferably identical, to that intended for use in patients. Vehicles are usually chosen to enhance absorption across the skin and this applies equally to the clinical situation as to the toxicity investigation. For *in vitro* investigation of dermal effects using skin replacement systems, the vehicle should be chosen to be compatible with the test system chosen.

For agrochemicals and food additives the most usual carrier is the diet, as this corresponds to the expected route of human exposure. Admixing exogenous chemicals with diet is usually straightforward, although it is crucial to establish that the final mix is homogeneous. In difficult cases the test substance may be dissolved in a solvent or food-grade oil before adding to the diet. With organic solvents caution must be exercised, as residues can persist despite efforts to remove them, acetone being a case in point. With dietary administration there exists the possibility that the diet may become unpalatable at high concentrations. In any case care should be exercised that the additions to the diet do not affect the nutritional status of the animals. The maximum inclusion rate for nutritionally inert test substances is generally taken to be 5 per cent, which is approximately equivalent to 2 g/kg/day in rats.

For food additives the inclusion level may be raised to 10 per cent but care has to be taken with nutrition of the animals. This factor is likely to be a problem in testing high concentrations of individual genetically modified foods, as it is unlikely that effects will be expressed at normal dietary inclusion levels. However, the relevance of effects expressed at unrealistically high dietary inclusion of such foods should be questioned before the study begins, there being no point in generating data that are irrelevant. As an alternative to diet, the drinking water may be used as a route of administration but this has a number of disadvantages over the diet, especially in tracking the amounts of water – and therefore chemical – ingested as distinct from that spilled.

With both water and dietary administration there is the ever present problem of recording the amounts consumed. With unpalatable diets there is usually a significant degree of 'food scatter' where the diet is discarded by the animals without consumption. Estimation of this, especially for low amounts, has usually been only semi-quantitative; the trend towards housing animals on sawdust bedding makes estimation of scatter practically impossible. With drinking water, evaporation of water spilled or lost through playing with the outlet means that there is no hope of estimating amounts lost. Without such estimation there can be no accurate calculation of dose levels in terms of milligrams per kilogram per day

Dietary administration of pharmaceuticals in long-term carcinogenicity studies is often used and is an attractive option in cases where the pharmaco-kinetics are such that admixture with the diet may produce a greater systemic exposure to the test substance than once a day dosing by the oral route. A more pragmatic reason is that this route of dosing is simple and less labour intensive than oral intubation (gavage). The calculations for dietary concentration required to achieve the desired dose levels are straight forward, the dietary concentration increasing with continued bodyweight gain by the animals. To calculate dietary concentrations (ppm) to achieve constant dose:

$$\text{Dietary concentration} = \frac{\text{Target dose (mg/kg/day)} \times \text{estimated mid-week bodyweight(g)}}{\text{Estimated food consumption (g/day)}}$$

To calculate achieved dose level from food consumption and dietary concentration:

$$\text{Dose (mg/kg/day)} = \frac{\text{Dietary concentration (ppm)} \times \text{food consumed (g/day/animal)}}{\text{Mid-week bodyweight (g)}}$$

Inhalation toxicity is a specialised branch in its own right due to the technical complexity of generating respirable atmospheres at precise concentrations and monitoring them. Due to the vast amount of equipment needed to generate, administer and then to dispose of waste air, it is an extremely expensive method of administration. A related route is intranasal administration that is increasingly popular for some drugs; in this case the vehicle used can prove to be irritant to the nasal epithelia, thereby compromising absorption.

Choice of test system

The test system should be selected on scientific grounds, bearing in mind its suitability for achieving the experimental objective and whether it is ethical to use it. Small amounts of test material only may be available, especially in the early development of a chemical and this may be a factor that influences choice of test species. If the objective is to study potential effects in a non-human species it is usual to use that species or to use an *in vitro* preparation from that species. Although it is politically correct to think in terms of moving away from animal experiments to studies in humans or to *in vitro* techniques, many *in vitro* methods require fresh tissue or cell preparations from animals; although animal use may be reduced, it is not eliminated. *In vitro* methods are particularly useful in screening a large number of chemicals during a process of lead candidate selection, usually for a specific activity or toxicity that is of interest.

The only viable rationale for choice of test system, in cases where the ultimate objective is to predict safety in humans, is to choose a test system that is sufficiently close to humans in terms of pharmacological susceptibility, metabolism, pharmacokinetics, pharmacodynamics and physiology. This is especially so for pharmaceuticals. However, it is highly unlikely that a perfect match will be available and therefore the choice of test system must be a pragmatic compromise. The factors to be considered are summarised in Box 3.1. In addition, there are also pragmatic factors to consider, including housing, diet, genetic homogeneity, lifespan, reproductive cycle and litter size and the size of individual and the amount of test material needed.

The question being asked in the proposed experiment will, in most cases, determine the type of test system. The shortest question – Is it toxic? – requires the most complex test system, as the range of possible interactions is so large that they cannot be encompassed in a simple *in vitro* preparation. On the other hand a question addressing a single defined endpoint – such as DNA damage – can be answered *in vitro* in a simple test system. Choice of *in vivo* test systems is usually straightforward, as the numbers of laboratory species are quite small, the mouse and rat, in various guises, being the favourites. Unless the more exotic transgenic strains are selected, they are also inexpensive and easy to maintain. A further factor in favour of the use of rodents is that because of their ready availability, ease of husbandry and price, it is relatively easy to design a statistically sound experiment without breaking the bank. Specific strains of rodent can be selected to answer questions of mechanism; for example the Gunn rat is deficient in glucuronosyl transferase and thus can be used in mechanistic

Box 3.1 Factors in test system selection

The following has been compiled with ultimate human use in mind; similar criteria can be used for other target species.

- Similarity of absorption, distribution, metabolism and excretion and pharmacokinetics to humans. Choice may be influenced by comparative studies of metabolism *in vitro*, especially using hepatocytes from possible test species and humans.
- Scientific justification. Using a test system without scientific reason is not sensible, although some regulatory guidelines may insist on strange choices on occasion.
- Genetic homogeneity. Inhomogeneity means that the system is likely to be more variable and that normality is more difficult to define; increased variability reduces the ability of the study to detect minor adverse change.
- Strain; outbred versus inbred, especially for rodents. These choices have been extensively examined by MFW Festing.[1,2]
- Availability, feasibility and cost. There is no point in commencing an extensive testing programme if the most suitable species is not readily available at sensible cost.
- Regulatory acceptance.
- Purpose of test and applicability of species. For a new veterinary drug for use in dogs, it is essential to carry out the evaluation programme in dogs.
- Validation. Investigations of genotoxicity normally require the use of validated cellular or bacterial systems or exposure of tissues such as bone marrow in rodents. Validation applies to newer *in vitro* systems in particular but also to any new *in vivo* tests such as the local lymph node assay in mice.

studies of toxicity due to phase II metabolism. For *in vitro* systems the choice is more complex and can be more driven by the question asked; for example, the potential for nephrotoxicity can be investigated in isolated nephrons or kidney slices.

As indicated previously, the simpler and more direct the objective of the experiment, the simpler the test system can be. For a broad investigation of toxicity for a new compound it is normal to use an animal system because whole animals have all the complex interrelationships in place between organs and tissues. Absorption from the gut and passage through the liver can result in metabolites that affect the kidney or other tissues. Such interrelationships cannot, at the present state of the science, be reproduced *in vitro*, although progress is being made in the construction of individual tissue systems. Liver bioreactors are under development for investigation of drug metabolism and the possibility for adaptation for toxicity screening will no doubt follow on from this work.[3,4]

A variation on the *in vivo/in vitro* theme is the use of *ex vivo* systems. In these animals are dosed once or twice with the substance of interest and are killed at an appropriate interval after administration. Tissues can then be removed for study *in vitro*. This type of system is used frequently in the unscheduled DNA synthesis (UDS) test, in preference to the exposure *in vitro* of hepatocyte cultures.

In comparison with animals, *in vitro* systems are usually inexpensive, quick to complete and tend to give simple data sets. However, they can be technically challenging and, as a consequence, may not be reproducible in inexperienced hands or from one laboratory to another. Animal test systems, in contrast, tend to be expensive, both in terms of the facilities needed to maintain animals and in study conduct and also tend to be slower in completion. They cannot be performed without permits or licences from governmental authorities, which cover both the facilities and the experimenters. In addition, the data sets produced can be very large and complex to interpret; a four-week rat study with 80 animals produces more than 10,000 individual data points. A research programme based on animals will be more expensive and less flexible than one based on *in vitro* techniques but, because of regulatory reliance on animal tests, this choice is not available for every study type.

One of the objects of toxicological study is to predict effects in humans. There has been considerable criticism of the accuracy of extrapolation of animal data to humans, although, as understanding of the various animal models improves with our understanding of their relevance to humans, this is becoming less of a problem. However, the extrapolation of results to humans becomes more difficult the further one moves taxonomically from humans or from a whole animal model. It is one thing to extrapolate from rats to humans, but quite another to use an *in vitro* system of liver slices from rats or, on an even less complex plane, a rodent hepatocyte culture, to achieve the same predictive power.

Although the best predictive model for humans would appear to be humans, this has difficulties, not least the ethical considerations. Some experiments were performed in convicts in the USA but these were not extended and attracted much criticism. By any of the above considerations, humans fail as a test system candidate. They are large, requiring huge amounts of test material which, in the early stages of development of a chemical, will probably not be available. They have a long lifespan and slow growth patterns, making assessment of toxic effects on growth difficult. They require and consume a varied diet, in large amounts, that is not easy to standardise (diet affects the absorption of chemicals). Investigation of reproductive effects is long winded due to the long period of gestation and low litter size. They are extremely heterogeneous genetically, meaning that normality is difficult to define. The data obtained from a randomly selected group could be so diverse as to be uninterpretable.

Above all, the moral arguments against the use of humans have been used in recent years to slow the acceptance of volunteer tests with pesticides conducted to investigate human metabolism and pharmacokinetics. Possession of these data would make risk assessment of selected pesticides much more secure and would help to kill off the concept of pesticides as demon chemicals that do nothing but harm. If people considered the chemical composition of a cup of coffee, they would look at pesticides very differently.

The test systems available for the various types and areas of investigation will be reviewed in greater detail below under the sections dealing with investigation of specific toxicities in the succeeding chapters.

Study design basics and confounding factors

To facilitate conduct and interpretation of the final data sets, it is best to keep the design of toxicological studies simple but robust. Design, whether of generic guideline protocols or of tailor-made experiments, should take into account the three Rs of reduction, refinement and replacement as well as any regulatory requirements. The presence in the testing laboratory of relevant historical control data relating to the test system to be used has to be considered in deciding the size of control groups.

The classic design for a toxicological investigation has three or more treated groups and a control group, which receives the same treatment regimen as the treated groups but without the test substance. Positive controls treated with reference compounds may be included to check the sensitivity of the assay (particularly in *in vitro* experiments). It is important to demonstrate exposure of the test system to the substance under investigation. This is not a problem *in vitro* where the test system is exposed to the test substance in the culture medium, usually as a solution. In animals, however, it is necessary to take blood samples for toxicokinetic analyses, toxicokinetics being the term used to describe pharmacokinetics at high dose levels. While collection at several time points after administration is not a problem in dogs or non-human primates such as cynomolgus monkeys, rats and other small animals are too small for this and it may be necessary to add groups of satellite animals to the study solely for this purpose. This means that the animals allocated to the study itself are not stressed to the extent that the toxicity of the test substance is exacerbated or masked. However, with increasing sophistication and sensitivity of analytical methods the use of satellite animals may not be necessary. Toxicokinetic data demonstrate the extent of exposure to the test substance and are vital in the full interpretation of the data that result from the study. A further consideration is the metabolism of the test substance and the toxicity or otherwise of the metabolites, as indicated by ADME – absorption, distribution, metabolism and elimination – studies that are conducted as a separate programme of experiments. The data from these studies should be considered in confirming the choice of test system.

If the test substance is carried in a particularly unusual vehicle, it may be necessary to have a further, negative, control that is treated with water or a similarly benign substance, to take account of any toxicity due to the vehicle. Although there may be statistical arguments for having larger numbers of control animals than in the individual treatment groups, it is normal toxicological practice to use equal numbers. Having said that, there are cases where larger numbers of controls are used, particularly in carcinogenicity bioassays where two control groups of equal size to the test groups are often used. Use of greater numbers of controls can help to obviate the effects of exiguous historical control databases.

In routine toxicological investigations the choice of controls is simple; a suitable number of cultures or animals is allocated to the control group or groups from the same stock set as for the remaining groups in the study. In epidemiological investigations, where the subjects of investigation are humans exposed to the substance under investigation, the choice of controls becomes much more critical and complicated. For such studies it is vital that confounding factors are avoided and that the correct comparators are chosen.

Although confounding factors are well known in epidemiology, they should also be considered in routine toxicological investigation. One such factor is high heart rate in response to restraining procedures for recording electrocardiograms in unanaesthetised animals. Unless an animal is accustomed to the procedure, the unfamiliarity with the situation will result in abnormally high heart rates, which can obscure a milder compound related effect, possibly associated with reduced blood pressure. Such effects can result in minor heart lesions that are not detected until histopathological examination;[5] the use of telemetric implants can avoid such problems, although their routine use in toxicity studies is unusual due to cost. Another frequent cause of confounding arises when blood samples for clinical pathology are taken immediately after extensive sampling for toxicokinetic investigations. As the controls are not normally subject to the same sampling regimen for toxicokinetics as the treated animals, the samples taken for clinical pathology will probably show an apparent treatment-related anaemia and associated effects. Experimental investigations should be timed so that they will not affect future examinations or be affected by previous procedures. Husbandry can also be a source of confounding factors, especially with regard to stress, which can have a variety of effects. As a result, care should be taken to avoid unnecessary levels of stress, which might complicate the interpretation of the data.

Correct housing is one means of avoiding stress in laboratory animals, and there is increasing emphasis on cage size and environmental enrichment. Group housing is generally considered to be the best husbandry system, but is not always appropriate if the benefits are negated by aggressive behaviour. For instance, male mice are usually housed singly because of fighting; lesions in group housed male mice have been shown to lead to subcutaneous sarcoma when allowed to persist, an effect that can be exacerbated by treatments that increase aggression.[6] This may give a false impression of carcinogenic potential.

Although husbandry is clearly an important factor in the maintenance of animal test systems, its equivalent should not be neglected for *in vitro* systems, where inappropriate storage or preparation of cell cultures can lead to test systems drifting from expectation.

In all toxicological investigation the quality of data that are generated are paramount. Poor data – incomplete, badly recorded or ill-chosen timings – will probably result in poor interpretation of the experiment. Good Laboratory Practice has made a huge contribution to the quality of data recorded in regulatory studies. Although it has been suggested that GLP and basic research do not mix well, the principles of GLP have a lot to offer to this area as well, as it should be a duty of all toxicologists to record data as accurately as possible. Secure interpretation can only be made from a complete set of appropriate data; in this it is probably better to over record slightly as recorded data can be dismissed as irrelevant after the event, but unrecorded data cannot be interpreted. Having said that, it is easy to get carried away on a wave of enthusiasm and record everything – it can be difficult to draw a sensible line between under and over recording – or to over burden the protocol with too much detail that endangers the interpretability of the final product.

Choice of dose levels or test concentrations

The correct choice of dose level is crucial to the successful completion of every toxicological experiment and is normally achieved by use of a small preliminary study. The normal procedure is to use a sighting or dose range-finding study or experiment, to assess the toxicity of the test substance in the same test system and under the same conditions as for the main study. Typically a small quantity of the test system is exposed to increasing doses or concentrations of the test substance until a reaction is seen that indicates that a maximum tolerated dose level (MTD) or concentration has been reached. For studies in animals, the MTD is either used as the high dose in the main study or is used to select a slightly lower level that is expected to result in some toxicity but also to result in the survival of the animals until the treatment period has been completed. In in vitro systems the maximum concentration is usually chosen according to degrees of toxicity seen; for example the highest test concentration in cytotoxicity studies for registration is usually selected as the one that causes 50 per cent toxicity in the test system. In the Ames test for bacterial mutagenicity, the thinning of background lawn – the minimal growth of bacteria resulting from a small amount of histidine in the culture medium – is taken as a measure of toxicity.

Because the sighting studies tend to use lower numbers of animals or test replicates than the main study, they are sometimes unreliable in their prediction of high dose, either over or under. A typical design for an in vitro study is to use a wide range (e.g. 1000-fold) of concentrations up a maximum of 5 mg/plate or 5 mg/ml, using two plates or cultures at each concentration. In animals it is usual to have an initial phase in a small group which is treated daily, with dose levels that are increased at twice weekly intervals, until effects are seen that indicate that an MTD has been reached. A second group of previously untreated animals is then dosed for 7 or 14 days at the chosen high dose to ensure that reactions are consistent; this second phase is important in ensuring that tolerance has not built up gradually in the animals receiving the rising dose levels. Having completed a sighting study, it is still possible to obtain unexpected results, either excessive toxicity or none at all when the main or definitive study is started. Although the three dose level design is calculated to mitigate the effects of the loss of the high dose or concentration groups, it is better to avoid this as far as possible. Some of the explanations for unexpected results are explored in Box 3.2.

Box 3.2 Troubleshooting dose range-finding results

Unexpected results may arise from a wide range of factors, including the following:

- Different age of animals used in the pilot and main studies. The metabolic capability of the liver in rats increases between about six and eight weeks of age and it is possible that a sighting study in seven-week-old animals will give results different to those in animals of 10 weeks, for instance if the test substance induces its own metabolism to a toxic metabolite that is not present in younger animals.
- Different strain or supplier. Responses vary from one strain to another and can also do so between suppliers.
- Dose range-finding data from another laboratory. There is no guarantee that the conditions in the original laboratory will be the same as in the facility chosen for the main study. In particular husbandry can be significantly different, leading to different absorption profiles.
- Differences in formulation or form. Significant differences may arise with changes in formulation; if solubility and absorption of the compound are poor, it is tempting to change the formulation to increase absorption. Changing to an isotonic parenteral formulation can result in very much quicker bioavailability and greater toxicity. Micronising is often used to enhance bioavailability and can lead to greater toxicity. If a new form or formulation is suggested, a short study should be performed to check consistency with the earlier work.
- Differences between naïve animals and those dosed over several days – where an animal is dosed at a low initial level that is gradually increased, tolerance to the test compound can develop that is not evident in naïve animals. Dosing naïve animals from the outset at the chosen MTD can result in unexpectedly high toxicity because they have not had the chance to acclimatise to gradually increasing dose levels.

Such short sighting studies are usual only in the early stage of development, or when there is a need to investigate a new formulation or form of test substance. A programme of toxicological investigation in animals normally progresses from sighting studies to two- or four-week studies and then on to studies of 13 weeks or longer. At each stage the results of the previous study are used to select dose levels for the next study. Successful dose level selection in this case depends on continuity of the factors discussed above. In other words, do not make radical changes to a formulation during a development programme without further sighting studies, use the same strain of test system throughout and so on. It is also wise to go through a toxicological programme systematically; data from a two-week study may well prove unsuitable for selection of dose levels for a 26-week study. In general animals can tolerate high dose levels of chemicals only for a short period but tolerate lower doses for much longer. Hence a high dose of 300 mg/kg/day selected for a four-week study might have decreased to 100 mg/kg/day when the dose levels are chosen for the chronic toxicity or carcinogenicity studies.

Duration of treatment

The process of harmonisation of testing requirements for pharmaceutical products – enshrined in the International Conference on Harmonisation (ICH) – has arrived at agreed maximum lengths of toxicity study in the conventional species, assuming that they are proven relevant to the target species (usually human). In rats this is six months and, in a second species (usually dogs), 12 months for new chemical classes or nine months for chemicals in which toxicity has already been evaluated in previous programmes. The difficulty lies in extrapolating effects seen at high doses in animals to those expected in humans at lower dosages. The numbers of animals used in testing will be small relative to the numbers of humans exposed to the chemical and it is important to be able to extrapolate the findings to the much larger human population to assess their relevance to humans.

Such extrapolation is dependent on a thorough understanding of the chemical's effects on the individual, whether animal or human (dynamic and toxic changes) and of the effects of the individual on the chemical (kinetics and biotransformation). Understanding these processes, dependencies and influences is key to successful prediction of effect in humans and then to the process of risk assessment that follows. The conduct of a carefully designed programme of toxicity studies in a range of test systems assists this understanding and makes risk assessments for human use more secure.

Chapter 4

Determination of toxicity
in vitro

Introduction

In vitro toxicology is an area that is expanding rapidly and has become so extensive that a detailed description requires a separate book. Furthermore, with its multiplicity of methods that for the most part have little current acceptance, beyond use in lead candidate selection or mechanistic explanation, detailed description of methods or test areas has not been attempted. The following is a broad review of *in vitro* technique, strengths, weaknesses and future potential.

Rationale for *in vitro* toxicology; strengths and weaknesses

There is considerable pressure to reduce and replace the use of animals in toxicological research or testing, for scientific, economic and political reasons. The goal is to reduce the use of animals, in a scientific manner, while ensuring product safety, i.e. to refine toxicological investigation so that human-relevant systems can be used for secure prediction of human hazard. *In vitro* systems have a lot of strengths but also, at their current state of development many weaknesses, which make them unacceptable to regulatory authorities when used to answer general questions. Their strength lies in the simplicity of their endpoints and their consequent use in the evaluation of toxicological mechanisms. Their principal weakness is that they are not readily able to respond to chronic exposure and they cannot easily replicate the interrelationships that exist in the body between the various organs and tissues. In particular they cannot (currently) give any indication of an effect that will accumulate over prolonged administration, such as progressive renal failure or neurodegenerative disease. However, they have a considerable role to play in lead candidate selection and in the evaluation of substance groups such as cosmetics where animals cannot be used. With new technologies such as combinatorial chemistry, there are increasingly large numbers of chemicals to screen for toxicity or efficacy to aid selection of lead candidates for development. Traditional methods are too slow and costly for this. For a series of compounds for which a particular mechanism of toxicity has been identified, this may be investigated *in vitro* and the least toxic compounds selected for development. The objectives of screening include:

- Acceleration of lead candidate selection.
- The early discarding of compounds which would fail later in the development programme, after considerable expenditure of animals, time and money. Reasons for failure include formulation problems, toxicity, poor efficacy and poor acceptability (dermal formulations should be neutral in colour – not bright yellow). Clearly some of these are not toxicological in nature but pressures to develop a compound may result in the best of a bad series being selected.
- Screening of members of a compound series for specific activity or adverse effects that may have a structure–activity relationship, for example screening of retinoids for embryotoxicity.

The pursuit of *in vitro* technique should be directed at development of test methods that are acceptable to regulatory authorities as replacements for animal tests and to focus attention on identifying toxicities *in vitro* that may be expected *in vivo*. For example, an *in vitro* screen may suggest potential for renal toxicity indicating the need for specific examinations in animal studies and, perhaps, influencing dose selection so as to minimise any suffering in test animals. The use of *in vitro* techniques can replace 'severe' procedures. Successful development of these methods will lead to reductions in animal use, through gradual regulatory acceptance and reduction of the numbers of compounds entering full development. Financial benefits should not be a sole reason for replacing animals but cannot be ignored as a factor.

Although *in vitro* techniques have many attractions, they also carry a number of significant disadvantages that makes them unsuitable (currently) for routine testing for regulatory safety evaluation. Test systems are limited to single cell type or organ (tissue slice or whole organ perfusion) and can be technically demanding and, as a result, difficult to reproduce between laboratories. Replication of *in vivo* exposure conditions may be difficult, especially for lipophilic or insoluble chemicals. Because the systems have a limited life expectancy they are not suitable for the examination of chronic effects, especially those that accumulate gradually over prolonged exposure. Many toxicities are multifactorial and dependent on interrelationships between tissues/organs that are not readily reproducible *in vitro*.

Validation of *in vitro* methods

Validation is a perennial problem with *in vitro* systems, although many would say that animal tests have not been properly validated. However, they are at least well understood and produce data that may be extrapolated to humans or another target species, which cannot be said so readily for *in vitro* data. Validation seeks to answer questions relating to the reliability and relevance of the method under evaluation. The European Centre for the Validation of Alternative Methods (ECVAM) and, in the United States, the Johns Hopkins

Center for Alternatives to Animal Testing (CAAT) have done a lot of work on the validation of new methods (see Appendix for websites). Validation should seek to answer questions of the following type:

- Is the biochemistry and mechanism *in vivo* and in the proposed *in vitro* system fully understood?
- Is the *in vitro* method reliably predictive for the endpoint *in vivo*?
- Where a surrogate marker of effect is used, what is the reliability of this marker of effects *in vivo*?
- What are the robustness, reproducibility and reliability of the method?
- Do the data mean what we believe they mean?
- Have the limits of method been investigated and defined?

There is an understandable tendency to validate methods with known chemicals; nephrotoxicity models are often validated with mercuric chloride or similar classic toxic compounds. Probably the best method of validation, following exploration of the method with known toxicants, is to use it in parallel with more conventional assays so that the data can be compared when both tests have been completed. Validation is likely to decrease with increasing complexity of endpoint and be less easy to achieve. Genotoxicity tests have been accepted because they investigate a relatively simple endpoint in a series of robust assays that can be readily transferred between laboratories and which are, for the most part, relatively simple to conduct.

Test types and test systems

The endpoints in *in vitro* systems are generally simpler than those in intact animals and include measures of cytotoxicity, a crude indication of toxicity without showing why, how or when. A development of this is to examine functional alteration or cellular damage, which can be assessed by measurement of enzymes or other analytes that leak into the medium from the cells. Isolated nephrons can be used to assess potential changes in renal function. The most varied endpoints are found in specifically designed mechanistic experiments, which are frequently conducted to explain the results of routine toxicity tests (Table 4.1).

Toxicity *in silico*

Much attention is currently focused on genomics, toxicogenomics and proteomics, which, respectively relate to the expression of genes in normality, gene expression following toxic exposure and protein expression as a result of gene activation. These have been termed toxicity *in silico* techniques because they are dependent on chemical reactions with molecules, such as DNA, bound to silicon microarrays, in contrast to more conventional *in vitro* methods that show a time-dependent response. This follows recognition that mechanisms of

Table 4.1 In vitro test systems

DNA probes	Microarrays
Subcellular organelles	Microsomes
Single cells – primary culture	Hepatocytes and hepatocyte couplets,
Single cells – cell lines	Tumour cell lines, Caco-2 cells, stem cell cultures
Tissue slices or organ components	Liver or kidney Isolated neurons or nephrons
Perfused intact organs	Liver or heart
Cultures reproducing tissue architecture and function; different tissue cultures interlinked to give a "circulation".	Liver bioreactors and similar systems. Potential for use of stem cells in these systems.
Embryo culture	Whole embryo or micromass
Fertilised eggs	Chicken eggs used for irritancy and corrosion prediction
Excised tissues	Bovine eyes used in ocular irritation studies

toxicity are reflected by the profiles of the genes expressed in response to the toxic insult; protein expression is consequence of gene activation. The use of DNA microarrays in which thousands of DNA probes or synthetic oligonucleotides are mounted on a chip in a known order and then hybridised with target DNA, is able to determine which genes are activated in target tissues as a result of a toxic exposure. It has been shown that the protein expression profile is associated with effect and mechanism of toxicity and that these profiles are broadly similar within each group of compounds which, in life, have similar of effects and mechanism. However, within each group, each compound has its own distinct profile of protein expression. By setting a desired profile or indicating thresholds for decision, compounds can be selected or rejected for further development.

The use of these techniques needs careful consideration of objectives before committing to a system that is likely to be expensive to buy and maintain and may be difficult to alter. Genomics offers the possibility of use of open or closed systems. In the former, the endpoint is not specified and all genes expressed can be highlighted as a pattern of spots on the array. In the latter, a specific number of genes, for instance a few hundred, may be investigated, giving a pattern of effect in these target genes. In contrast to genomics, protein expression can (currently) only work as an open system in which all proteins are examined. Because of the vast amount of data that are generated using these techniques, pattern recognition software is important in interpretation of the data.

Protein and gene expression both change with time, and the number of genes expressed a few hours after exposure may be an order of magnitude greater than that at one hour. Both proteomics and genomics offer a snapshot of the effects of the compound at a particular time point and do not reliably show the past or the future. Choice and consistency of time point is therefore important in ensuring that the data generated contain enough information – but not too much – to achieve the experimental objective. The study of proteins expressed is a reflection of what is happening in the cell, whereas the pattern of gene expression is a reflection of possibility. Both techniques are, however, necessary to give a full picture of what is occurring.

Genomic and proteomic expression both produce patterns of effect that may be associated with particular toxicities. This principle is also exploited in the use of nuclear magnetic resonance spectroscopy, which can be used to reveal the amounts of small molecules (up to a molecular weight of 600) in a biological fluid, especially urine. The readouts from this can carry 3000 vertical lines, each specific for a particular chemical such as citrate or hippurate. The problem is that there will be simultaneous changes in the quantities of many endogenous metabolites, quite apart from those due to the test compound. Sorting these data and then using appropriate software to plot them is an important part of the process. One aspect of this technology, which has been around for a long time, albeit without the pattern-recognition software to make it more universally useful, has been the name given to it – metabonomics. If there is not much debate about the utility of the technique, there is a fair amount of speculation on how to pronounce it correctly.

A significant strength of these pattern-based techniques is their potential, when used as open systems, to show changes that may indicate toxicities due to novel mechanisms. However, they cannot show what the mechanism of toxicity is and further investigation, which could be prolonged, would be needed. The problem here is that compounds showing novel patterns of change are likely to be dropped from development and not investigated further unless the pattern is common to the members of a promising series of compounds. This may represent a missed opportunity for examining new mechanisms of toxicity that could be of significance in humans. Many successful, but toxic, compounds with acknowledged benefits might have been dropped from development if such techniques had been used for them. Such knowledge might prevent some of the more unpleasant surprises of chemical development and marketing but, equally, is probably responsible for the rejection of compounds which may have benefit despite toxicity.

In cellular culture, the use of stem cells holds out the prospect of developing different human tissues from a uniform stock of cells and the possibility of co-culturing these tissue cells to give an indication of interactive effects between tissue types. However, there may be a problem, in a mixed culture, in differentiating the direct effect of the compound from indirect effects that may be due to metabolites. The basic tenet, that chemicals can induce a particular profile of protein expression, is a useful one. The profiles produced by investigational chemicals may be compared with those from a library of known toxins, as an indication of anticipated effect. The weakness of this, and similar systems, is that they are critically dependent on the size and content of the database against which the profiles are compared. Inherently, it is unlikely that new types of toxicity can be predicted by this type of database-dependent system, because their discovery is dependent on their presence in the database for previous compounds. Much trouble is caused by unexpected or novel effects, which become apparent following significant human exposure and which are not predicted by routine screening techniques. The possibilities for comparing members of a series is very good, however, if the effects of the first few members have been adequately characterised.

The interest in these technically demanding and expensive technologies is based on their perceived potential as methods of early rejection of compounds from development. The savings in time, laboratory space, animals and expense could be significant. However, for medicines at least, it should be appreciated that many successful drugs have significant toxicities that were found in preclinical development. In so far as drug development is an art, part of this art is to assess the relevance and impact of these effects and to judge if the drug can be used beneficially in appropriate patients. The basis on which compounds are rejected or selected must be chosen in advance otherwise indiscriminate rejection may limit the development of effective chemicals – medicines or pesticides – in the future.

'Traditional' *in vitro* toxicology

These complex, technically difficult systems offer a greater precision of mechanistic assessment than the older, less complex cell-based systems which are used for estimation of toxicity. These older techniques are usually based on cytotoxicity (death) or leakage of cell contents into the culture medium – for instance lactate dehydrogenase. These assays include the neutral red assay and trypan blue exclusion, which works on the basis that a live cell can exclude the ingress of trypan blue whereas dead cells take it up. Primary cell cultures have several advantages in that they usually retain more of the typical capabilities of the cell *in situ* than cell lines, although these capabilities decay fairly quickly, usually over a few hours. Another disadvantage is that, for cells such as hepatocytes, in the process of producing a single cell suspension, the blood–bile duct polarity of the cell is lost. This important aspect of hepatocyte function can be maintained by the use of hepatocyte couplets, in which the biliary side of the cells is maintained in the middle space between two hepatocytes.

Isolation of functioning tissue units such as nephrons or axons is a useful way of examining specific tissue function, which can be extended by the use of tissue slices or perfused organs. These techniques have the advantage that the architecture of the tissue is maintained, allowing the possibility of microscopic examination of the preparation at the end of the exposure period.

The use of culture methods to produce blocks of cells that have some of the characteristics of the original tissue is also a technique with considerable potential. Hepatocytes can be induced to maintain functionality for several weeks when mounted in an appropriate matrix of collagenous material. There is then the possibility that such tissue blocks could be placed in connected incubators linked through a circulatory system, offering the potential for studying interactive effects.

Future utility

One of the areas of particular interest with *in vitro* techniques is their potential to replace mammalian tests in areas such as pharmacology and quality testing. The prime example of this is the LAL test, which exploits the sensitivity of amoebocytes from *Limulus*, the horseshoe crab, to detect pyrogens in solutions for infusion; it is significantly more sensitive than the rabbits it replaces. Pharmacological models increasingly use *in vitro* techniques, such as the use of human cloned potassium channels for assessment of the potential for prolongation of the QT interval of electrocardiograms. Other applications of *in vitro* techniques are discussed under the relevant sections below, particularly reproductive toxicity, genotoxicity and irritancy and corrosivity. The last two have frequently been associated, in the past, with unacceptable animal suffering, particularly in the eye irritation tests in rabbits. As a result there has been considerable effort expended in finding viable alternatives, the challenge being to reproduce the complexity of the situation in the living eye in the context of *in vitro* simplicity.

Pitfalls

The basic challenge with any *in vitro* technique is interpretation of the data in relationship to the animal from which the system was derived and then, if needed, to humans. The absence of interaction between organs or tissues and the static nature of many (older) systems means that some effects are seen that would be absent in life. Also the transient nature of most *in vitro* systems means that chronic administration and the detection of progressive effect is not possible. These test systems are often technically demanding and difficult to reproduce from one laboratory to another. An additional factor to consider is the sheer volume of data that are produced by some of the new techniques and the consequent requirement for suitably validated pattern-recognition or data-plotting software. Where the software 'cleans' a data set to simplify a data plot, there should be confidence that the correct data are being excluded, otherwise useful information may be lost. As already pointed out above, the choice of time point can be critical in achieving data that can be analysed to best advantage. In the absence of good validation work, the significance of the differences seen may be misinterpreted and erroneous conclusions drawn. If the mechanism is not understood correctly and the meaning of the data is not clear, there is no point in doing the test, except as part of a validation exercise. It is clear, in these cases, that these unproved systems would be totally unsuitable for toxicity prediction or safety evaluation.

Overview

In vitro techniques have enormous potential that will be realised with increasing effect, leading to gradual regulatory acceptance of validated tests that have been shown to have relevance to prediction of human hazard. Their basic weakness – and strength – is the limited number of endpoints that can be covered in a single system in comparison with a whole animal, in which all the inter-relationships between tissues and organs are intact. However, ethical pressures together with the increasing constraints of cost and time will drive development of these techniques forward. Ultimately, they will come to play a more central role in safety evaluation.

The future of *in vitro* toxicology was reviewed in 1997 by a working party of the British Toxicology Society in a report on *in vitro* toxicology published as *Human and Experimental Toxicology*, Volume 16, Supplement 1 (1997). A report prepared by ECVAM (the European Centre for the Validation of Alternative Methods) entitled 'Alternative (Non-animal) Methods for Chemicals Testing: Current Status and Future Prospects' was published in the journal *ATLA* (Volume 30, Supplement 1, July 2002). This 'non-animal' based report recommends tests such as whole embryo culture, for which animals are required, albeit not treated *in vivo*.

Chapter 5

Determination

General and reproductive toxicology

General toxicology

In broad terms, general toxicology is something of the poor relation of toxicology. It can be seen as lacking the glamour or intellectual rigour of other areas of toxicological investigation because it sets out to be a catch-all; to paraphrase Gerhard Zbinden, it looks for everything but hopes for nothing. However, it is central to safety evaluation of novel chemicals, as effects that may be seen in other more specialised areas can also be detected or supported by well-designed general toxicity studies.

Test systems for general toxicology

The large majority of test systems for general toxicity are animal-based, due to the need to demonstrate toxicity elicited after repeated administration over long periods, something which *in vitro* systems are not able to do convincingly at present. A further factor militating against such systems is the multiplicity of endpoints examined in a classic study and the limited number of such possibilities in a cell culture that lacks the complex interactions between tissues seen in whole animals. For a complete picture, general toxicology also requires an estimation of the absorption, distribution, metabolism and elimination (ADME) of a compound and of the pharmacokinetics following single and repeated administration. With pharmaceuticals particularly, it is important to choose one species that is as close to humans as possible in terms of ADME; two such similar species would be better but as one is almost always the rat, this luxury is not always possible. The use of comparative *in vitro* metabolism data and preliminary *in vivo* data should allow a scientifically justifiable choice of test species to be made. In practice the test species are chosen from a relatively limited pallet of possibilities, restricted by toxicological conservatism and regulatory acceptance, as indicated in Table 5.1. The advantages and disadvantages of each system are summarised in Box 5.1.

Table 5.1 Test systems for general toxicology

Rodent	Non-rodent
Rat	Dog
Mouse	Non-human primate
Hamster	Minipig
	Rabbit

Box 5.1 Characteristics of test systems for general toxicology

The following attributes for the main test species are given in no particular order and without guarantee of completeness:

- *Rats/mice* Easy to house; small, meaning that relatively little test substance is needed; well understood with ample historical control data; multitude of strains; short life spans; good regulatory acceptance; traditional; few ethical problems associated with their use; genetic consistency; statistically robust designs are relatively easy to achieve at sensible cost; not necessarily good models for humans; metabolism tends to be rapid and systemic exposure lower than in humans; males have greater metabolic capacity than females, which often leads to sex-related differences in toxicity.

- *Hamsters* Alternative to rat or mouse but rarely used except in specialist studies and some carcinogenicity bioassays; few historical control data; the species to use when all other rodent options are exhausted.

- *Beagle dogs* Reasonable size to work with; good natured; well accepted and now the only dog available in the UK for laboratory experiments; well understood; ample historical control data; good regulatory acceptance; can react badly to compounds such as non-steroidal anti-inflammatory drugs; low workplace handling risk; usually weigh between 10 and 15 kg, needing large amounts of test substance; large areas needed for stress-free housing and husbandry.

- *Minipigs* Similarity of skin to humans makes them suitable for dermal studies; kidney structure similar to humans; not a mainstream species but with increasing regulatory acceptance; omnivorous diet gives similarity to humans; large – 'mini' can mean up to 50 kg with a norm of about 30 kg, with consequent effect on test substance requirements; not as easy as dogs to dose or to take samples from; some metabolic peculiarities, particularly in sulphation.

- *Non-human primates (NHPs)* Species used at present normally cynomolgus monkey, previously baboon or rhesus monkey, marmoset used in some circumstances; supposedly closer to humans in terms of ADME but not always; good regulatory acceptance; historical control data are now more consistent as a result of captive breeding, which can give some control over viral status depending on source; size generally between 2 and 5 kg (cynomolgous monkey) or 250–600 g (marmoset); small size of marmosets means lower compound requirement (good for biotech products) but this alone cannot justify selection; wild-caught animals have problems of unknown age, origin, disease or parasite profile and give inconsistent historical control data; complex to keep, group housing gives optimum results; can transmit fatal zoonoses to humans such as hepatitis B, and viruses such as rabies, Ebola and Marburg; more expensive and less available than dogs; small size of marmosets may necessitate use of satellite groups for pharmacokinetic determinations; marmosets are subject to stress and diet factors; intense ethical and government pressure against use of any NHP.

Ferrets were suggested, at one time, as an alternative to dogs, because they have a similar gut microflora to humans. However, they offer more problems than solutions and I have never seen a general toxicity study in ferrets. Rabbits are the species of choice in short-term dermal toxicity studies but not for other routes of administration.

The age of the animals used should be considered. Young animals tend to metabolise chemicals somewhat differently to adults and this can lead to unexpected results due to age-related differences in metabolic capabilities, especially in rodents. Similarly with dogs, it is quite normal to use immature animals at about five or six months old; the consequence of this is that reproductive toxicities, such as testicular atrophy, may not be apparent in shorter studies. For practical reasons of age and safety of handling staff, primate studies are usually conducted with immature animals of about two to three years old. It is possible to obtain mature monkeys but they are expensive and difficult to handle safely, a factor of some importance, given the sometimes fatal diseases that they can pass on either through a bite or through faeces or urine.

Study designs in general toxicology

Studies in general toxicity include the shortest and the longest studies in toxicological investigations, the only others of comparable length being the peri- and post-natal development reproductive study and the two-year carcinogenicity bioassay. The shortest study is the single dose acute study, which is intended to characterise severe toxicity following a single large dose. The original objective was to calculate the LD_{50} or median lethal dose at which 50 per cent of the treated animals died; this was established statistically from the results of several treatment groups of up to 10 animals of each sex. The results were not always reproducible as acute toxicity may be significantly affected by many factors, such as heat, which have less influence at lower doses. Although the LD$_{50}$ test itself is no longer conducted, the concept is retained as a useful indicator of toxicity ranking; the figure can be estimated approximately from the data from the initial sighting studies, usually in terms of a dose greater than xxx mg/kg. In an acute study the animals are dosed once and observed for 14 days, which is both a strength and a weakness. Some toxicity expressed in the period immediately following administration, for example liver toxicity seen with carbon tetrachloride, may be completely repaired by the end of the 14 days. However, 14 days may allow any slowly developing toxicity to be expressed; this can be seen with cytotoxic anti-cancer chemotherapies. The basic designs for general toxicity studies are summarised in Table 5.2 (see also Basic study designs in chapter 3, page 67). The observations and measurements indicated in this table are discussed below.

Table 5.2 Summary of basic designs for general toxicology

	Species	Acute (single dose)	4 weeks	13 weeks	26 weeks
Group size[a]	Rodent	5 m+5 f[b]	10 m+10 f (Rev 5m+5f in 3 groups)[c]	10 m+10 f (Rev 5m+5f in 3 groups)	15 m+15 f (Rev 5m+5f in 3 groups)
	Dog	Not used	3 m+3 f (Rev 2m+2f in 2 groups)	4 m+4 f (Rev 2m+2f in 2 groups)	4 m+4 f (Rev 2m+2f in 2 groups)
Clinical pathology	Rodent	Not done	Wk 4+end rev.	Wk 4 or 6, 13, rev.	Wk 13, 26
	Dog	Not done	Wk 0, 4+end rev.	Wk 0, 4 or 6, 13, rev.	Wk 0, 13, 26, rev.
Ophthal- moscopy	All	Not done	Wk 0, 4, end rev	Wk 0, 13, rev	Wk 0, 13, 26, rev.
Necropsy	All	All groups	All groups	All groups	All groups
Histopath- ology[d]	Rodent	Gross lesions	Control+high dose+affected tissues at low and mid dose groups.		
			Affected tissues only in Reversibility groups.		
	Dog	Not done	All animals are examined.		

Notes: m, male; f, female; rev, reversibility studies; Wk, week.
[a]Except in acute studies there are usually three treated groups and a control – see text).
[b]Groups of 2 m+2 f used for dose selection.
[c]Reversibility studies usually controls, mid and high dose for rodents, controls and high dose for dogs (or mid and high dose only – see text); examinations normally conducted in final week.
[d]In addition, organ weights are recorded on all except acute studies. In-life observations on all studies include clinical signs, bodyweight and food consumption.

Study duration

The duration of studies in safety evaluation is largely fixed by toxicological convention and increases as the programme progresses, from 14- or 28-day studies, to 13 weeks, to 26 weeks (rats) or 39 or 52 weeks in non-rodents. The basic design of all these studies is the same, namely a control and three treatment groups. These receive dose levels that are based on a high dose expected to cause toxicity, a low dose calculated to be a high multiple of expected human exposure and an intermediate dose level at an approximate geometric mean of the other two. One of the objectives is usually to determine a no observed effect level (NOEL) or a no adverse effect level (NOAEL), from which safe exposure levels for humans may be estimated. A typical dose level choice could be 10, 30 and 100 mg/kg/day. With increasing study duration the number of animals tends to increase from 10 per sex per group in rats in 14- or 28-day studies to 15 per sex per group or more in the longer ones. In addition the longer studies will probably include animals allocated to recovery or reversibility studies to assess the regression of effects when treatment is withdrawn. In practical terms this means that 18 weeks should be allowed for a 13-week study in rats, divided into one week for acclimatisation to the study room, 13 weeks for treatment and 4 weeks without treatment. For non-rodents the study durations are the same but animal numbers are lower for reasons of ethics, space and cost. Typically a 14- or 28-day study in dogs will be conducted with three dogs per sex per group and a 13-week study with four per sex per group, with additional animals allocated for reversibility studies (see below).

Parameters measured in general toxicology

General toxicity studies are relatively non-specific screens for adverse effects that are not necessarily predictable but which are likely to arise in known ways or manifestations. For this reason the measurements that are conducted in these studies are very similar across programmes and study type. Where toxicity of an unexpected or new type is seen, it is often investigated in specifically designed mechanistic studies. The normally conducted measurements and observations are discussed briefly below. They can be broadly divided into three categories, in-life observations, clinical pathology and post-mortem investigations.

In-life observations

Of the investigations summarised in Box 5.2, clinical observation and measurement of growth and food consumption are usually the most informative. Effects on the eyes are rare but this is an examination that is common to all regulatory guidelines, in deference to the importance of ocular effects in humans. Although examination of the other senses would also seem sensible, it is difficult to achieve, the only other occasionally examined being hearing, usually by means of a whistle or other sudden noise. A deeper investigation of the nervous

Box 5.2 In-life observations and measurements in general toxicology

- *Clinical observations* following administration are the most basic investigation and give information of the effects of the compound that may be expected at high doses in humans. Subjective indications of ill-health, such as headache or nausea, are not readily assessable in animals; however, lack of activity or abnormal posture may be a consequence of these. Salivation at or immediately after dosing is seen frequently in oral toxicity studies and may simply reflect the expectation of dosing or taste of the test substance.

- *Food consumption and bodyweight* are non-specific indicators of toxicity that may be affected by many factors such as general malaise, pharmacological action, sedation or other neurological effect. They act as critical early indicators of effect before other examinations are employed to investigate further.

- *Water consumption* can be measured if there is suspicion that kidney function is affected. It should be noted, however, that water consumption will tend to be lower if food consumption is also reduced.

- *Ophthalmoscopy* is performed before treatment and at the end of the treatment and, if appropriate, reversibility periods.

- *Electrocardiography* is useful for assessing unwanted or pharmacological effects on the heart and can be allied with *blood pressure* measurements. Although routine in non-rodents, it is only practicable in rats if sophisticated computerised systems are used. Blood pressure measurement is normally indirect by use of a pressure cuff on the tail but can be direct from an artery by use of a pressure transducer. These measurements are more satisfactorily achieved by telemetry but this is an expensive add-on to toxicity studies.

system can be achieved through neurological examination, a relatively simple estimate for neurotoxicological potential, which can be performed in most species. Other in-life examinations relevant to the expected effects of the test substance may include measurements of testicular size and semen sampling or examinations such as electroencephalograms or electroretinography. The last two are rarely used and are of questionable utility in general toxicology.

Clinical pathology

The next group of investigations is performed on blood, urine or faeces to assess the effects of treatment on the function and status of a number of major organ and tissue systems. This may give early warning during a long study of toxicity that is not apparent from in-life observation or may support these findings. Clinical pathology investigations are relatively simple and give quantitative data, which are amenable to statistical analysis. Interpretation of variation from controls or historical control data depends on the inter-relationship of observed differences, the presence of dose relationship and of other changes in the study.

Haematology examines the numbers and morphology of the erythrocytes, platelets and leucocytes in the peripheral circulation:

- *Erythrocyte parameters*   Haemoglobin, red cell count, haematocrit, absolute (calculated) indices (mean cell volume, mean cell haemoglobin, mean cell haemoglobin concentration), reticulocyte count. Cell morphology.
- *Leucocyte parameters*   Total and differential white blood cell counts. Morphology.
- *Coagulation*   Prothrombin time, activated partial thromboplastin time, fibrinogen concentration, platelet count.

These measurements give insight into the condition of the bone marrow and the presence of peripherally induced anaemias. The coagulation measurements give some indication of the condition of the liver in that prolongation may mean that there is reduced synthesis of coagulation factors due to changes in hepatic synthetic capacity. These examinations may be extended by examination of smears to determine any effects on the bone marrow.

Clinical chemistry is intended to examine the function of several organ systems, particularly the liver and kidney, through determination of the activity of enzymes and of measurement of a number of analytes such as urea, proteins and electrolytes:

- *Enzymes*   Alkaline phosphatase, alanine and aspartate aminotransferase, lactate dehydrogenase, gamma-glutamyl transpeptidase, leucine aminopeptidase, creatine kinase.
- *General analytes*   Urea, creatinine. Glucose, total protein and differential protein electrophoresis, albumin, A/G ratio. Cholesterol, triglycerides. Total bilirubin.
- *Electrolytes*   Sodium, potassium, chloride, calcium, phosphate.

Liver function is indicated by changes (usually increases) in the activities of several enzymes that are more or less specific for differing functional changes; the concentration of the various proteins is also useful in this respect. Kidney function is shown by the concentrations of urea, creatinine and electrolytes. There is no reliable enzymatic indicator for kidney damage in the plasma but several enzymes may (occasionally) be assayed in the urine, for instance alkaline phosphatase and *N*-acetyl glucosaminidase. Other tissues or organs may be assessed through the activity of other enzymes such as creatine kinase for heart-related effects, aspartate aminotransferase for changes in musculature (in the absence of change in alanine aminotransferase as together these two enzymes are markers of liver toxicity). Changes in alkaline phosphatase and lactate dehydrogenase may be further assessed through isoenzyme studies to indicate if the liver or another tissue is the prime organ of effect. Some enzymes are more appropriate than others in the various species used. Marmosets have low peripheral activities for alanine aminotransferase, rats have low gamma-glutamyl transpeptidase, and in other non-human primates, the plasma activity of alkaline phosphatase and lactate dehydrogenase tend to be more variable and consequently less useful than in other species. In non-human primates leucine aminopeptidase is usually used instead of alkaline phosphatase.[1]

Urinalysis is the main in-life window on kidney function, through examination of urinary electrolyte concentrations (used with volume to calculate total output), stick tests and microscopic examination of sediment obtained after centrifugation. It is either quantitative or semi-quantitative:

- *Quantitative* Volume, osmolality or specific gravity, pH, electrolyte concentrations (Na, Cl, PO$_4$, Ca).
- *Semi-quantitative* Appearance/colour. Stick tests for: protein, glucose, ketones, bilirubin, blood.
  Microscopy of the deposit left after centrifugation.

Unlike blood it should be collected over a period of hours, preferably overnight and so requires special collection cages in which the animals can be isolated. It is possible to allow access to water over this period but one of the functions of urinalysis is to determine the ability of the kidneys to produce concentrated urine.

Post-mortem examinations

At the end of the study the animals are killed humanely and subjected to a thorough post-mortem (autopsy or necropsy) in which a range of organs is weighed and the tissues examined *in situ* and after removal. Up to 50 organs or tissues may be retained in fixative against histopathological processing and microscopic examination (Table 5.3). The purpose of these examinations is to detect morphological effects that may correlate with other changes seen in-life or in clinical pathology. Changes that may have long term consequences for the animal should also be found, such as endocrine-induced hyperplasias that might develop into tumours in later life.

Organ weights indicate effects due to atrophy, for instance in the testis, or of adaptive hypertrophy, which may be seen in the liver following administration of enzyme inducers or peroxisome proliferators such as diethylhexylphthalate. Some organs are weighed routinely but the data do not necessarily reveal much that is useful due to variability of post-mortem blood loss, lung weight being an example. The weight of the uterus is greatly affected by the stage of sexual cycle

Table 5.3 Organs and tissues that may be retained after post-mortem

All gross lesions	Pancreas
Adrenals[a]	Pituitary[a]
Aorta	Prostate
Bone (sternum)	Rectum
Bone marrow smear	Salivary gland
Brain[a]	Sciatic nerve
Caecum	Seminal vesicles[a]
Cervix	Skeletal muscle
Colon	Skin
Duodenum	Spinal cord – cervical, thoracic, lumbar
Eyes/optic nerves	Spleen[a]
Heart[a]	Stomach
Ileum	Testes/epididymides[a]
Jejunum	Thymus[a]
Kidneys[a]	Thyroids/Parathyroids[a]
Liver[a]	Tongue
Lungs (with mainstembronchi)[a]	Trachea
Lymph node mesenteric submandibular	Urinary bladder
Mammary gland or site	Uterus[a]
Oesophagus	Vagina
Ovaries[a]	

Note: [a]All these organs are weighed; paired organs should be weighed separately.

at the time of kill and this should be taken into account when examining the weights. A further variable that must be considered is bodyweight and this can be corrected for by expressing the organ weights as a percentage of bodyweight. This becomes important when there is a significant difference in bodyweights between controls and treated animals. The weights of some organs follow bodyweight fairly closely (e.g. the liver); others tend to remain constant despite fluctuations in the animals bodyweight, the brain being a good example of this.

Macroscopic appearance of the tissues as determined at necropsy is an important indication of effect and may be the only pathological evidence of change. Any abnormalities are noted and the tissue retained for microscopic examination. It is important that this examination is carried out by experienced technicians and that the information is accurately recorded. This is the link between the in-life observations, particularly information on the presence of tumours noted at clinical observations, and the pathological examination of the tissues sections.

Microscopic appearance assessed in stained sections cut from fixed tissue is the final examination of the study. Microscopic examination is used to detect any subtle or obvious differences between the control and treated animals which may have arisen as a result of treatment with the test material. These changes may correlate with other evidence, for instance from gross findings at post-mortem or clinical pathology. The normal fixative is 10 per cent neutral buffered formalin, although Davidson's fluid is used for the eyes and occasionally the testes. If it is intended to carry out testicular staging (i.e. assessment of all stages of spermatogenesis present) Bouin's fluid is often preferred. The normal stain used is haematoxylin and eosin but specialist stains may also be employed, for instance Oil-red-O (on frozen sections) for lipid or periodic acid Schiffs (PAS) for glycogen. The use of electron microscopy (EM) is infrequent in routine toxicity studies, it being more applicable to mechanistic studies. The fixatives commonly used for EM are glutaraldehyde and osmium tetroxide and it is important that the samples are as fresh as possible. Although it is possible to carry out EM studies on formalin-fixed tissue, results are inferior and they become more unreliable with increasing sample age.

Reversibility or recovery studies

In studies of 13 weeks or longer it is normal to include subgroups of animals, that receive the same duration and dose levels of treatment as the other animals on the study, but are retained to assess the reversibility of any toxicity seen during the study. The usual length of such treatment-free periods is four weeks, which is normally enough to show the regression of treatment-related effects, either completely or in part. However, there may be reasons for using a longer period to achieve reversal of effects seen. These may include the toxicokinetics of the test substance or the type of lesion seen in the test animals. For chemicals with long elimination half-lives it is possible for clearance to be delayed for several weeks. As the continued presence of the test substance in the tissues or plasma may prolong the adverse effects of treatment, it is important to ensure that a period is allowed for recovery after complete elimination of test substance. For certain types of lesion, usually those seen microscopically, a longer period without treatment is required simply because they take longer to regress. Amongst such changes are pigment deposition in the liver, e.g. haemosiderin or intracellular inclusions that have accumulated due to slow metabolism of their constituents. One example of the latter type is the accumulation in male rat kidneys of the complex of $\alpha2$-u globulin with compounds such as trimethyl pentanol, the metabolite of trimethyl pentane. Three months is normally the longest recovery period in routine use. Longer periods may be used but become increasingly difficult to justify; if a change is not reversible in three months, this may indicate the possibility of undesirable persistence of effect in humans.

The numbers of animals allocated to reversibility studies is also largely defined by convention. In studies using rodents the usual number is five males and five females allocated to each group, including the controls, although such animals may be omitted from the group treated at the lowest dose level. In studies with non-rodents, reversibility animals are typically included in the control and high-dose groups and occasionally at the intermediate level. The usual number is two males and two females, numbers being restricted for ethical reasons. The omission of animals for reversibility studies from the intermediate and low-dose groups can be a weakness if there is excessive toxicity at the highest dose resulting in early termination of that group. However, it is usually possible to make an estimate of the expected reversibility of effects seen, based on knowledge of type and extent of changes seen in the high-dose animals. Thus, adaptive change such as hepatocyte hypertrophy in the liver due to induction of hepatic enzymes is usually readily reversible, whereas other change may be expected to persist. Fibrosis consequent upon extensive necrosis in the liver would be expected to be irreversible, although function may not be seriously impaired if the lesions are not too extensive. For these reasons it is possible to have reversibility animals for non-rodents in the mid- and high-dose groups to indicate any dose response in recovery from toxic change. To track reversibility in rats, animals for reversibility studies should be included in clinical pathology examinations at least at the end of the treatment period and at the end of the treatment-free period. This is not an issue with non-rodents.

Examinations for specific toxicities

There are several areas of toxicity that do not merit their own special category of investigation, unlike genotoxicity or carcinogenicity, but which may be incorporated into general tests for toxicity. These include investigation of toxicities in the immune, respiratory and nervous systems and in the skin. The problems inherent in these systems and investigations are sketched out below.

Immunotoxicity

As with other organ systems, the function of the immune system may be enhanced or suppressed by xenobiotic chemicals. Unlike most other organ systems, the immune system is not a discrete organ but an interrelated set of tissues distributed throughout the body. It includes the thymus, bone marrow, Peyer's patches, spleen, lymph nodes and other lymphoid tissues. An effect on one part of this system may have contrary effects on other parts; consequently interpretation of small change in one area is made more complex by the difficulties of predicting the impact on other parts of the system. This complicates study of immune responses to xenobiotics, with the added problem that, in general, animals are poor models for human immunotoxicity, particularly autoimmune reactions and hypersensitivity. With such a diffuse system, the best approach is to obtain a broad overview and then, if significant change is seen, to focus on the areas of interest in specific mechanistic studies. Accordingly, it is generally recommended that a tiered approach be adopted, the first tier being contained within the conventional toxicity tests. These examinations include differential leucocyte counts in peripheral blood, plasma protein fractions and the weights and/or microscopic appearance of the lymphoid tissues. The distribution of lymphocyte subsets can also be examined by homogenisation of tissues and flow cytometry. However, these investigations may not give a definitive answer as to whether there are changes that are truly indicative of a significant effect on immune function. The immune system is not static through the lifetime of an organism. The thymus involutes or atrophies with age and this is quite normal; however, acceleration of involution relative to controls or expectation may well imply an immunotoxic effect. A further layer of complexity is added when it is considered that such atrophy is also a response to stress, although this is usually accompanied by changes in the adrenal glands. Immunotoxic investigations are additional to the normal assessment of skin sensitivity reactions, which are particularly useful for assessing workplace hazards and risk; these tests are discussed in greater detail in chapter 7. Extended testing may include assessment of antibody responses, cytokine production and susceptibility to infectious agents in mice, the intention being to define the cell population affected and any dose-response relationship. With a full set of data an assessment of possible effect in humans may be made.

Neurotoxicity

The nervous system is toxicologically significant because of the far reaching effects of change, which is often irreversible. Whereas other tissues, such as the liver, have extensive repair capabilities following toxic insult, this is absent or very small in the nervous system. Also in contrast to other tissues the nervous system has a more limited functional reserve, meaning that a 15 per cent reduction in nervous function is likely to be much more significant than a similar reduction in renal or hepatic function. Detection of effects in the nervous system requires a range of special techniques that are often technically complex and require specialist interpretation. However, much can be done in a routine toxicity test as a first tier of neurological assessment. Clinical signs, combined where appropriate with a functional observation battery, can lead to detailed neurological examination for reflexes, grip strength, co-ordination, gait, etc. Electroencephalography may prove useful, although the benefits over a thorough neurological examination conducted by a veterinary surgeon should be considered first. Similarly, ophthalmoscopic examinations may be supplemented by electroretinography, a rarely used method of assessing the electrical response of the retina to light impulses; it is time-consuming and technically demanding both in conduct and interpretation. Assessment of the senses is very limited in general toxicology. Hearing may be tested using a whistle or other noise but the assessment is crude, as it is based on Preyer's reflex (the ears pricking forward). The loss of hair cells from the cochlear is associated with hearing loss and to detect this, the use of scanning electron microscopy is recommended. The other senses, smell, taste and touch, are not investigated routinely in toxicity testing due to the difficulties in assessing these functions in laboratory animals.

In the blood, measurement of cholinesterases may indicate toxicity due to certain pesticides; however, after chronic administration rats can show large decreases in activity without clinical evidence of effect. Organophosphates, which inhibit cholinesterases (as do carbamates), are classically associated with delayed onset neuropathy, which has been tested routinely in chickens. This is the species of choice for assessment of the target enzyme for this condition, neuropathy target esterase. Much emphasis is placed on histopathology, where the use of special fixatives and stains with appropriate microscopic technique can be very informative.

Respiratory toxicology

Essentially this is the field of toxicity resulting from inhalation of toxicants. Pulmonary toxicity as a result of systemic exposure, following administration by oral or parenteral routes, is not a common finding, paraquat being a prime example. The use of inhalation as a route of administration becomes important in assessing workplace hazards and, clearly, for medicines given by inhalation. Technically, inhalation is in a field of its own due to the problems of generating the correct atmospheres, administering these safely to the animals and wasting them to the outside through suitable filters.

The basic objective is to generate a respirable, uniform atmosphere from the test substance. It is important to determine the physical characteristics of the atmosphere generated and to calculate and sustain the correct rate of generation to achieve the desired dose or concentration. A relatively large proportion of inhaled material is eventually swallowed, giving a significant oral component to the toxicity elicited. Rats are usually exposed for up to 6 hours/day, restrained in tubes fixed onto a central cylindrical chamber so that only their noses protrude into the atmosphere that flows through the apparatus. Whole-body chambers can be used, although these use larger amounts of test material and result in dermal and oral exposure. Dogs and non-human primates are dosed through the use of masks.

Intranasal administration is relatively straightforward and can be performed using droplets or an aerosol of test solution. Vehicles should be chosen with care to avoid local irritation. Although the rat is used as the rodent species in intranasal studies, the nasal turbinates of non-human primates are generally considered to be a better model for humans than the dog.

Dermal toxicity

Dermal administration is used less frequently than other routes but is relevant to the workplace and topical medicines. Species used include the rat, rabbit and minipig, the last because the skin structure is close to that in humans. Careful choice of vehicle is essential as this has considerable influence on absorption of the test substance. In pharmaceutical toxicology, the formulation must be the same as or as close as possible to the clinical formulation to avoid any effects due to the vehicle. The potential toxicity of any excipients should be investigated by the use of sham-dosed controls in addition to a group that receives the vehicle only. Occlusion of the application site for several hours by wrapping the site in an impermeable dressing enhances absorption of the test substance and prevents ingestion. This is normal practice in acute studies and up to 28 days but is not recommended in longer experiments. Due to the absorption characteristics of the skin, the concentration of the test substance and the area of the dosing site tend to be more important than the dose in milligrams per kilogram, especially as dermal toxicity studies are usually undertaken in part to assess local irritation or other effects due to the test article/vehicle combination.

Pitfalls in general toxicology

The major pitfalls in study conduct, which result in spurious results, are related to the timing of the various examinations. Electrocardiograms (ECG) can be expected to show two types of basic effect – pharmacological and toxicological. The pharmacological effects, wanted or unwanted, should be related to the presence of the test substance or an active metabolite and are generally seen in the few hours after administration. If effects are present 24 hours after dosing in treated animals, it may well be an indication of toxicity unless the elimination of the test substance is prolonged. The timing of ECG examinations is therefore important, based on what is required of the study. With current interest in QT prolongation, it makes sense to look at an ECG at the time of peak plasma concentration; examination after 24 hours should confirm the absence and transience of any effect. ECGs are usually only recorded in non-rodents that are not sedated. The process of restraint and application of electrodes is, at the first experience, a stressful process resulting in increased heart rate and blood pressure. It is useful to accustom the animals to the procedure by taking two or more recordings before the definitive measurements. Despite this, it is likely that heart rate and blood pressure will still be higher than normal and this can mask effects of the test substance. To avoid this kind of error, the use of telemetric implants is recommended. With these internally implanted devices, it is possible to record a number of parameters such as locomotor activity, electrocardiograms, heart rate, arterial blood pressure, respiration and body temperature, although not all at the same time. Collection of these data from unrestrained animals gives a better indication of variation from normality than when in the presence of an observer or under restraint. In animals it is possible for cardiotoxicity to develop in response to excessive pharmacology and this must be taken into account in analysis of the data; toxicity without evident pharmacological cause needs careful interpretation.

In non-rodents the timing of collection of blood samples for toxicokinetics relative to collection for clinical pathology is also critical; in rats this is not such a problem because separate animals are generally used to avoid collection of excessive volumes of blood from the same animals. Samples for clinical pathology should always be collected before those for toxicokinetics if the same animals are to be used. The controls are not usually subjected to the same sampling regimen for toxicokinetics as the treated groups, although it should be noted that there is increasing requirement for analysis of control samples in toxicokinetic studies. Varying sampling regimens and stress between controls and treated animals may introduce confounding factors. This could include a mild anaemia, found at clinical pathology, which is not present in the controls but is not treatment-related. In two-week studies, with intensive toxicokinetic sampling in non-rodents, there may not be sufficient time between day 1 samples and clinical pathology and day 14 toxicokinetic samples for complete recovery. As it is usual to take blood samples immediately before the start of the treatment period from dogs or non-human primates, the sampling stress on the animals becomes significant and complicates interpretation of the clinical pathology data.

Although it is desirable to show toxicity, to give an estimation of the dose-response curve for a test substance, this is not always possible. In some cases this is due to genuinely low toxicity even at high doses; here it is necessary to demonstrate absorption and adequate systemic exposure. Some drugs intended to have a local action in the lumen of the gastrointestinal tract may not be absorbed but this is probably beneficial. For low-toxicity compounds that are not absorbed after oral administration, it may be necessary to use the intravenous route to elicit toxicity if that is considered essential. In contrast, there are instances where the acute pharmacological action is so intense that it becomes a toxicological effect in its own right. In these cases, anaesthetics and narcotic drugs being good examples, it may be impossible to demonstrate any toxicity apart from the excess pharmacological action.

Poor choice of form or formulation can be a pitfall in any toxicity study. Particle size can be a limiting factor in absorption and thus in toxicity; micronising a test material or changing the carrier system or vehicle can cause a radical increase in toxicity. Such changes should be avoided in the middle of a programme unless some form of sighting study is conducted with the new form or formulation to ensure continued lack of effect.

Another factor to consider is the correct choice of examination for the test species being used. This is particularly true with clinical pathology where there are significant differences between species in the plasma activity of some enzymes. For instance alkaline phosphatase is very variable in cynomolgus monkeys and leucine aminopeptidase is often preferred for that reason. Marmosets have very low activities for alanine aminotransferase and gamma-glutamyl transpeptidase is very low in rats.

In the final analysis, correct study design and interpretation will avoid the majority of these pitfalls and will facilitate interpretation of the whole data package. When reviewing a study report, it is important to understand where such problems can arise and to allow for them in your interpretation, bearing in mind that the pitfalls seen may not be included in the above analysis.

Reproductive toxicology

General principles in reproductive toxicology

The intention in studies of reproductive toxicology is to assess the potential for adverse reproductive effects in humans due to exposure to chemicals, whether as a result of intentional – drugs and food additives – or unintentional exposure in the case of pesticides and other chemicals. In contrast to general toxicology, which has a very broad approach to toxicity testing, the endpoints in reproductive toxicology are much more defined and there are specific stages to examine and evaluate. The reproductive process and its various stages are illustrated in Figure 5.1.

Despite this relatively simple definition of endpoints, reproduction is immensely complex and can be affected in many ways. Toxicity can occur during any part of the process and the various tests are designed to examine every stage of the cycle in digestible chunks. However, there is enormous scope for different effects on reproduction. There may be indirect or direct effects on the gonads, which have dual function as the source of the gametes and of sex hormones, the secretion of which is controlled by the pituitary. After gametogenesis, variations in behaviour, fertilisation or effects on the processes of gestation can also influence the final outcome. The net result of this is that presence of an effect at one stage of the sequence does not necessarily pinpoint the origin of that effect;

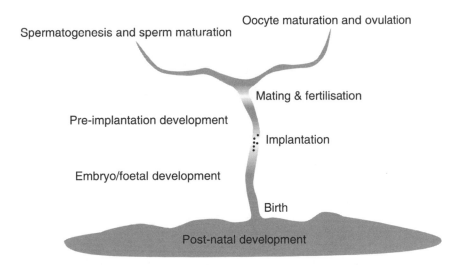

Figure 5.1 The river of reproduction
Source: Newall, Derek, 1999 – used with permission.

consequently further investigation is needed to elucidate mechanisms and facilitate risk assessment. Where effects are seen it may become necessary to break the process down further to determine the location of the effect, in terms of time and place. This element of timing is unique to reproductive toxicity, especially with respect to teratogenicity. For example, thalidomide was associated with reproductive effects when given in weeks 4 or 5 of human pregnancy. From the time of implantation until closure of the palate, the organs develop in the fetus according to a well-defined pattern and timing. Accordingly, treatment of a pregnant rat with a teratogen on day 8 of gestation will produce a different spectrum of effects in comparison with treatment on day 12 (Figure 5.2) Timing of treatment is also important in spermatogenesis, where single treatment may affect only one stage of the spermatic cycle. It is increasingly recognised that the visible processes of organogenesis are matched by biochemical changes that have profound influence on the toxicity of compounds in the fetus or neonate in comparison with an adolescent or an adult.[2-4]

Pregnancy is associated with a wide range of physiological changes that affect the ADME of chemicals. Total body water and lipid are increased, associated in the former case with an increase in plasma volume. Because the total red cell population increases to a lesser extent than plasma volume the effect is to reduce the red cell count to near anaemic levels. There is an increase in the extracellular space which, with the increase in total body lipid, increases the

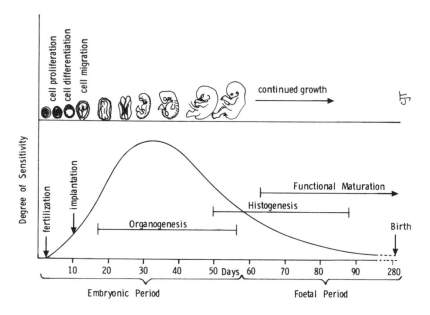

Figure 5.2 The stages of human embryogenesis.
Source: Timbrell, J. Principles of Biochemical Ecotoxicology. London: Taylor & Francis, 2000.

available volume of distribution of chemicals. The body lipids accumulate over the early part of the gestation and are used in the latter part. Thus, where there is accumulation of lipid-soluble chemicals into the adipose tissue, rapid release late in gestation can lead to increased plasma concentrations, which have the potential for adverse effects in the mother and fetus. Plasma concentrations of albumin, important in reducing the free concentration of chemicals in the plasma by binding, are lower in pregnancy, partly due to the increase in plasma volume and partly due to decreased total body content.

Examples of reproductive effects with particular substances include testicular atrophy seen with the fumigant dibromochloropropane, teratogenicity with vitamin A or alcohol, transplacental carcinogenesis with diethylstilbestrol and many more. Indirect effects through hormonal imbalance are also a frequent cause of reproductive toxicity and specialist studies may be needed to investigate these. Until recently, reproductive toxicity was relatively resistant to mechanistic explanation, in contrast to other toxicities, although the numer of elucidated mechanisms is increasing.

Test systems for reproductive toxicology

The thalidomide tragedy had a huge influence on the choice of test species for assessment of reproductive toxicity, leading in particular to the use of the rabbit, which was sensitive to its effects. As indicated in Table 5.4, the rat, rabbit and mouse are the principal test systems for examination of reproductive toxicity. Although the non-human primate and minipig are used in studies to evaluate effects during gestation (developmental toxicity studies) they are used only in special circumstances. In general the placental structure of animals used in assessment of reproductive toxicity is not the same as in humans, although this may not be a factor that is always significant. A summary of the various test systems that are in reasonably regular use is shown in Box 5.3.

Overall there is no escaping the general acceptance, especially by regulators, of the rat, rabbit and, to a lesser extent, the mouse as models for reproductive toxicity. They have the advantages of availability, size, length of reproductive cycle and a level of understanding that is not so clear for the other systems. For

Table 5.4 Stage of reproductive cycle and preferred test systems

Stage of cycle	Test system
Fertility and mating	Rat or mouse
Organogenesis – *in vivo*	Rat or rabbit. Alternatives are mouse, minipig or non-human primate
Organogenesis – *in vitro*	Whole embryo culture, limb bud assay
Late gestation, parturition and early development	Rat or mouse

Box 5.3 Characteristics of test systems for reproductive toxicology

- *Rat and mouse*   The reproductive cycle is completed relatively quickly; they do not hesitate to mate in laboratory conditions; relatively large litters are produced after a conveniently short gestation (about 20 days); inexpensive and easy to maintain; there is a wealth of historical control data. However, the rat produces a very large number of sperm in comparison with humans and, consequently, a relatively large reduction in sperm number or quality is necessary before effects are seen. Rats are the preferred rodent species for use in studies of embryotoxicity.

- *Rabbit*   The rabbit is a reasonable size and reproduces readily in laboratory conditions; gestation is relatively short at about 30 days; litter size is generally good; there is good historical control data for a number of strains. Disadvantages include their intolerance of compounds such as antibiotics or with chemicals that disturb their alimentary canals, including several vehicles, such as oils. They are not used in other reproductive studies but they are ideal for longitudinal studies of the sperm cycle.

- *Minipig*   The use of the minipig is increasing in teratogenicity studies and there may be a future for them in fertility studies. They have a clear advantage when the rabbit cannot be used due to rabbit-specific effects, although the mouse is the known alternative; gestation at about 113 days is long and litter size small (five or six). If they are used as the non-rodent species in the general toxicity studies, the reproductive studies can be done in the same species. However, they are large (about 35 kg) and so require large amounts of test material and more extensive housing. They require skill in dosing and in sample collection. They are particularly suited to dermal studies.

- *Non-human primates*   Used occasionally as an alternative non-rodent, but expense and availability limit their use. The usual species is the cynomolgus monkey; although marmosets have been investigated as an alternative, they are not used in regulatory toxicology. The rhesus monkey has been used but is a seasonal breeder, while the cynomolgus can breed at any time of year due to a menstrual period of about 30 days. Litter size is small and gestation is long with a high miscarriage rate, meaning more animals are needed. The testicular physiology of the cynomolgus testis is said to be a good model for humans and fetal malformation frequencies have been quoted at around 0.5 per cent. Normal practice is to remove the fetuses via caesarean section and then to allow the mother to recover for re-use in another study. Phylogenetic proximity does not mean necessarily that they are good models for humans in terms of ADME.

> • *Alternatives*   There are a number of *in vitro* systems for assessment of
> teratogenicity but none have been validated sufficiently for regulatory
> purposes. Whole-embryo culture is one of the best of these and has
> particular use when screening members of a series of compounds that
> are known to come from a teratogenic class, for instance retinoids. In
> this case the assay may be used to aid selection of lead candidates for
> development from a teratogenic series. The micromass assay is a
> variation on the whole-embryo culture theme, which uses primary cell
> cultures from the limb bud or brain. There is also an assay that uses
> *Hydra* but use of this has not been pursued. Chick embryos have also
> been used occasionally.

all models it is essential that there be a large amount of in-house historical
control data to facilitate interpretation of the study data. In addition, this database has to be kept up to date by performance of new studies in order to
compensate for drift in the strain of animal used.

The various alternative models indicated in Box 5.3 are useful as screening
methods in candidate selection. However, none of these *in vitro* systems has yet
been accepted by regulatory authorities as a satisfactory alternative to whole
animal experiments. They lack the complex interrelationships that exist
between the mother and the fetus and between the various tissues and dynamics
in each. Other systems that might appear to have value in teratogenicity testing,
such as metamorphosis in amphibians or invertebrate larval stages, have not
been widely investigated, although the fruit fly, *Drosophila* has been used in some
experiments. Other possibilities include fish and chick embryos, the latter
having been investigated as a screening system. Another possibility for the
future is the nematode *Caenorhabditis elegans*; the complete cell lineage for this
900-cell organism has been elucidated. Care is needed in the collection of data
and interpretation of these assays. There are also systems based on fragments of
reproductive tissues (e.g. isolated seminiferous tubules), which can be used to
investigate functional aspects of particular parts of the reproductive system,
including the effects of one cell type on another. These specialised studies may
be technically demanding and not readily transferable from one laboratory to
another in a reproducible manner. These alternatives were reviewed in 1997 by
a British Toxicology Society working party.[5] A positive result does not necessarily stop development of a chemical but merely emphasises the possibility of
reproductive effect, leading to an appropriate change in study timing.

Reproductive effects may also be assessed in the course of general toxicity
studies through records of oestrus in non-rodents, plasma hormone analysis,
organ weights and histological examination. Testicular staging, in which the
presence of the various stages of spermatogenesis is assessed, is a possible addition
to routine toxicity studies of four weeks or longer. Although many chemicals

will show effect within four weeks, some may take longer and treatment for at least one full spermatogenesis cycle is desirable. In practice this means a 13-week study.

Study designs for reproductive toxicology

As indicated, the process of reproductive toxicity assessment is broken up into manageable chunks, addressing fertility, embryonic development or fetal toxicity (teratogenicity) and peri- and post-natal development including maternal function. A full programme in rats will cover the 63 days before mating in the males and may run into two generations, with continuous treatment of all animals up to weaning of the final litters. Such studies are lengthy and produce vast amounts of complex data.

Basic design

As with general toxicology the standard design is for three treated groups with an untreated control. In the same way, doses are chosen after an appropriate set of sighting studies (for the rat the general toxicity studies are generally adequate for this, although it may be wise to perform a sighting study in pregnant animals to confirm dose choice). In rabbits it is also usual to perform a small sighting study in non-pregnant animals and then to confirm in a few pregnant animals.

The chief design driver in reproductive studies is the stage of the cycle under examination. This determines length and timing of treatment and, to a large extent, the type of examination undertaken (Figure 5.2). Specialist design becomes necessary if, for any reason it is not possible to carry out a normal study due to the expected effects of the test substance; in this case the studies have to be broken up into individual stages. The designs of three main types of reproductive study are summarised in Box 5.4.

The duration and timing of the treatment period is relatively fixed. In rats the spermatogenesis cycle lasts 63 days. However, even with significant testicular toxicity rats can be successful sires due to the large numbers of sperm produced. Histological examination is a good method for detecting effects in the testis and data can be compared between species to give an indication of whether any changes are specific to the rat. For this reason pre-mating treatment in fertility studies is generally 28 days, with the possibility of increasing this to 63 days if effects are expected. In embryotoxicity studies, the treatment period is chosen to last from implantation until closure of the palate, which is approximately day 15 of gestation in the mouse, day 16 in the rat and day 18 in the rabbit. However, it should be noted that the day of palate closure can vary slightly between strains and this should be accounted for in the study design. Following closure of the palate, there is a treatment-free period until just before natural parturition when the dams are killed and their uterine contents are examined. In minipigs treatment is from day 11 to 35 with examination of uterine contents on day 110

Box 5.4 Outline designs for example reproductive studies

Note that these are examples only and should not be taken as the only option. Guidelines such as those for ICH (see website given in the Appendix) give preferred designs according to chemical class and use.

- *Rabbit (Oral Gavage) Developmental Toxicity Study* Four groups of 20F. Time-mated (=day 0). Dosed days 6–18 of pregnancy. Clinical observations daily. Bodyweights on days 0, 3–18, 22, 25 and 28 of pregnancy. Food consumption – daily days 3–6 then every 2 days. Post-mortem examination on day 28 of pregnancy – parental females examined, gross abnormalities retained; fetuses – external, visceral and skeletal examination then retained.
- *Rat (Oral Gavage) Fertility & Embryonic Development Study* Four groups of 25M+25F. Dosed for: (a) males – 28 days pre-mating, through mating and to necropsy; (b) females – 14 days pre-mating, through pregnancy to day 17 of gestation. Clinical observations daily. Bodyweights: males twice weekly, females twice weekly pre-mating then daily to necropsy. Food consumption – males weekly, females weekly pre-mating then at appropriate intervals during pregnancy. Post-mortem examination on day 20 of gestation; parental animals – males testes and epididymides retained; gross abnormalities retained; fetuses – external, visceral and skeletal examination.
- *Rat peri- and post-natal development study* Four groups each of 25 mated females treated from day 6 of pregnancy to day 20 post-partum; 20M, 20F selected from F_1 per group (not treated) and reared to sexual maturity and mated; necropsy day 13 of gestation. Examinations are similar to those on other studies and may vary according to protocol.

---

of gestation. The treatment period in pre- and post-natal development studies is from day 6 of gestation to weaning of the litters; males are not treated.

Mating

There are three methods of obtaining pregnant animals for reproductive studies, by natural mating, artificial insemination or by buying in time-mated animals from a supplier. Which is used depends largely on the personal preferences of the laboratory performing the study. Natural mating, preferably using one male to one female, has the advantage that proven males can be used and that the sire of each litter is known; this means that particular abnormalities can be traced back to specific animals. Although successful and simple, natural mating requires the maintenance of an adequate stock of reproductively proven males.

Artificial insemination uses pooled semen from several animals and so the sire cannot be identified for each litter. Time-mated animals from suppliers are increasingly used and provide a good source of pregnant animals at reasonable reliability; these animals are mated naturally, offering the same advantages as in-house mating without the need to maintain stud males.

Group sizes

The ICH pharmaceutical guideline on Detection of Toxicity to Reproduction says that there 'is very little scientific basis underlying specified group sizes in past and existing guidelines nor in this one'.[6] Numbers of animals per study are chosen to give a satisfactory number of litters for evaluation and have been suggested as providing the best compromise between insensitivity in terms of detection of low incidence effects and large numbers of animals, which may not increase the statistical sensitivity of the test. As always in toxicology, if the effect to be demonstrated is one with a high incidence, fewer animals are needed than for a rare event. It is, however, unusual to embark on a reproductive study with the sole intention of investigating a single effect. In an embryotoxicity study the typical number of animals per group is 24 rats or 20 rabbits. Minipig studies inevitably use smaller numbers, for example 12 females per group, which results in nine or ten litters of five to six. In rats, if the study includes investigation of more than one generation, it is likely that more animals will be needed to ensure that there are sufficient F_1 litters at each treatment level from which to choose the males and females for mating to produce the F_2 or subsequent generations.

Parameters measured in reproductive toxicology

Measurement of food consumption and bodyweight and recording of clinical signs is common to all study types *in vivo* and recording of clinical signs that may be treatment related. Record of litter size together with sex and weight is also a feature of all reproductive studies. Clinical pathology is not normally performed and histopathology may only be carried out on selected adults and offspring in multi-generation studies. Each arm of the reproductive study programme has its particular parameter measurements that may be loosely grouped as based on fertility, embryonic development and pre- and post-natal development, which includes examination of maternal function up to weaning; these are listed in Table 5.5.

Fertility

The origin of the gametes is a factor in the sensitivity of the sexes to reproductive toxins. In the female the ovarian germ cells are present before birth and decrease with age, being a pool of finite size that can be depleted but not replenished. In the male, spermatogenesis is a process that is continuous from

Table 5.5 Reproductive parameters

Fertility	Embryonic development	Pre- and post-natal development
Both sexes: Time to mating **Females:** Litter size Fetal sex Number and position of implantations Number of corpora lutea **Males:** Computer-aided sperm assement (CASA) Sperm counts Sperm motility Sperm morphology Sperm quality Testicular weights Retention of epididymides Histology where appropriate	**Females only:** Litter size Number and position classified as early resorptions, late resorptions, dead fetuses or live fetuses Number of corpora lutea Weight of gravid uterus and placentae Fetal weights and sexes (live foetuses) Foetal abnormalities – external, visceral and skeletal	**Dams:** Length of gestation Onset and duration of parturition Observe through lactation, necropsy at weaning **Litters:** Number of pups, external malformation, bodyweights Survival Opening of eyes and pinnae, pupil and righting reflex, startle response. Learning test in swimming maze, post weaning. Ophthalmoscopy, Preyer's reflex, locomotor activity Sexual development and mating with necropsy of females on day 13 of gestation – numbers of corpora lutea and of position and numbers of implantations

the point of sexual maturity, a factor that allows recovery according to the extent of the toxic insult. In a fertility study mating behaviour is assessed by recording the time taken to successful mating. Lack of mating can be investigated by pairing unmated females with successful males from the same group, while unmated males are paired with untreated females. The number and distribution of implantations in uterine horns, classified as early resorptions, late resorptions, dead or live fetuses, is recorded to assess effects *in utero*, together with the numbers of corpora lutea in the ovary. Pre-implantation losses are calculated by subtracting the number of implantations from the number of corpora lutea. For the males, assessment of sperm quality is increasingly recommended by sperm counts, motility, morphology and quality. Testicular weight is a sensitive indicator of male effect and can be backed up by histological processing and examination. Computer Assisted Sperm Assessment (CASA) generates a large amount of data, which may not yet be fully understood, making interpretation difficult; it is, however, enthusiastically supported by regulatory authorities, presumably in the questionable belief that volume of data gives added security in assessment of prospective safety. The use of this technique should be balanced against what can be revealed by alternatives such as testicular staging in routine toxicity studies.[7]

Embryonic development

Fetal weight gives an indication of maternal or placental function and of any retardation in development that has taken place. Smaller fetuses may have skeletal variations from controls that are a product of slower development rather than direct teratogenicity. The fetuses are assessed for abnormality by visceral or skeletal examination. Visceral development can be assessed by Wilson's sectioning of fetuses fixed in Bouin's fluid (not in rabbits), but this has increasingly been replaced by or combined with microdissection. Dissection of other foetuses may also be performed before the carcasses are cleared with potassium hydroxide and stained with Alizarin red, which stains bone red for skeletal examination, and alcein blue for cartilage. Not all the parameters listed in Table 5.5 are universally applied; for instance placental weight is rarely affected, although some classes of drugs have been known to produce differences from controls, notably some cardioactive substances. The weight of gravid uterus is useful for assessing effects on carcass weight, by subtraction of the uterus weight from the complete bodyweight immediately before necropsy.

Structural congenital abnormalities that impair or potentially impair the survival or constitution of the fetus are classified as major abnormalities. Other defects are classified as minor abnormalities. Commonly observed variations in the degree of ossification from that expected of a day 20 gestation fetus, together with common variations in the extent of renal pelvic cavitation and ureter dilation are recorded as variants. In some fetuses, an extra 'wavy' rib may be seen; the significance of these has been widely debated down the years but they are now considered to be without developmental significance. Embryofetal examinations in the rabbit are similar to those described above for the rat, with the exception that the head is treated and examined separately. All rabbit fetuses are dissected and cleared for skeletal examination.

Peri- and post-natal development

This type of study is among the most complex toxicity studies conducted and can be made more complex by the addition of extra generations and longer treatment periods. In the simpler of these studies, treatment ceases when the F_0 females give birth. In multi-generation studies, usually conducted with agrochemicals or food additives, treatment may be continued throughout the study until termination of the F_2 pups. It is possible to continue such studies into a carcinogenicity assessment by continued treatment of the F_2 generation, although such studies are rare, due to complexity and expense. Mating performance is assessed in a similar manner to fertility studies. For the dams of the F_0 and subsequent generations the records of length of gestation and onset and duration of parturition are probably self-explanatory. The performance of the dams through lactation, coupled with the survival of the pups and their bodyweight gains during lactation are also an indication of maternal function. In the studies where parturition is examined, the survival of the pups to day 4 post partum is checked. At day 4 the litter size may be reduced, where necessary, to four females and four females to obviate effects on post-natal development that may be attributable to large or uneven litter sizes. The pups are examined for external abnormalities and their development is charted according to the time of achievement of a series of physical, sexual and sensory milestones – opening of eyes and detachment of pinnae, eruption of incisors, vaginal opening and balanopreputial separation, pupillary and righting reflexes and startle response. Learning ability is usually tested in a simple Y- or E-shaped swimming maze after weaning. An open field test is performed looking at general activity and exploratory behaviour; locomotor activity is assessed by performance on a rotating rod. Reproductive function is assessed by mating of the F_1 pups.

Pitfalls in reproductive toxicology

Although fertility studies are usually performed in rats, this should not be taken as the only method to assess male fertility. The rat produces approximately four times as many sperm per gram of testis than a man and is correspondingly less sensitive to effects on spermatogenesis. The mouse produces about three times more sperm than the rat. The use of data from routine toxicity studies in conjunction with those from reproductive studies gives an overview of testicular effects and so of the necessity for more specialised mechanistic studies. The rat is a robust species in which most compounds can be investigated in a wide range of vehicles, including oils. The rabbit's gastrointestinal physiology, however, means that it is unable to cope with compounds or vehicles that disturb the physiological balance or osmotic environment in the gut. In essence, this means that antibiotics should be tested in other species such as mouse, minipig or non-human primate and that lipid-soluble substances must be used as a suspension in an aqueous vehicle, with attendant problems of suboptimal absorption.

Compound type is also a consideration. As indicated, rabbits are sensitive to antibiotics and hormonally active compounds may be inappropriate in rats or rabbits where the ovaries are responsible for maintaining hormonal control of gestation; in humans and primates this is carried out by the placenta. Selection of an inappropriate species may result in toxicity at doses so low that they approach expected human exposure or dosing levels. This situation, which gives no margin of safety over human usage, is unsatisfactory and makes safety evaluation difficult; in these cases the risk/benefit of the drug and indication for which it is intended should be considered. An alternative to these species is the cynomolgus monkey, although its use should be carefully considered against that of alternatives such as the minipig.

Various aspects of the reproductive process mean that it is subject to disruption by substances such as hormone derivatives or cytotoxic agents. With compounds such as these it may become necessary to break the studies down into specific stages either to minimise the length of the treatment period or to investigate particular parts of the reproductive cycle. For instance, the fertility study usually requires mating of treated males with treated females; in some cases it may be necessary to treat both sexes but to mate them with untreated partners. Effects on maternal function may be investigated by fostering the offspring of treated females on untreated females and vice versa. In dietary multi-generation studies toxicity in the dams may be encountered during late lactation when there is a marked increase in food consumption.

Transplacental carcinogenesis, as shown by diethylstilbestrol, is an uncommon effect – or at least has not been demonstrated to be detectable over normal background incidences of cancers – and is unlikely to be demonstrated by routine reproductive studies as the effects do not become apparent until the offspring are adult. However, multi-generation studies go some way towards addressing this problem. Where there is some retardation of fetal development, for instance due to lowered maternal food consumption or another indirect effect of treatment, there may be variations from control values, particularly in weight and/or skeletal development. These are not teratogenic effects, merely an indication of indirect toxicity. In similar ways, neurologically active compounds may affect maternal behaviour or lactation and have indirect effect on pup survival through reduced maternal care. These compounds may also have indirect effects on fertility if they affect mating behaviour to the extent that mating is delayed or completely unsuccessful.

Chapter 6

Determination

Genotoxicity and carcinogenicity

Genotoxicity

General principles in genotoxicity

The intention in testing for genotoxicity is to determine the potential for damage to DNA and thereby to highlight any effects that might, with administration or exposure, lead to an increased incidence of tumours or birth defects through heritable effects in the germ cells. In the latter context it is worth considering that changes in chromosomal number are usually fatal in laboratory animals but not in humans, where conditions such as Down's syndrome are associated with an extra chromosome but do not lead to abortion. The genetic changes associated with some cancers are given in Table 6.1.

Though individual genetic disorders are rare, collectively they comprise over 15,500 recognised genetic abnormalities and affect about 13 million Americans. For instance 3–5 per cent of all births result in congenital malformations and 20–30 per cent of all infant deaths are due to genetic disorders, while 11.1 per cent of paediatric hospital admissions are for children with genetic disorders and 18.5 per cent are children with other congenital malformations. In adults, 12 per cent of hospital admissions are for genetic causes and 50 per cent of mental

Table 6.1 Genetic associations with cancers

Proto-oncogene	Activation by	Chromosomal change	Associated cancer
c-myc	Genetic rearrangement	Translocation: 8–14, 8–2, or 8–22	Burkitt's lymphoma
c-abl	Genetic rearrangement	Translocation: 9–22	Chronic myeloid leukaemia
c-H-ras	Point mutation		Bladder carcinoma
c-K-ras	Point mutation		Lung and colon carcinoma
N-myc	Gene amplification		Neuroblastoma

Note: Data provided by Mike Kelly, Oxford Glycosciences.

retardation has a genetic basis. Amongst chronic adult diseases, 15 per cent of all cancers have an inherited susceptibility and 10 per cent of the chronic diseases (heart, diabetes, arthritis) which occur in the adult populations have a significant genetic component. Given this context the assessment of the potential for new or existing chemicals to cause genetic damage is an important area of toxicological testing. This is the main area of toxicological investigation in which *in vitro* testing has been accepted, principally on the basis of the relatively simple endpoints that are examined in these tests.

Testing for genotoxicity or mutagenicity, in a regulatory context, became much more frequent in the early 1970s when Bruce Ames developed the bacterial reversion assay or Ames test. This simple test, using specially derived strains of *Salmonella typhimurium* for which histidine is an essential amino acid, determines the ability of a chemical to produce mutations that allow the bacteria to grow in the absence of histidine. The basic hypothesis was that carcinogenesis originated through damage to DNA and chemicals that damage DNA are more likely to be carcinogenic than those that do not. The problem with this is that, while there is good correlation between mutagenesis and carcinogenesis, not all carcinogens damage DNA directly and these are not readily detected by current methods that determine direct toxic effects on the DNA. The attraction of genotoxicity testing is that it offers a method of assessing carcinogenic potential that is quick, inexpensive, usually *in vitro* and can be performed early in the development of a chemical. This contrasts with the traditional approach which is the use of long studies in rodents that take a minimum of two years to complete, are expensive and conducted later in development. With the realisation that the simplistic Ames test system examined only one endpoint in bacteria and resulted in a number of false positives, an increasingly large number of tests were developed to examine the effects on DNA in other ways. A more recent development has been that of determination of structure–activity relationships and the computerised prediction by expert systems of mutagenic potential through the presence in the test molecule of structural components or groups that have been associated with mutagenicity in other compounds. These are discussed in more detail later in the chapter on prediction (chapter 10).

Testing for genotoxicity acknowledges that there are basically two levels of effect – at the gene and at the chromosome. At the former level, mutations are sought that lead to localised changes at one or a few bases in the DNA, thereby changing the coding for the protein produced by the gene. A change from one base to another, or the misreading of a chemically altered base, may lead to a different amino acid being inserted into an otherwise normal protein; this is a point mutation. When a base or base pair is inserted or deleted this is known as a frameshift mutation, as the reading frame of the code is changed, leading to an abnormal protein product. At the level of the chromosome the changes are broadly in terms of structure or number; there may be changes in number due to effects on mitosis or meiosis and translocations, rearrangements, breaks or gaps, which indicate an effect on the chromosomes themselves. DNA or chromosomal damage is detected directly or indirectly. Direct evidence comes from the induction of genetic change, such as the ability of Ames test bacteria to divide in the absence of a previously essential amino acid, or by examination of chromosomes in metaphase where breakages and abnormalities are evident under the microscope. Indirect evidence of genetic damage may be obtained by measurement of DNA repair in tissues. This is easier to detect in tissues that do not normally divide and is used in the assessment of unscheduled DNA synthesis (UDS) in hepatocytes.

The majority of chemicals are not directly genotoxic and one disadvantage of a bacterial system *in vitro* is that the bacteria lack the enzymes that are responsible in mammals for the activation of chemicals to toxic metabolites. Consequently, a metabolising system was devised that uses the microsomal fraction from homogenised rat liver, which contains the majority of xenobiotic metabolising enzymes; this is known as S-9 mix. For normal regulatory purposes, this is prepared from the livers of rats treated with an enzyme-inducing agent, such as repeated doses of β-naphthoflavone and/or sodium phenobarbitone or Arochlor 1254. In some cases, S-9 mix may be prepared from other tissues such as kidney or with the use of other inducing agents. One factor to consider is that S-9 has its own intrinsic toxicity and that incubation of mammalian-derived cells should be limited to a few hours. S-9 mix is rich in the microsomal elements of metabolism typified by cytochrome P450, which carry out the initial reactions (phase 1) of metabolism. It has much less of the phase 2 metabolism systems, which conjugate the metabolites with endogenous molecules to make them more polar and thus easier to eliminate. This is unlikely to be a significant problem much of the time as these conjugates are unlikely to be mutagenic in their own right. However, it means that the test system may be exposed for an unrealistic time to active metabolites that might otherwise be removed by conjugation.

Test battery and study design

In assessing the genotoxicity of a new chemical it is normal to use several tests that examine different endpoints or mechanisms of effect, in recognition of the limited scope of individual tests. The types of test used are typically a bacterial mutation test – usually the Ames test – an evaluation of chromosome damage in mammalian cells, an *in vivo* test for chromosomal damage, such as the micronucleus test in rodents, and possibly a test for gene mutation in mammalian cells. The general composition of the chosen test battery is largely determined by the type of chemical and the regulatory authorities at which it is aimed. The nature of the chemical may also influence the choice of tests, for instance excessively bacteriotoxic materials, such as antibiotics, are not suitable for bacterial assays although some guidelines may still require them. For an antibiotic, two tests using mammalian cells, one for gene mutation (e.g. mouse lymphoma L5178Y TK±assay) and one for chromosomal damage (e.g. CHO assay) with a micronucleus test *in vivo* might be recommended as a basic test battery. For a compound known to disrupt cell division, test design is critical and harvest times and exposure concentrations must be carefully chosen; however, mammalian cell mutagenicity would still be possible. In every case the choice of tests should be made on a rational and scientific basis, bearing in mind the regulatory guidelines for the class of chemical. In the event of a single positive result that is of borderline biological significance, the test battery may be expanded to include studies of DNA interaction, damage or repair such as UDS or the comet assay. However, when responding to a positive result with additional testing, it should be noted that increased numbers of ill-chosen tests may not clarify the picture and may simply serve to produce interpretative uncertainty.

The design of genotoxicity studies follows the broad pattern of other toxicity tests, using a control and several increasing concentrations of test material. In a typical Ames test there could be a control and five concentrations of test material up to a maximum of 5 mg/plate. There should be at least three plates for controls and at each test concentration and positive controls using known mutagens should be run at the same time to ensure that the bacteria are responding as expected. The positive controls are chosen according to the strain of bacteria and whether they need metabolic activation through S-9 mix or are directly mutagenic (Table 6.2). Benzo(a)pyrene or 2-aminoanthracene are used with S-9 mix to demonstrate sensitivity to metabolically activated mutagens but are not the only choices available.

As with other branches of toxicology, the choice of exposure concentration or dose level is of crucial importance. This is normally achieved through the use of dose range-finding studies to assess toxicity. In the Ames test, toxicity is assessed by addition of a small amount of histidine to the agar medium, allowing a small amount of growth, which is seen as 'background lawn'. At toxic concentrations of test substance this background lawn is thinner than in the controls. This

Table 6.2 Direct-acting positive controls used in the Ames test

Strain	Direct acting mutagens (no S-9 mix)
Salmonella typhimurium	
TA1535, TA100	Sodium azide
TA97Aa	9-Aminoacridine
TA98	2-Nitrofluorene
TA1537	9-Aminoacridine
TA1538, TA98	2-Nitrofluorene
TA102	Cumene hydroperoxide, mitomycin-C
Escherichia coli	
WP2, WP2 uvrA	4-Nitroquinoline-N-oxide

Note: Compiled from several sources.

leaves a reduced number of bacteria available for mutation and, as a result fewer mutant colonies are formed, which may give a false impression non-mutagenic effect. In experiments with cultured mammalian cells a degree of toxicity is considered desirable as this demonstrates exposure of the cells. However, cytotoxicity itself can give rise to false positive findings of genotoxicity, either due to the apparent chromosomal damage visible when there is a high proportion of dead or dying cells or due to chance clonal selection of mutant cells when high levels of toxicity are used in a mammalian gene mutation assay. Positive results at toxic concentrations should be interpreted with caution. The maximum level of desirable toxicity at the highest concentration is around 50 per cent in the chromosome aberration assay and around 80 per cent in the mouse lymphoma L5178Y TK± assay. It should also be noted that genotoxicity has not only been shown at concentrations where the test material is insoluble but that dose responses have been observed past the concentration at which precipitation occurs and that, accordingly, insolubility is not necessarily a valid criterion for choice of the highest concentration. If other criteria, such as the pH of the medium or osmolarity, do not limit the concentration of test substance the usual maximum concentration is set at 5 mg/plate, 5 mg/mL or 10 mM.

For genotoxicity tests in animals, doses are chosen according to the known acute toxicity of the test substance. The route of administration is chosen according to the expected route of exposure in humans but is normally oral or by intravenous or intraperitoneal injection. For *in vivo* tests, such as the micronucleus test in rodents, it is necessary to prove exposure of the target cells (normally bone marrow) to the test substance, by analysis of plasma samples. Additional animals may be necessary for this. Although it may be reasonable to assume that intravenous injection is associated with target cell exposure, where compounds are precipitated or rapidly transformed in the plasma, this assumption may be misplaced. Exposure is less certain with intraperitoneal injection and even less so with oral dosing. However, it is generally assumed that the plasma concentrations of the test substance give a good indication of the concentrations to which the target cells in the bone marrow or liver are exposed, as these tissues have a good blood supply.

The duration of exposure is also a factor to consider in study design, although to a very large extent this is indicated in the guidelines and literature. Due to its toxicity, exposure of mammalian cells with S-9 mix is generally shorter than without it; in a human lymphocyte study this can mean 3 instead of 24 hours. In whole animal experiments the number of doses is a factor to consider; generally single administration of a high dose is used although several doses may be used in some cases. The cells of interest may be sampled or harvested at different times after administration to take account of different times of onset of effect. Taking the micronucleus test as an example, it is normal to harvest bone marrow cells on at least two occasions, for example 24 and 48 hours after dosing; a harvest at 72 hours is recommended in some guidelines. An older design involved giving two doses and sampling on one occasion only.

Test systems and tests

There is an extensive history of genotoxicity test systems, including the use of mice in the mouse coat colour spot test to assess mutation due to radiation and the dominant lethal assay also in mice, both of which were developed in the late 1950s and 1960s. The use of the fruit fly, *Drosophila melanogaster*, has a longer history in mutation research but has fallen out of favour. These tests depended on anaesthetising the flies at intervals to check effects. The potential disadvantages of imperfect anaesthesia and the escape of the flies into the open laboratory or their death, together with the technical demands of difference recognition, may have had some influence in the decline in its use. The stress associated with chasing an expensive experiment around a laboratory with a butterfly net could not be expected to increase its popularity with toxicologists.

Progress in the acceptance of new tests for genotoxicity is slowed by the multitude of test systems under development and by the consequent dilution of effort for really promising lines of research. The spectre of validation for new tests or test systems is a constant problem, collaborative studies usually being conducted by a number of laboratories. These multi-centre studies are expensive and cumbersome to organise, and may show up a lack of reproducibility in the more technically demanding assays. Following validation there is the task of gaining regulatory acceptance and persuading companies developing new chemicals to use them. Sometimes assays have gained credibility in industry through their use as screening assays, before gaining acceptance from regulators.

Many genotoxicity assays are conducted *in vitro* using unicellular organisms that have been produced with particular characteristics for the purposes of the test endpoint and which may be subject to insidious genetic drift. As a result, test system characterisation is an important factor in the conduct of these tests, in a way that is not seen *in vivo*. Whole animals have a much longer lifespan than microbial or cellular systems and therefore change more slowly, over a period of years rather than months. The rate of change in any animal species or strain is usually not large enough to cause problems and a single change is unlikely to invalidate an experiment. With single cell preparations, either bacterial or mammalian-derived, the generation times are quicker and there is the possibility that the cells may lose the characteristics that are vital to correct performance of the test. For instance the strains of *Salmonella* used in the Ames test have been modified in various ways to make them more sensitive to carcinogens. Modification has been performed to enhance absorption via a rough coat or to increase sensitivity to UV light or antibiotics. These characteristics are essential for the correct function of the tests and, because they are not immediately visible or verifiable by conventional biochemical testing, they must be checked in the stock cultures at regular intervals. The primary requirement for the Ames test is that the *Salmonella* or *E. coli* strains used should not grow in the absence of histidine or tryptophan respectively. The presence of rough coat can be ascertained through absorption of a high molecular weight dye and the consequent lethality. Sensitivity to UV light is checked by irradiation; in addition the antibiotic resistance of some strains has been increased and is tested with the appropriate antibiotic. Finally the relative sensitivity to known mutagens is checked in every study against expectation from laboratory background data ranges. Failure to complete these checks may produce unreliable results. This requirement may be less stringent for primary cultures of cells, such as hepatocytes, which are derived from animals of known strain and biochemical profile, which can themselves be characterised by conventional means.

Test systems for the evaluation of genotoxicity may be divided broadly into the categories in Table 6.3, which also lists the main tests in which they are used. Due to the multiplicity of test systems only the major ones used in regulatory toxicology are discussed here, with references to tests or systems that may not be considered to be mainstream.

Bacteria

Bacterial mutation assays were amongst the first *in vitro* toxicity tests to gain regulatory acceptance and the reversion assay using strains of S. *typhimurium*, the Ames test, has become the most widely conducted genotoxicity assay, with the addition of E. *coli* in deference to Japanese wishes. The test is based on mutant *Salmonella* strains that cannot grow without histidine but which can be reverted to wild type by mutation, when they are able to synthesise their own

Table 6.3 Principal genotoxicity test systems

Mutation event	Test systems	Tests
Bacterial reverse mutation	Salmonella typhimurium,	Ames test for reversion to histidine independence
	Escherichia coli	Ames test for reversion to tryptophan independence
Mammalian mutation *in vitro*	CHO or V79 Chinese hamster cells	Mutation at HGPRT[a] locus
	Mouse lymphoma L5178Y cells	Mutation at TK[b] locus
DNA damage *in vitro*	CHO or V79 cells	Chromosome aberration
	Human peripheral lymphocytes	Chromosome aberration
	Primary cultures of rodent hepatocytes	Unscheduled DNA synthesis or COMET assay
DNA damage *in vivo* or *ex vivo*	Rat and mouse	Micronucleus test or UDS or COMET assay

Notes: [a]Hypoxanthine guanine phosphoribosyl transferase
       [b]Thymidine kinase

histidine. After a period of incubation with the test material, with or without S-9 mix, the colonies of revertant bacteria are counted. Each strain of bacteria used has a normal background incidence of mutation and a dose-dependent increase from this is taken to be evidence of mutagenic effect, which should be reproducible in a second experiment. Normally four strains are used, selected from TA 100 and TA 1535 which detect base substitution, TA 98 and TA 1538 which detect frameshift mutations and TA 97 and TA 1537 which detect single frameshift mutations. TA 102 may also be used but is not generally required by regulatory guidelines. The same principles are applicable to E. coli, which is used to comply with Japanese guidelines and detects base substitutions; usually a single strain such as WP2 uvrA is used. These strains are dependent on tryptophan and mutations are revealed by the presence of colonies growing in the absence of tryptophan.

Salmonella and E. coli may also be used in forward mutation tests and in DNA repair tests in which repair-deficient bacteria are mutated to repair-competent, which are able to form colonies that can be counted.

Mammalian cells in culture

Mammalian cells may be used in mutation assays and in chromosome damage or aberration tests, also known as cytogenetic assays. The most commonly used mammalian cells are the Chinese hamster-derived cells – CHO (Chinese hamster ovary) and V79 lung-derived cell lines, the mouse lymphoma L5178Y cell, and primary cultures of rodent hepatocytes or human peripheral lymphocytes. The cell line cultures have advantages in that they are easy to culture reproducibly but, in contrast to primary cultures of cells from tissues such as liver, they have little metabolic activity and tend to have abnormalities of chromosomal number (aneuploidy). The Chinese hamster lines cells tend to grow in sheets which can make intercellular communication easier in some circumstances, leading to transfer of cellular components that may negate any mutation in the receiving cell. Therefore, the plating density of the cells needs to be controlled. These lines have particular use in chromosome aberration assays but may also be used for detection of mutations, for example at the HPRT locus. The mouse lymphoma L5178Y cell, which uses the TK locus, is more sensitive to mutagens than the Chinese hamster-derived cells; they can grow in suspension culture and thus do not have the problem of intercellular communication. In addition it has been suggested that this cell line can be used in the detection of chromosomal abnormalities and mutations through differences in colony size, although the reproducibility of this has been questioned. This, using an appropriate protocol, potentially gives the cells a much broader scope than the Chinese hamster-derived lines for which mutation and chromosome damage are assessed in separate tests. If the TK assay is used, the size of colonies produced may indicate whether the damage is due to clastogenicity or mutation. There is the possibility that these cell lines may undergo some genetic drift in different laboratories, a factor which may ultimately lead to some inconsistency and irreproducibility of results.

Human peripheral lymphocytes are also used and have the advantage that they are from a relevant species and are also primary culture cells. They are used only for the assessment of chromosome aberration; these tests tend to be more expensive than those using cultured cell lines. It is important to ensure that the donors of the blood from which the lymphocytes are separated are free of viral infection, non-smokers, not too old and not on medication that may be expected to affect the assay results. As stated earlier, it is important to demonstrate cytotoxicity in these assays and positive controls are routinely used to demonstrate that the test system is valid. Once again it is important to conduct a second experiment to confirm the results of the first.

The basic principle in mammalian cell mutation assays is to induce mutations that confer resistance to toxic nucleotide analogues. Metabolic activity in these tests is provided by S-9 mix. The cells are exposed for up to 24 hours without S-9 or up to 6 hours with and are then cultured without the test substance to allow for phenotypic expression of mutation. Then they are cultured with the appropriate selective agent to check for the formation of colonies.

In chromosome aberration tests the cells, which may be human peripheral lymphocytes, are exposed to the test substance for up to 24 hours and may have a treatment-free period. They are then treated with a spindle poison, which arrests the cell division in metaphase. Metabolic activation is again provided by S-9 mix. The cells are taken onto microscope slides and stained. An appropriate number of metaphases, which may be 100 cells from two or three culture replicates at each of three treatment concentrations, are scored for the presence of chromosomal aberrations, which are seen as gaps, breaks or exchanges and abnormalities of number. Although numerical abnormalities due to polyploidy and endoreduplication may be seen with other cell lines, aneuploidy is easier to detect in human cells. A chromosomal gap is an area in which the stain has not been taken up and where there is minimal misalignment of chromatid(s). A chromosomal break is defined as an unstained section accompanied by a clear misalignment of the chromatid(s). General opinion is that gaps are not as significant as breaks but they are reported anyway, usually as separate totals to the other aberrations. More extreme disruption may be seen and this is also reported. Cytotoxicity is determined by reductions in mitotic index for human lymphocytes. For cell lines a variety of methods to assess cytotoxicity are available, including viable cell number, colony-forming ability and MTT assessment of mitochondrial activity.

Hepatocytes isolated from rats may be used in a range of assays, such as unscheduled DNA synthesis (UDS), which assesses repair that takes place following damage to DNA. The extent of DNA repair is assessed through the incorporation of tritiated thymidine into the nuclei of cells exposed to the test substance. The isolated hepatocytes are allowed to attach to glass microscope slide coverslips where they are exposed to the test substance; they are then exposed to medium containing tritiated thymidine and, after fixing and drying, with photographic emulsion. The cells are stained and the number of grains in the nucleus are assessed microscopically. There is also a method of measurement that uses liquid scintillation counting of the activity, however this does not allow the exclusion of cytoplasmic grains from the total counted and so is less sensitive but also less time consuming.

Cultured cells can also be used to assess sister chromatid exchange (SCE), in which sections are exchanged between the chromatids of a chromosome pair; however, the *in vitro* SCE test suffers from a high background incidence, which limits its sensitivity. SCE correlates well with genotoxicity and carcinogenicity but is not fully understood. It can be assessed from cells obtained from cancer patients or workers exposed occupationally to chemicals, where it may indicate increased effects on the DNA.

Ex vivo *systems*

In these systems an animal is treated and, after an appropriate interval, tissues such as the liver are removed for further treatment *in vitro* followed by examination. This approach is used in another design of UDS assay and in the Comet assay. The advantage of this approach is that the chemical is administered to a whole animal and is subject to the normal processes of metabolism and elimination before its effects are examined in the target tissues. In the *ex vivo* UDS assay the livers are removed from the animals at a suitable time after dosing and sections or slices are treated with tritiated thymidine. The slices are fixed and then treated in a similar way to the cells in the *in vitro* method described above.

The comet, or single cell gel electrophoresis assay, is potentially a powerful means of detecting DNA damage in cells from animals that have been treated with suspected carcinogens. The basic principle is to electrophorese the DNA from a single cell nucleus, damaged DNA having a greater spread of travel (tail) than control or undamaged, the shape of the electrophoresis pattern giving the assay its name. The assay is simple and can be performed rapidly but may not characterise the type of damage that has occurred. Unlike many genotoxicity tests it can be applied to any tissue believed to be a target for the test substance. The assay can be carried out after a single administration or could be included in routine toxicity studies as an indicator of DNA change and, by implication, of potential carcinogenicity. However, it should be seen as one element of a set of data collected to examine genotoxicity or carcinogenic potential and not be taken, by itself, to be a clear indication of hazard. It is likely that regulatory acceptance of this test will increase.

In vivo *systems*

Mice and rats are used for examining the potential of chemicals to cause chromosomal damage by examination of bone marrow cells either by scoring of metaphases or, more usually, micronuclei in erythrocytes. Standard strains can be used in these routine tests, which are performed by administration of a dose near the limit of tolerance. Bone marrow is harvested from the femur 24 and 48 hours after a single administration and, in some designs, at 72 hours. Another design has two administrations 24 hours apart and one harvest 24 hours after the second administration. Chromosomal damage is assessed in bone marrow smears by the presence of micronuclei, which are fragments of damaged chromosomes or whole chromosomes left behind when the nucleus is extruded following the final cell division in normal erythrocyte maturation. Up to 2000 polychromatic erythrocytes from each animal are assessed for micronuclei. The test can assess chromosome damage and spindle defects. Toxicity may be indicated by the ratio of polychromatic (early stage) erythrocytes to normochromatic (late stage) erythrocytes (PCE:NCE). A decrease in the ratio may be due to either prevention of early stage development or replacement of dead bone marrow from peripheral blood. Therefore a decrease in the PCE:NCE ratio indicates bone marrow toxicity and thus exposure. Opinions and guidelines tend to differ in the choice of an all-male design or one that uses both sexes and on the numbers of erythrocytes that should be scored. In the event of a negative result it is important to demonstrate exposure to the test substance, especially if the route of administration is oral or intraperitoneal. Consequently it may be better to build these examinations into the original experiment with the same batch of animals, rather than do a separate experiment at a later date which might not be equivalent in every respect to the original test. However, this uses more animals and does not comply with the three Rs.

In addition mice have been used in sister chromatid exchange assays (see above) and in the mouse spot test and in the dominant lethal test, which detect mutations. However, these tests are more extensive in terms of animal numbers and take longer to complete than other assays and are not routinely used. In the former test pregnant females are treated on day 10 of gestation and the offspring are checked for the presence of relevant spots of colour difference in the coat which imply the presence of mutation in the coat colour genes of pigment cells. In the dominant lethal test the effect of a prospective mutagen on the germ cells is assessed by single or sometimes limited repeated administration to males which are then mated with a fresh untreated female each week for a complete spermatogenic cycle. After two weeks gestation the uterine contents are inspected for implantations and implantation losses and fertility index. The presence of increased implantation loss implies that a mutation has occurred and the week in which the effect is noted indicates the stage of the spermatogenic cycle that is involved.

Transgenic mice are also used occasionally in mutation assays and it is likely that this will increase as validation of the various models proceeds and regulatory acceptance increases. Such systems have the advantage that they are *in vivo* and the chemical is subject to the dynamics of tissue interrelationships, metabolism and elimination, in contrast to the tests conducted *in vitro*. They have the disadvantage that the animals are expensive and may need specialist care.

Pitfalls in genotoxicity

The absence of toxicity is a major concern in genotoxicity assays as it is often taken to mean that the test system was not adequately exposed to the test substance. This may be due to inherent insolubility of the test substance, making high concentration exposure difficult or impossible. However, as genotoxicity has been shown in the insolubility ranges of some substances, restricting test concentrations on the basis of solubility is not usually an option. Equally, it should be pointed out that there should also be a lack of toxicity at lower concentrations as toxicity itself may produce positive results in some test systems. In the Ames test, toxicity may lead to reduced colony counts, not through lack of genotoxicity but through a reduction in the number of viable bacteria able to demonstrate a response. With substances that are particularly bacteriotoxic, low achievable concentration may make the Ames test inappropriate.

An absence of response in positive controls may indicate that the test system was not what it was supposed to be and the characterisation of the cell or bacterial line should be checked, together with the laboratory background data accumulated from previous experiments. Poor characterisation of test system is a factor to bear in mind in looking at any set of unusual test data.

In chromosome aberration tests in mammalian cells *in vitro*, damage seen only at high concentrations may indicate that the harvest times were inappropriate; different harvest times in the second experiment may help to clarify effects seen. In a similar way, the use of a pre-incubation assay in the bacterial reverse mutation (Ames) test can provide alternative metabolic conditions in the second experiment. The use of different conditions in the second experiment following a negative or equivocal first experiment provides a more robust study with less chance of a false negative result. Osmotic pressure or pH outside normal limits is also a source of invalid data and should be considered in the design of studies. In some cases, biologically irrelevant effects can be produced by choice of an inappropriate test system.

In tests *in vivo* there is a problem if the test material has marked pharmacological effects at low doses that preclude high dose testing. In these cases it may be impossible to produce a high enough exposure at the target cells. A similar lack of exposure may be seen in substances that are absorbed to a negligible extent. In these cases a parenteral route may help to increase target cell exposure; however, intraperitoneal injection may not be appropriate and intravenous injection may be difficult due to low solubility. This becomes problematic when an *in vitro* test has indicated a positive result that cannot be verified *in vivo* due to toxicity, poor absorption or poor solubility. One approach is to consider the use of additional tests such as UDS, but the best administration route for this test is oral as this is the route most likely to be associated with the highest possible concentrations in the liver, where the target cells are. In the final analysis a negative result *in vivo* achieved as a result of low-level exposure does not offset a positive result *in vitro*.

The possibility of false positives should be considered. This is the chief reason for conducting a second experiment for *in vitro* assays, the object being to confirm the reproducibility of the first set of data, a factor that is particularly important where a marginal effect is examined. In the mouse micronucleus test excessive stress may lead to a small increase in micronuclei.

One area of fundamental importance is the purity of the test substance, as impurities have been associated with genotoxicity. A positive result with an impure early production batch of chemical may not be relevant to the effects of future batches. Equally it should be borne in mind that a change in synthetic pathway during development may introduce new impurities that have not been properly tested in previous genotoxicity assays.

Care should used, in responding to a positive result, that additional tests are chosen that will help to explain the data produced rather than simply add to them. In data sets relating to older chemicals, it is possible to see the large numbers of tests that have been conducted to investigate positive results in early testing; these effects have been known to disappear when there has been a change in production methods. The initial response to a positive result should be to ask if it is biologically relevant and how it has arisen. With this inform-ation it is then possible to design a set of investigations that will explain the initial data set.

Carcinogenicity

General principles in carcinogenicity

Cancer is a degenerative condition of old age which is seen at high incidence in animals and in approximately 30 per cent of the human population. Further-more it is a tremendously diverse condition, affecting practically every tissue in the body and, in terms of individual tumours, occurring at widely differing rates; for example, in humans, lung and breast cancer are common but haemangio-sarcoma is rare. As life expectancy increases the background incidence of cancer will also tend to increase. The principle in carcinogenicity assessment is to screen chemicals for the potential they might have to cause or be associated with an increased incidence of cancer in humans. This process, which is wider than any single study, looks for structural similarities between the chemical and known carcinogens and examines all the data from genotoxicity tests, metabo-lism and pharmacokinetics and the data from long-term testing in animals, usually rats and mice. The intention in these latter tests is to look for relevant tumour increases in animals or to look for mechanisms that may be expected to result in human tumours at a significant rate. These assessment methods are obligatory before a chemical is allowed to come into regular contact with humans through marketing. For existing compounds – natural or synthetic – there is the possibility of epidemiological study to elucidate relationships between observed tumours and human exposure.

Most known human carcinogens are genotoxic and it is reasonable to assume that a chemical that is found to be clearly genotoxic in appropriate tests, including those conducted in vivo, is likely to be carcinogenic in humans. The problem with testing for carcinogenicity in rodents is that this tends to show that the test material is or is not carcinogenic in rodents; as such, careful extrapolation to the human situation is necessary before the risk of human carcinogenicity can be properly assessed. This extrapolation requires the careful assessment of all the available data and, possibly, the performance of additional mechanistic studies to explain any effects seen in animals or in vitro tests. The absence of carcinogenic effect in rodent tests should not be taken as definitive proof that a chemical will not be carcinogenic in humans. Equally the presence of an effect in rodents, for a non-genotoxic chemical, is often not taken as evidence that there will be a similar effect in humans. The contradictory nature of these two positions calls into question the utility of the carcinogenicity bioassay and there is, in fact, a growing acknowledgement that this is an unsatisfactory form of test, which will in time be replaced when satisfactory alternatives have evolved.

Carcinogenicity may be simply defined as the process of conversion of normal cells so that they can form tumours. However, this simple definition masks the complexity of the process, which is multi-stage and multi-factorial. At its most basic level, genotoxic carcinogenesis is a three stage process – initiation, promotion and progression. Initiation is where the initial change in DNA takes place and is fixed; promotion is the initial division of these cells to form a focus of less differentiated cells and progression is where the focus of cells grows to become a tumour. Each of these stages is itself subject to a wide range of influences, which makes testing for the individual stages extremely difficult if not actually impossible. This picture is made more complex when the intricate mechanisms of non-genotoxic carcinogenesis are considered. Where genotoxic carcinogenesis is the endpoint of direct effects on the genetic material – DNA and/or chromosomes – in terms of quality or quantity, non-genotoxic carcinogens act by producing changes in the expression of the genetic information. For instance changes in the basic mechanisms of cellular control of programmed cell death (apoptosis) and division or simply increasing cell turnover can lead to cancer, without an initial direct effect on DNA. A further distinction between genotoxic and non-genotoxic effect is that the former, once fixed by cell division, is irreversible, whereas the latter can be reversed by withdrawal of the stimulus. Furthermore, carcinogens in humans can rarely be said to be acting alone. Human DNA is subject to a high background of 'normal' damage due to environmental influences, independent of any specific xenobiotic chemical. When an additional potent carcinogen is added to this, the effects may be more than simply additive; chemicals to which we are exposed routinely in the course of everyday existence may serve to promote the effects of chemicals encountered at work or elsewhere. The carcinogenicity of mixtures, such as cigarette smoke, is bound up in the world of these interactions. In fact, smoking has a marked upward effect on the risk of cancer in workers who were employed in the asbestos industry or uranium mines. Conversely, a reduced incidence of cancer is associated with high levels of antioxidant or other protective chemicals, typically contained in a diet rich in fruit and vegetables.

In regulatory toxicology, the lifespan study in rodents has been the gold standard of assessment for many years, although this is changing gradually. The objective of these studies is to detect increased incidences of tumours in the treated groups that can be ascribed to the test substance. Although tumours may be caused by chronic inflammation or physical mechanisms such as implants, radiation or fibres, the main emphasis here is on assessment of chemical carcinogenesis. However, the whole area of carcinogenicity assessment is under review as the relevance and utility of data provided by classic two-year study are increasingly questioned. This section sets out to provide a review of current methods and those that may supersede them.

Test systems for carcinogenicity

The normal species in which lifespan carcinogenicity is assessed are the rat, mouse and, rarely, the hamster. The hamster is used very little in these experiments, particularly because of the lack of background data; also, where temperature control was less than perfect, the prospect of an entire study going into hibernation in cold weather was less than ideal. Other species may be more appropriate than these but are usually ruled out by long lifespan and consequently increased study length, housing requirements or expense.

The usual approach has been to conduct bioassays over a 24- or 30-month period in rats and mice. The mouse has a long history in carcinogenicity testing; it was skin-painting experiments in mice that demonstrated the tumour promotion properties of phorbol esters, and they have also been used in photocarcinogenicity testing. However, the use of the mouse is increasingly questioned.

Historically, several strains of rodent have been favoured over others but each has its pros and cons. The choice of strain was greatly influenced by the US National Toxicology Programme (NTP) which tended to use F344 rats and B6C3F1 mice. The former has a high incidence of testicular tumours and leukaemias and the B6C3F1 mouse is associated with a high incidence of liver tumours. Other strains have been used successfully, notably the Sprague–Dawley CD and Wistar rats and CD-1 mice, each of which has its own tumour profile.

Growth, survival and tumour profile are inextricably entwined and have caused problems in the past. It has been noted, especially in studies where an unpalatable test substance is mixed with the diet, that lower food consumption in the treated groups is associated with lower tumour burden and longer survival, when compared with contemporary controls. The Sprague–Dawley derived CD rat was used extensively until it was found that it was becoming increasingly overweight, with a consequent reduction in lifespan (see chapter 2, page 48) so that fewer than 50 per cent of animals survived until the end of the treatment period. As this is one of the criteria of a successful carcinogenicity bioassay, there was a move towards other strains. One of the advantages of the F344 rat was that it was somewhat smaller than the CD, with better survival, eating less food and requiring less test material.

The chief disadvantage of using a strain with a high incidence of a particular tumour is that it is difficult to show a small increase in tumours in the affected tissue, especially as the normal incidences can vary significantly between studies. In the final analysis, the choice of strain should be influenced by strains usually used in the laboratory that is expected to carry out the tests; or choose the laboratory that uses the strain you prefer. This is a pragmatic decision based on the fact that the historical control data at the laboratory are important in the interpretation of the data; an apparently significant but small increase in testicular tumours may be dismissed as being within historical ranges. Such dismissal is even more authoritative if no dose relationship is present. Although there is good sense in using the strain of rat that was used in the general toxicity testing this is not always possible and is, in any case, not possible with the mouse, which is not often used in general toxicity.

It has been suggested[1] (see Box 3.1 also) that several strains should be used in a single study, which could be expected to address differences in response between strains. The problem with this is that the numbers of animals needed to show a weak carcinogenic response is large for statistical reasons. Hence, in order to detect a weak effect in only one strain, a large number of animals would be necessary in each strain, increasing the size of the study beyond practicable means, although Festing[1] indicates that this would not be necessary. Furthermore, if a chemical is carcinogenic in only one strain of several tested, it becomes necessary to question the relevance of the result to the human situation. Given these considerations, if there was a reason to expect significant metabolic differences between strains, it would probably be better to choose a strain specifically for the carcinogenicity studies, based on closeness of metabolic relevance to humans. By the time it is necessary to perform the carcinogenicity studies the information necessary for this choice should be largely present. However, such deliberation is rare and more pressing concerns are the more obvious characteristics of the chosen strain, such as survival and tumour profile.

Test systems that allow demonstration of a carcinogenic response in a shorter time than the standard two-year bioassay would appear to be attractive. The transgenic option, which can be completed in six months, is popular with US regulatory authorities but is greeted with some scepticism in Europe. In these studies, the importance of various genes in carcinogenesis, for example the *p53* or H-*ras* gene, is exploited by using strains of mice that are partially or wholly deficient in the gene of interest. This protocol has a clear application in assessing genotoxic carcinogens, but for non-genotoxic mechanisms the same drawback as with the lifespan study exists, namely that the assay may produce responses that are irrelevant to humans. One aspect of such assays to be wary of is the potential for all animals eventually to have a particular tumour, including in the control group. This very much reduces the utility of the assay as it reduces comparators to tumour number or size in treated animals in comparison with the controls or to time of observation of the first tumours. Overall, there are probably better ways of assessing carcinogenic potential and these will become more important as the mechanistic bases of non-genotoxic carcinogenicity are elucidated.

Study design and methods of assessment

The basic design of the classic rodent bioassay is another toxicological constant, defined by years of practice and regulatory acceptance. The norm is to treat three groups each of a minimum of 50 males and 50 females for at least two years, a treatment period which may be extended to 30 months if survival indicates that this is necessary. Frequently there are two control groups, giving 100 males and 100 females; this becomes more important where there is weak in-house historical control data. The numbers of controls must be decided based on the data available at the laboratory and on the preferences of the regulatory authorities at whom the study is aimed.

The route of administration is normally oral by intubation or admixture with the diet (see chapter 3 for more extensive comment), which has the advantage of being simple and cost effective. Oral intubation or gavage has the advantage for pharmaceuticals that this is most likely to be the route of administration in patients. However, where oral intubation gives poor systemic exposure this may be improved by dietary administration where the animals eat over an extended period. For agrochemicals or food additives the most appropriate route is usually in the diet. Poor palatability of diet offered can reduce food consumption and consequently affects tumour profile and survival. There are occasional studies which are carried out by administration in the drinking water; however, it is extremely difficult to estimate spillage, making calculation of exposure very inaccurate. Other routes of administration include dermal or inhalation; the former is relatively simple, the latter highly complex and, due to the amounts of high-cost equipment required, extremely expensive.

Although the classic bioassay approach uses both sexes of two species, there have been various attempts to get acceptance of a reduced protocol that uses male rats and female mice. Clearly this is useful for picking up male rat-specific carcinogens, for instance those acting via α-2u globulin. However, the ability to pick up such specific mechanisms does not necessarily make the assay results relevant to humans.

One type of carcinogenicity assay that does not fit well with more normal designs is the photocarcinogenicity study, a fairly straightforward concept which is not at all straightforward in its execution. The object of these studies is to determine the potential of the test substance to cause cancer in the presence of sunlight. Generally they involve dermal dosing of mice followed by exposure to UV radiation for known durations and known intensities, the latter being difficult to monitor, as the light sources tend to degrade with use and to become less intense. The studies can last between six and twelve months. Problems arise when all the animals, including controls, show skin tumours, which reduces the useful data to earlier onset and individual burden of tumours rather than incidence. Also there has been a lack of consistency in design, strain of rodent, numbers of animals and in the UV exposure system used, meaning that comparison between protocols is extremely difficult and that the results are more difficult to reproduce.

Choice of dose levels

Correct dose level is critical in these studies, especially for regulatory acceptance. Generally, it is required that the high dose be chosen as a maximum tolerated dose (MTD) that is responsible for toxicity that will not shorten an animal's survival other than by carcinogenicity. It is important that exposure should be for the lifetime of the animals; reduced survival due to toxicity reduces time of exposure and so lessens the opportunity for tumour formation. However, it should also be recognised that increased survival could be associated with higher tumour burdens due to the natural incidences being higher in old age; tumour profile may also be affected. A 10 per cent reduction in bodyweight gain is considered to be acceptable evidence of toxicity but care should be taken to ensure that this reduction is not simply due to indirect factors such as poor palatability of diet offered. The lowest dose level is chosen as a suitable multiple of expected human exposure, based on anticipated pharmacokinetics or expected daily intakes either as food additives or as residual pesticides on foods.

The use of the MTD has been widely criticised, especially on the basis that the doses thus selected are often unrealistically high. Pharmacokinetics and metabolism at high dose are frequently unrepresentative of those at lower doses; in addition a general relationship between toxicity and carcinogenicity cannot be drawn for all classes of chemicals. A further consideration is that most human carcinogens, which are mostly genotoxic, are carcinogenic at less than the MTD. Other criteria for dose choice have been suggested, such as pharmacokinetics and systemic exposure (AUC) or metabolism.

Parameters measured

Measurement of food consumption and bodyweight gain should always be carried out and are, obviously, critical in dietary studies for calculation of achieved dose levels (chapter 3). In studies with administration of constant concentrations – typical in agrochemical studies – the achieved dose will fall as the study progresses due to the animals' growth and the fact that food consumption will tend to remain similar throughout the study. In the estimation of dose levels in these studies it is important to reduce scatter of food as far as possible or to be able to make a reasonably accurate estimate of this, as this has a significant impact on the accuracy of the dose calculations. Young animals tend to play more than old animals (and scatter more food) and unpalatable diet will be scattered more as the animals dig into it looking for something better; this is usually more of a problem in the early weeks of a study.

Clinical observations, especially for palpable swellings, which give an indication of the time of onset of tumours and their location, are routine. From these data and those collected at necropsy the tumour burden for each animal can be assessed, as it is possible for treatment to produce a greater number of tumours in individual treated animals than in the controls. Skin tumours would be a good example of this type of effect as they are easily seen clinically or at necropsy and each would be sampled and examined. In some cases, the onset of a tumour type may be accelerated by treatment although the overall incidence of tumours may remain very similar to that in the control group. This is particularly important with tumours that are present in the test strain at high incidences, such as mammary tumours in Sprague–Dawley rats.

Histological processing of a wide range of tissues and their examination is the primary endpoint of a carcinogenicity study; this would normally include examination at least of a blood smear and, more usually, haematological processing of a blood sample. It is important to ensure that the pathologist has experience of reading these studies and is using terminology that is consistent with that used by other pathologists. In contrast to other types of toxicological data, which may be graded for severity, a tumour is either present or absent and there can be heated debate between pathologists over the diagnosis of a tumour or group of tumours. At such times reliable, independent peer review of the sections is vital, although this does not always solve the problem. Unlike numerical data which are wholly objective and can be examined according to whether they were obtained with correct technique, pathologist opinion may be partly subjective and is very much dependent on factors such as skill of histological sectioning and processing and on the experience of the pathologist. Also, unlike a set of numbers, which can be accepted or transformed for analysis, the same set of slides may be examined by several pathologists, each of whom can express subtly different opinions on them. The problem with this is that while there may be one favourable opinion pointing to an absence of effect, there may be two others – one non-committal and one indicating carcinogenic effect. It is not possible to ignore the unfavourable opinions and all must be reported.

Because animals die at different times during the study – typically, mortality will increase in the last 26 weeks of treatment – the time of exposure of the individual animals to the test substance may differ significantly. Also the animals may die early as a result of toxicity or causes unrelated to treatment, reducing the time of exposure to the test substance and therefore potentially reducing the final incidences of tumours that might have formed later. Reduced survival, for instance due to nephrotoxicity, may be associated with a similar or lower incidence of a tumour type than in the controls, which may give a false negative in respect of carcinogenicity. For this reason the data resulting from the microscopic examination are processed to give an age-related adjustment to tumour incidences.

Other systems for carcinogenicity assessment

The process of carcinogenicity assessment is progressive and not solely reliant on the results of the bioassay studies. It has been pointed out above that the causes of cancer are multi-factorial and that the results of a rodent bioassay may not be relevant to humans if they indicate a non-genotoxic mechanism. Equally, testing a confirmed genotoxic chemical in a two-year bioassay is an irrelevant waste of animals. In view of this, the assessment process to determine carcinogenic potential should itself look at as many different aspects as possible of the test material and its effects. This is reviewed in Box 6.1.

Box 6.1   Additional means of assessing carcinogenic potential

The following are used in addition to the data from classic lifespan bioassays:

- *Molecular structure*   This can be computer driven (see chapter 10) and is known as QSAR (Quantitative Structure Activity Relationship) or, without the quantitative aspect, simply as SAR. It is well established that certain molecular groups or structures are associated with carcinogenicity and their presence acts as an early indication of carcinogenic potential.
- *Genotoxicity studies*, as discussed above, also indicate if the substance is likely to interact with DNA and so be associated with increased cancer incidence.
- Data from *routine toxicity studies* should be reviewed. At the simplest level, the presence in the liver of foci of altered uptake of either haematoxylin or eosin, the stains routinely used in histological processing and examination, can indicate the presence of altered cells which may be the precursors to tumour development. These foci can be investigated by the use of techniques to visualise the presence of various enzymes such as gamma-glutamyl transferase or the placental form of glutathione transferase, both of which may also be indicative of tumourigenic foci.

- Examination of *hormonal levels* in the plasma may also indicate changes that may lead to increased tumour incidences. This type of effect can also be assessed by microscopic examination of the various endocrine organs such as the pituitary, thyroid or adrenal glands.
- *Other investigations* of tissues and data from routine toxicity studies should be considered. The comet assay may give useful data when conducted at the end of studies to assess DNA damage in target tissues, such as the liver or gastrointestinal tract. Other tests which could be performed include proteomic investigations, to examine the levels of proteins that are expressed due to genetic changes, for instance in the *p53* gene, deficiency of which is seen in many human tumours. DNA adduct studies could also be used to indicate effects on the DNA that might suggest a degree of carcinogenic potential.

Beyond the extension of investigations in routine toxicity studies there are a multitude of proposals that are based on accelerated protocols to study tumour incidences. These are generally based on a faster time to tumour and may involve transgenic animals or surgical techniques such as partial hepatectomy. With the latter technique, the theory is that the fast reparative proliferation in the liver would provide an environment that favours the early emergence of tumours. The less expensive option of causing hepatic damage with carbon tetrachloride did not take off in any significant way. The use of transgenic animals is examined in Box 6.2 and Table 6.4.

Box 6.2 Transgenic animals in carcinogenicity assessment

The use of transgenic animals in carcinogenicity is popular in the USA but less so in Europe and their use has been examined in a major study co-ordinated by ILSI.[2] These models have been extensively reviewed by RW Tennant.[3–5] Treatment periods are about 26 weeks, using groups of 15 males and 15 females, having significant effects on the statistical power. The following is an assessment of the data presented by Cohen *et al.* using seven models and 21 compounds,[6] summarised in Table 6.4.

- Non-genotoxic non-carcinogens were all negative in these models.
- All known non-genotoxic rodent carcinogens, dismissed as not relevant to humans by mechanism or human data, were negative.
- Peroxisome proliferators did not give consistent results.
- Genotoxic carcinogens were positive or gave equivocal results. Phenacetin is a weak mutagen with a possible mechanism of carcinogenicity in humans associated with non-genotoxic effects, leading to cell proliferation, to which weak mutagenicity may contribute.

- Hormonal carcinogens gave mixed results.
- Peroxisome proliferators gave mixed results but were mostly negative.

The question should be asked if these studies are simply a shorter method of producing tumours that have as much relevance to humans as those produced in a full-length bioassay. Results are clearly dependent on model choice.

In conclusion, model choice is critical and there is no guarantee that selection of a model according to class of chemical will be viable as you could, theoretically, choose the model according to the result you want – and do you really want to show that your pet compound is carcinogenic?

Table 6.4 Comparative data from transgenic models

	rasH2	TgAC Dermal	TgAC Oral	p53 +/−	XPA −/−	XPA−/− p53+/−	Neonatal mouse
Genotoxic human carcinogens							
Cyclophosphamide	E	E	+	+	+	+	+
Mephalan	E	E	+	+	+	+	+
Phenacetin	+	N	N	N	N	N	N
Immunosuppressants							
Cyclosporin	E	+	E	+	+	+	N
Hormonal carcinogens							
DES	+	+	N	+	+	+	N
Estradiol	N	+	N	E	E	+	2N 1+
Rodent non-genotox carc – human non-carc (human data)							
Phenobarbital	N	N	N	N	N	N	N
Clofibrate (perox. prolif)	+	+					
Reserpine	N	N	N	N	N	N	N
Dieldrin	N	N	N	N	N	N	N
Methapyrilene	N	N	N	N	N	N	N
Rodent non-genotox carc – human non-carc (mechanism)							
Haloperidol	N	N	N	N	N	N	N
Chlorpromazine	N	N	N	N	N	N	N
Chloroform	N	N	N	E	N	N	N
Metaproterenol	N	N	N	N	N	N	N
WY-14643 (perox. prolif)			E		+		
DEHP (perox. prolif)	+			E			
Sulphamethoxazole	N	N	N	N	N	N	N
Non-genotoxic/non-carcinogens							
Ampicillin	N	N	N	N	N	N	N
d-Mannitol	N	N	N	N	N	N	N
Sulfisoxazole	N	N	N	N	N	N	N

Source: Compiled from Cohen, SM *et al.* 'Alternative models for carcinogenicity testing', *Toxicological Sciences* 2001; 64: 14–19.
Note: N=negative, E=equivocal, +=positive, perox. prolif.=peroxisome proliferators.

Carcinogenic assessment is one of the areas in toxicology with the greatest scope for change in the way it is carried out. As the mechanisms of cancer generation become clearer in both general and specific senses, more methods of examining for these mechanisms will become apparent. Although identification of relevant mechanisms that can be reliably investigated will continue to be slow, it may be expected that there will be gradual acceptance of new protocols and investigations. This aspect of carcinogenicity is discussed below.

Pitfalls in carcinogenicity studies

Inevitably with these studies there is considerable potential for pitfalls that have great significance for individual studies and the future of chemical safety evaluation. These can occur in any aspect of the study, starting with design and finishing with the conclusion.

The design of the classic bioassay is much dictated by tradition and regulatory preference and, with careful consultation, it should be relatively easy to avoid mistakes in this area. The possible exception to this is housing. Authorities in the USA have tended to prefer single housing for rats and mice, whereas Europeans tend to house them in groups of up to five of the same sex. Rats are social animals and are less stressed when housed in this way. However, male mice tend to fight and the injuries can reduce survival and compromise the validity of the study, especially if the test substance increases aggression. For this reason male mice are housed singly. The design of cages and the use, or not, of bedding, also provide some dilemmas. In studies where the test substance is mixed with the food, the amount of food discarded is a useful indication of palatability and is a critical factor in maximising the accuracy of calculation of achieved dose levels. It is difficult to produce a sensible estimate of food scatter where the animals are housed in solid bottom cages with sawdust bedding. Such estimates are much more secure when the cages have mesh floors suspended over absorbent paper (although these cages are not generally used for mice). It is now considered that sawdust bedding is better as it is not associated with granulomatous lesions on the feet, which can lead to early sacrifice of the animals.

Dose level choice is critical in these studies and correct design of the dose range-finding studies is vital, as is the careful interpretation of their results. Poor palatability of food in dietary studies can lead to lower bodyweight gain in comparison with the controls; but it is doubtful that a 10 per cent decrease in bodyweight due to this would be accepted as evidence of toxicity. This could mean that the MTD had not been reached and that, accordingly, the study objective was not achieved. Although the MTD is accepted as a method of dose level choice, it is better to have other support for this, for instance pharmacokinetics. Equally it should be reiterated that poor survival, due to excess toxicity or to characteristics of the chosen test strain, may also produce an invalid study.

Once the study has been designed and any controversy produced has been overcome, the most contentious issue is the way in which the data are evaluated and interpreted. Faulty collection of the data will confound accurate interpretation. This includes incorrect estimation of food consumption and poor recording of clinical observations, particularly those relating to palpable masses, which affects the estimation of time of onset of tumour formation. This can be important where the tumour concerned is seen at high incidences and earlier onset may indicate treatment-related tumorigenesis. Inevitably, this leads us to the conduct of the necropsies and accuracy of recording of existing masses or tumours and their relationship to the clinical record. Once all the tissues have been sectioned and slides prepared, their evaluation is possibly the cause of more controversy and debate than any other part of the study. While toxicological pathology is clearly a science, it is a science with a high 'art' content. Terminology can differ between pathologists and interpretation of the sections can differ widely. For age-related analysis of the data it is important that correct decisions are made as to whether a tumour was fatal, probably fatal, probably incidental or incidental. Skewing these decisions can produce different interpretations of the data. One way round this is to ensure that the peer review of the sections is without reproach. In the event of disagreement, particularly in studies that are contracted out, a second or third pathologist opinion may not help the overall conclusion, as the original report will always stand as a valid alternative opinion.

One histopathological trap, especially where there are treatment-related increases in necropsy findings, is the tendency to examine more sections from treated animals than from the controls. The tissue typically affected in this respect is the liver, for which it is normal to examine two sections from different lobes in every animal. If necropsy shows a lesion in another lobe from those sampled routinely, that lesion is sampled in addition to the scheduled sections; discovery of a tumour in the additional section will increase the tumour incidence in that particular animal and in the treatment group as a whole. In strains where there is a high incidence of liver tumours this has the effect of biasing the incidences upwards and can suggest a treatment-related increase in tumour incidence, where there is none.

In addition to these factors, there are others which have less impact but which can still be significant. The presence of high incidences of common tumours in control animals will tend to blunt the analysis of the data. Accordingly, the presence of good background data, or at least two control groups, is crucial in evaluation of the results. Complications are also introduced when the mechanism of toxicity is not present in humans, as is usually the case with non-genotoxic carcinogenesis.

In shorter studies in rodents or in studies *in vitro*, the same basic precautions in study design, dose level choice and evaluation have to be observed, with the added complication that the technical conduct of the study has to be consistent with practice in other laboratories. This is particularly the case with the more complex *in vitro* assays such as the comet assay. However, perhaps the biggest pitfall in this type of study is in the understanding of the changes seen and their interpretation. If the origins of the data and the mechanisms of their generation are not understood, it is not possible to draw a supportable conclusion.

Overview of the future of carcinogenicity assessment

If it is accepted that the results of the classic rodent bioassay are of dubious relevance to humans it becomes necessary to examine other methods of assessment of carcinogenic potential. Overall it is relatively simple to detect genotoxic chemicals using established methods without use of a full-length rodent bioassay. Equally, it has been shown that detection of non-genotoxic carcinogenesis in rodents is relatively easy. The challenge is to detect non-genotoxic carcinogenesis that is relevant to humans. Having said that, it is increasingly apparent that there are elements of promotion in cancer that are due to non-genotoxic chemicals or mechanisms, even with chemicals that are strongly genotoxic. It is also apparent that there is no simple battery of tests currently in existence that will reliably predict human carcinogenicity. It is usual to consider the results of a range of tests in order to assess carcinogenic potential, however it is clear that there is considerable scope to develop new tests that examine mechanisms of carcinogenesis that are not currently covered.

One of the first techniques that can be applied to assess carcinogenic potential is the use of an expert system to examine structure–activity relationships in the molecule. There are several such systems available and they are discussed in greater detail in chapter 10; however, it should be noted that they are principally of use in detection of structural groups associated with genotoxic carcinogenesis. This is due to the inherent reactivity of these agents or their metabolites and the presence of DNA as a common target. In the case of non-genotoxic carcinogens, attribution of effect to structural aspects of molecules is much more complex, due to the very wide range of mechanisms through which such carcinogenicity can be expressed. Where a particular structural group is associated with a particular non-genotoxic effect – for instance peroxisome proliferation – there is a possibility that this may be entered into computer databases for detection in future structures. However, the extent of the problem is underlined by the extent of the structural diversity of compounds that are associated with peroxisome proliferation.

Table 6.5 sets out a number of factors or effects that are important in non-genotoxic carcinogenesis and looks at how these effects may be detected. Additional mechanisms that can be investigated include changes in receptor interactions which may be assessed through changes in the activity of tyrosine kinases. A proportion of these events can be covered in routine toxicity studies, either within the current set of examinations or by extending those examinations to take in new endpoints. Examples include immune suppression, as seen with cyclosporine, hormonal imbalance or using the comet assay to assess DNA

Table 6.5 Processes or mechanisms in carcinogenicity and markers of effect

Mechanism or endpoint	Marker	Where or how assessed
Immune suppression	Leucocyte differential counts, plasma immunoglobins, histology of lymphoid organs, T-cell activity. Loss of host resistance	In routine toxicity studies and in specific indicated studies
Chronic cell damage. Increased oxidative damage	Histopathological change. Lipid peroxidation, decreased glutathione concentrations, etc. Lipid breakdown products.	Metabolite studies, *in vitro* studies, antioxidant concentrations. Routine toxicity studies. Proteomics or genomics
Changes in intercellular communication	Test for gap junction patency	*In vitro* cellular systems. Staining for connexin shows gap junctions
Inhibition of tubulin polymerisation	Function of spindle formation in mitosis or meiosis – aneugenesis	Tests under development
Cell proliferation	Hyperplastic foci Proliferating cell nuclear antigen (PCNA)	In routine toxicity studies and in proliferation responsive cell lines
Hormonal	Hormone levels, e.g. thyroid hormones or oestrogens	In routine toxicity studies
Chronic inflammation	Histological examination, sometimes backed up by clinical observations	In routine toxicity studies
Faulty DNA repair	Altered function	*In vitro* in specific bacterial assays
Alterations in apoptosis, especially inhibition	Histological examination. Overexpression of *p53* gene	In routine toxicity studies *in vitro* tests and genomics. TUNEL assay
Promotion	Alterations in gene expression and precancerous lesions or foci	In routine toxicity studies or in specific promotion studies. Genomics
DNA damage *in vivo*	DNA adducts, DNA synthesis	Urine. Comet assay. Unscheduled DNA synthesis
Changes in gene expression	Protein levels	Proteomics *in vivo* or *in vitro*

damage in target tissues. Extension of routine histological processing and examination to include immunocytochemistry for specific markers of precancerous change is a relatively simple and cost-effective method of increasing the database for assessment of carcinogenic potential.

Although there are clearly simple extensions to routine testing, there are areas of non-genotoxic effect that will also become routine as the tests are developed, such as the function of intercellular gap junctions, which are essential for communication between cells. This communication has various roles in areas as diverse as cardiac function and embryonic development; in carcinogenesis the gap junctions are responsible for the exchange of small molecules that inhibit cell division – so-called contact inhibition. Where this communication is disrupted, uncontrolled proliferation can result. High-dose administration of carbon tetrachloride has been associated with reductions in connexin and gap junction communication. The formation of a functional spindle apparatus is critical to successful mitosis or meiosis and this is disrupted by compounds that inhibit polymerisation of tubulin. Inhibition is reflected in aneugenesis – abnormality of chromosome number or structure – and this may be detected in cytogenetic assays, although more specific tests are under development. Other examinations oriented towards the detection of proliferation include proliferating cell nuclear antigen (PCNA) and changes in apoptosis. Inhibition of apoptosis is an important mechanism for non-genotoxic carcinogenesis, the process of which is becoming better understood. Apoptosis can be induced in cell lines by changes in the culture media, for instance removal of fetal calf serum, and may be assessed through induction of enzyme markers, which are known factors in the process of programmed cell death.

Numerous other *in vitro* systems have been investigated for detection of non-genotoxic carcinogens, such as the Syrian hamster embryo (SHE) cell transformation assay. The usual potential limitations of differences in metabolism and elimination *in vitro* exist in these assays. However, there is considerable scope for incorporation of oncogenes or inactive tumour suppressor genes and these tests will develop further. An examination of changes in the thyroid, kidney and liver of rodents following exposure to non-genotoxic carcinogens[7] concluded that there was no specific single alert for carcinogenesis in these organs but that careful choice of a range of markers could prove to be predictive, when time of evaluation and class of chemical was taken into account. The relevance of new assays to human carcinogenesis must be established for them to have their own credibility, rather than relying on the possibly flawed data from rodent carcinogens.

There does not appear to be any sensible way at the moment of monitoring the early stages of progression, other than by the appearance of tumours. It is possible that protein analyses, particularly in urine using nuclear magnetic resonance spectra, may be of use here.

Proteomics and genomics, discussed under *in vitro* toxicology above, will become more powerful as their science develops. This can be used to assess the concentrations or levels of different protein products of genes, particularly oncogenes and proto-oncogenes or of the genes themselves. The study of protein expression and the association of particular proteins with carcinogenesis would be a useful investigation to be added to standard toxicity studies. This sort of investigation may also have some relevance to examination of human samples in clinical trials of pharmaceuticals or in surveillance of patients after marketing has been authorised.

There are also factors in carcinogenicity that are not readily tested in toxicity studies as they are of relevance to the individual rather than to the population as a whole. These include the roles in carcinogenesis of viruses, diet and caloric intake and genetic susceptibilities such as those predisposing individuals to breast cancer or to the skin cancer xeroderma pigmentosum, due to faulty DNA repair following UV irradiation. Ultimately genomics will become crucial in assessing an individual's chance of developing cancer, particularly where there is a family history of a particular type of cancer.

In the future it is probable that there will be an overall assessment of the results of a battery of tests which should be chosen according to the class of chemical being investigated. This assessment will begin with a computer-based assessment of the structure of the chemical and its possible or probable metabolites, which will also be predicted. Although pharmacokinetic prediction is not particularly reliable at the moment, when based solely on structure and calculated partition coefficient, the role of physiological-based pharmacokinetic models will grow. From these initial assessments, the design of the toxicity studies may be adjusted to test the early predictions and, as the database develops, the study designs can be further refined. Specific *in vitro* tests will then be conducted to examine for common carcinogenic mechanisms or for those considered relevant to the test chemical. It is also probable that this battery will not include two-year bioassays in rodents except in special circumstances. The mechanisms of toxicity, which can be investigated in a focused manner *in vitro*, will become more important a priori rather than being examined after the toxicities have been expressed. The overall effect of this would be expected to reduce the numbers of animals used in box-checking studies and to increase the relevance and focus of information in the database, allowing an assessment of carcinogenic potential in the target species, usually humans. An attractive side effect of this increased focus is likely to be a reduction in the development times of chemicals by at least two years.

Chapter 7

Determination

Irritation and sensitisation

General principles

The skin is the largest organ in body, up to 2 m^2 and forms one of the three most significant routes of exposure, with oral and respiratory, especially in a domestic or occupational setting. The agents involved come from numerous sources but can be industrial chemicals, pharmaceuticals or agrochemicals and their intermediates, or chemicals encountered in routine domestic existence, amongst which cosmetics are a significant inclusion. The most typical dermal reaction is inflammation, characterised by redness, swelling and heat, in response to irritants, sensitising agents or phototoxic substances; corrosive agents can produce disfiguring burns and excessive UV irradiation is associated with skin cancer.

In testing programmes, dermal irritation and sensitisation are often considered together as they are not usually central to a development plan, but are clearly of interest in an occupational or domestic context. Statements on irritation and sensitisation are essential in Material Safety Data Sheets that accompany chemicals sold to industry. There is some lack of consistency in nomenclature for the allergic form of skin irritation, contact hypersensitivity or allergic contact dermatitis being used according to source.

There is a clear distinction between dermatitis due to irritation and allergic contact dermatitis. The former is associated with a dose- or concentration-dependent reaction that is due to direct interaction of the chemical or mixture with local skin constituents; the response is usually immediate, localised and requires similar concentrations in subsequent exposures to elicit a similar effect. This form of dermatitis is distinct from the burns that are due to corrosive chemicals such as strong acids or bases. In contrast, with allergic contact dermatitis there is a period during which relatively large amounts of the chemical may be tolerated without any obvious effects; this reaction-free period can last for years. After this initial period, sensitivity develops (in susceptible individuals), which may produce severe reactions triggered by minute amounts of the substance. There is usually a clear difference in effective concentrations between a pure irritant and one that has induced contact sensitivity.

Whereas a relatively simple set of chemical reactions determines irritation, allergic contact dermatitis is driven by a complex set of processes. These start, typically, with the passage of a hapten (a complex of a small exogenous molecule with an endogenous protein) into a Langerhans cell in the epidermis where it is processed and passed to a regional lymph node for presentation to T lymphocytes. Interleukin 1 (IL-1), produced by the Langerhans cell stimulates the T cell to produce cytokines, which cause sensitised T cells to proliferate and act in the production of the clinical signs of sensitisation at the site of exposure.

Contact dermatitis is a major cause of occupational ill-health and is an area of concern to toxicologists assessing exposure limits for the workplace; allergic contact dermatitis is less common but is, perhaps, of greater significance because of the very low exposures that are needed for a significant response. Phototoxicity is also a potential problem; for instance the presence in celery of psoralens has been associated in celery pickers with extensive skin reactions brought about by sunlight-induced reaction of the psoralens with DNA, inhibiting DNA repair. Certain cosmetic ingredients have also been associated with phototoxicity and with more mundane forms of dermatitis.

Factors in dermal toxicity

Toxicity in the skin is affected by factors such as local humidity/moisture, temperature, local injury, exposure to light, local concentration and location and area exposed. Increased temperature and moisture, as found when the treatment site is occluded by a bandage, act to increase the local reaction. Location on the body is significant because the skin differs in thickness from one area to another and this affects the reactions seen, the head and neck being more sensitive than the palms of the hands or soles of the feet. The local concentration and the area of exposure are more important in determining the extent of local reaction than the dose expressed in terms of miligrams per kilogram; concentration also determines extent of sensitisation but not of subsequent allergic reactions. Although it is possible to produce dermal toxicity as a result of systemic exposure through the blood system, this is relatively unusual. The skin also has significant metabolising capability that can result in the production of sensitising or photo-reactive molecules.

Physicochemical factors that affect dermal toxicity include lipophilicity (indicated by the partition coefficient), molecular weight, pK_a, the pH of any solution and the ease with which it reacts with local proteins to form haptens that could result in allergic sensitisation. Small lipophilic molecules are more likely to be absorbed than large lipophobes and reactive molecules are more likely to be associated with hapten formation than unreactive ones.

Ocular irritation studies have been a regular source of controversy over many years and are now moving slowly towards the use of *in vitro* systems. However, the simplicity of the alternatives counts against them in comparison with the structure and complex processes of the human eye and, as a result, no single test has proven to be an acceptable alternative. The potential for ocular toxicity should be assessed from physicochemical data relating to the chemical and from the results of *in vitro* screens before animals are used to confirm lack of irritation. It is now generally accepted that if a chemical is shown to be a dermal irritant then exposure of the eye is unnecessary.

Test systems

Test systems for irritation and sensitisation can be divided between the traditional – rabbit, and guinea pig – and the new – *in vitro* systems for irritance and corrosivity studies and mice for assessment of allergic sensitisation. The rabbit has been used for many years in the assessment of dermal and ocular irritation, although it is generally considered to be a more sensitive model in comparison with human skin. It is now being replaced gradually by *in vitro* systems; negative results in such a test can then be confirmed with a small *in vivo* study. As with the eye, the processes of dermal irritation in humans are complex and are therefore difficult to reproduce *in vitro*. There are a number of skin equivalents using dermal keratinocytes, which can be used to assess some aspects of ocular damage. The assessment of corrosivity is theoretically easier *in vitro* in view of the simpler nature of the damage caused (i.e. direct reaction with skin components) and a number of *in vitro* systems have been developed to assess this endpoint. One such test measures the reduction in electrical resistance across a sample of skin in response to exposure to corrosive substances. The leakage of enzymes such as lactate dehydrogenase into the incubation medium can also be used as a marker of toxic effect.

The guinea pig has been the traditional choice for conduct of dermal sensitisation studies but, with increasing acceptance of the local lymph node assay, is set for replacement by mice. There is currently no generally accepted *in vitro* method of assessing hypersensitivity reactions; as with carcinogenicity it seems probable that no single *in vitro* test will give a reliable assessment of sensitisation and the complex processes involved.

For ocular irritation studies the rabbit is still the *in vivo* model of choice, although systems such as the chick chorioallantoic membrane (CAM) test or systems using enucleated bovine or chicken eyes can be used to identify severe irritants. The best approach appears to be the use of *in vitro* systems in a tier of tests that culminates, for chemicals believed to be non-irritant, in the use of a limited number of rabbits.

For cosmetics or their ingredients, the development of *in vitro* methods is a priority because, in Europe, testing these substances is no longer allowed, making the evaluation of new ingredients by traditional methods impossible.

Study design and parameters measured

Allergic sensitisation in guinea pigs

There are a large number of protocols using guinea pigs, based essentially on two designs, the maximisation test of Magnusson and Kligmann and the Buehler test. Both involve dermal treatment of guinea pigs at relatively high, irritant doses to achieve sensitisation, followed after 14–28 days by a challenge at a different site using a non-irritant dose to assess any allergic reaction. The basic Buehler test uses dermal application to one flank on two occasions in the sensitisation phase followed by a dermal challenge on the other flank up to four weeks later. The application site may be occluded by wrapping the animal in a dressing that keeps the site warm and moist. The maximisation test uses a more rigorous protocol during the sensitisation phase in which the immune response is enhanced by intradermal injection of the test substance with and without Freund's adjuvant. In addition, irritants such as sodium lauryl sulphate may be used before the challenge dose in order to induce mild inflammation. In both tests, response to treatment is assessed by scoring for erythema and oedema 24 and 48 hours following the challenge dose.

Allergic sensitisation in mice

The mouse ear swelling test (MEST) gives a more quantitative measure than the subjective scoring of the guinea pig tests. Topical application to the abdomen, after preparation by intradermal injection of adjuvant and tape stripping for four days, is followed after 10 days by a challenge dose to one ear, using the other ear as a vehicle control. The thickness of the ears is measured at 24 and 48 hours after challenge, a 20 per cent increase over the control ear being taken as a positive result.

In the local lymph node assay (LLNA) sensitisation is assessed by incorporation of tritiated thymidine into proliferating lymphocytes in the lymph nodes draining the site of topical application. Topical application to the ears over three consecutive days is followed five days later by intravenous injection of tritiated thymidine; 5 hours later the animals are killed and the draining lymph nodes are removed for preparation of single cell suspension for counting. This test, which has been accepted by the United States FDA, uses fewer animals than the guinea pig tests and uses a quantitative endpoint.

Dermal and ocular irritation

In animals, dermal tests are based on application of the test material to the shaved backs of rabbits for up to 24 hours under an occlusive dressing, to prevent ingestion and to maximise the response. Following removal of the dressing, the response is graded at intervals up to 72 hours or until no further response is seen. Erythema, oedema, skin thickening, exfoliation, cracking or fissuring, necrosis and ulceration are assessed and scored relative to control values. Non-irritant substances may then be assessed in an eye irritation test, in which 100 mg or 100 μl of the test substance are instilled into the conjunctival sac of one eye of one or more rabbits, the other eye being used as a control. Reaction to treatment is observed and scored at appropriate intervals; if intense irritation is seen the eyes are immediately irrigated to remove the chemical.

The CAM test has been used as a screen to identify severe irritants before the use of animals. In this test the response of the blood vessels in the chorio-allantoic membrane of fertilised chicken eggs is assessed after a brief application of the test chemical. Vasodilation and haemorrhage are scored, in comparison with controls and known irritants, at intervals after washing off the chemical. Scoring is based on the intensity of reaction over time following treatment; this period may be as short as 5 minutes.

Pitfalls in irritation and sensitisation

Observation of the reaction to treatment in the guinea pig sensitisation and rabbit dermal irritation tests is not fully quantitative and requires a degree of subjective judgement and, by implication, skill and experience in scoring the results. With the gradual adoption of quantitative methods such as the LLNA, this problem is being overcome. With the dermal and ocular irritation tests in rabbits the visible clinical signs are readily scored but clinically relevant signs such as itching, pain and other invisible effects cannot be assessed other than by inference from the behaviour of the animal.

Although no single *in vitro* test is likely to replace animal studies, their use will inevitably increase, particularly by the use of batteries of tests to assess the individual processes that make up each overall human endpoint. It should be noted that if the data from a test are poorly understood, supplementing them with more uninterpretable data will not enhance the overall assessment. A plethora of mechanistic work from poorly chosen tests will merely confuse.

Chapter 8

Determination

Environmental toxicology
and epidemiology

Environmental toxicology and ecotoxicology

General principles

The environment may be loosely defined as the surroundings and conditions in which we live; environmental toxicology is the study of toxic chemicals within that environment and the effects that they have on humans and populations. Ecotoxicology is specifically the study of environmental toxins on the flora and fauna that make up an ecosystem. The former has an implied human slant, while the latter is oriented more towards the effects of chemicals on the natural ecosystem studied as a whole.

There are similarities between the pharmacokinetic behaviour of compounds in ecosystems and their behaviour in individual organisms; both are governed by the interaction of the physicochemical characteristics of the chemical with the subject. The overall response is affected by the extent and duration of exposure and by the way the chemical is handled in the subject – in this case the ecosystem. In ecotoxicology the main subjects for studying effects are populations (individual species), biocoenoses (communities of associated species) and whole ecosystems comprising a larger number of species, habitats and functional features. In contrast to toxicology, where variability is limited to differences within one species or controlled differences in experimental technique, ecotoxicology deals with much greater diversity due to the presence of many species interacting in an essentially uncontrolled manner. These interactions eventually achieve equilibrium in a delicate balance, which is a function of interdependencies between the different components of the ecosystem. Effects on one species or group of species (e.g. insects) can have significant effects on a whole ecosystem. Changes in the ecosystem lead to adjustment and re-equilibration which may have far reaching effects out of proportion to the size of the original change. In the Gaian concept of James Lovelock, the earth is seen as a single organism which regulates (and heals) itself. There may be truth in this, but on current performance we are outdistancing the reparative processes and are in danger of compromising our own existence; at which point the healing process may begin.

Pollution, routes of entry and environmental ADME

There is much heated debate about pollution and what constitutes pollution or a pollutant. A potentially useful definition of a pollutant is that of a chemical that has exceeded normal background levels and that has the potential to cause harm – always remembering that the potential for harm increases with concentration. Definitions of pollution refer to noxious chemicals discharged into the environment and it has been suggested by some that pollution started when primitive humans lit the first fires. It is probably better to consider pollution as an excessive discharge into the environment that persists or accumulates to the extent that it causes harm. This may be considered on a local or national level as appropriate. Pollution as a result of fires, particularly coal fires, was noted before AD 1500 in London and efforts were made to restrict the use of coal at intervals subsequently, culminating in the clean air acts in the UK in the second half of the twentieth century. For all the furore at the time and subsequently, it is unlikely that these localised and transient episodes of coal fire-induced smog have had any long-term adverse effects on the environment as a whole. Discharge into the environment as a result of industrial activities is easier to define as harmful in the long term. This would include unintentional discharge from mining reservoirs of water with high levels of heavy metals or other pollutants. These elements are present naturally in the environment but at lower, generally non-toxic concentrations; sudden high levels carry significant risk for water supplies, fisheries and ecosystem well-being. In environmental or ecotoxicology there are two major aspects for investigation: the environmental fate of a substance, i.e. what happens to a substance once it is introduced into the environment, and the ecological effects on the environment or ecosystem that follow its discharge.

In common with general toxicology, there are several routes by which a chemical enters an ecosystem and there are different compartments analogous to the organs in the body of an animal, into which the chemical may be distributed. Following entry to the environment, the fate of a chemical can be described by the processes of ADME (absorption, distribution, metabolism and elimination) in a broad analogy to similar processes in individual animals. As in animal pharmacokinetics, the chemical may be sequestered into individual compartments; in animals this might be the bone or adipose tissue, in the environment it might be a clay soil. In either case, sudden acceleration of release can result in harmful concentrations.

The major compartments of the environment may be summarised as water, air, soils and flora and fauna (wild and domestic). Chemicals enter these via many diverse routes, including (intentionally) by agrochemical spraying or illegal discharge, or (unintentionally) as air pollution from industrial fires, smoke stacks or vehicles or as run off into waterways from industrial sites or intensive farms. Many routes are not considered at the evaluation stage and can have had unexpected effects. For example ivermectin, an antiparasitic chemical given to cattle, is excreted in the faeces and increases cowpat life by killing the insects responsible for their degradation.[1,2]

The system into which a chemical is discharged – air, soil or water – is important in determining the significance of the discharge and the extent to which it can be distributed through the ecosystem. In terms of distance of transport, the greatest distances are found with air, while water has the greatest capacity for movement in terms of volumes. Discharge into soil will ensure the lowest distance and the lowest volume of transport. While both soil and water have great potential as sinks for pollution, water pollution has the greatest potential to threaten populations due to the ease with which substances are transported.

As indicated above, clay soils have a high capacity for adsorption of some chemicals, which become tightly bound; as a result, their adverse actions are attenuated. Of course, in time they will be slowly released from the clays into the rest of the ecosystem, giving a prolonged low-level exposure, of organisms or a prolonged opportunity for degradation. Peat soils, on the other hand, do not have such adsorptive capacity, a contrast that was noted after the Chernobyl accident.[3] The differences in binding of caesium-137 between the clay soils in the lowlands and the acid peat soils in the hills affected the amounts that were available and this was reflected in the radioactive content of crops and livestock. In contrast to organic chemicals, metals – particularly heavy metals – are not degraded and detoxification is dependent on their removal, irreversible binding or dilution. Complex molecules may be broken down and eliminated from the ecosystem at greater or lesser rates according to chemical class. Simple carbon compounds are easily biodegradable but halogenation may well prolong this process into years, as seen with molecules such as the dioxins and organo-chlorines such as DDT.

One important factor to consider in ecotoxicology is the ability of some chemicals to concentrate as they progress up the food chain until concentrations at the higher levels become toxic. This is the effect seen with the organochlorine DDT, long banned from the 'developed world' but use of which is still widespread elsewhere. The long half-life of DDT and its metabolite DDE, due to high lipid solubility and slow metabolism, result in increasing concentrations up the food chain until there is a clear effect, most easily seen in carnivorous birds. In the peregrine falcon, eggshell thickness was diminished with increasing DDT exposure to the extent that breakages in the nest increased and the population declined.

Factors in testing for environmental effect

With the realisation that environmental release of chemicals can have far reaching effects, whether of unusually large amounts of endogenous (natural) substances or synthetic chemicals, has come the acceptance of the need for testing for potential adverse effects on the environment. The emphasis on such testing is inevitably on compounds intended for agricultural use as pesticides but there have been initiatives to test pharmaceuticals for their environmental impact and there is a continuing debate about the environmental effects of oestrogenic compounds.

The problem of testing for ecotoxicity is that the scope for subtle change is much greater than in a single organism or test species and it is impossible to test every aspect of an ecosystem except in very large and complex experiments ('mesocosms' or field trials). The objective of ecotoxicity testing is to predict the behaviour of a chemical in the ecosystem and to assess the potential for adverse effects in the situations under which it will be released. The major difficulty with this objective is the enormous diversity of the environment and the selection of representative test systems. Inherently, one species of fish cannot be considered to be completely representative of all other fish. Equally, an aquatic herbivorous invertebrate cannot be representative of an aquatic herbivorous mammal, although both are at the same trophic level in ecological terms. Because bees are not harmed by an agrochemical, it should not be assumed that it will be non-toxic to other, less obviously beneficial insects. In any case, what is a 'beneficial insect'? Imbalance of any sort should be discouraged.

It seems probable that in the longer term the ecotoxicological impact of genetically modified crops could be much more significant than their immediate adverse effects on consumers. At this point the extent of or scope for interaction of chemicals and the natural world, of which we are a part, becomes of concern. The precise definition of ecotoxicity therefore becomes important. Clearly, if there are widespread effects on beneficial (or desirable) insect populations due to insecticidal gene expression in crops, this is a toxic manifestation of the crop and can be classified as ecotoxicity. Loss of a species is a clear-cut event, with imponderable impact; if an effect is limited to a shift in populations of plants or animals due to cross-breeding it may be more difficult to describe it as toxicity, although such an event may indeed be entirely adverse environmentally.

In assessing the potential for environmental effects there are two roughly definable areas of investigation; those that are dependent on the physico-chemical properties of the material that determine environmental fate and those that examine the potential for ecological effects. The first has to consider:

- physicochemical characteristics – partition coefficient (water and oil solubility), adsorption and desorption characteristics, volatility;
- fate and behaviour – relative persistence, liability to abiotic degradation, final fate, rate and route of elimination.

The potential for ecological effect is investigated via:

- effects on bacteria and other degrading organisms including assessment of biological oxygen demand;
- effects on higher organisms, such as bees, earthworms, fish and birds, with extrapolation from laboratory species to environmentally relevant organisms.

Although such assessments are made before the release of novel chemicals, there is the continuing need for monitoring after sales of the chemical have started. Such studies are the ecological equivalent of epidemiology and have similar weaknesses and uncertainties, unless the effects are unusual and clearly attributable to exposure to the suspect chemical. Thus, the thinning of eggshells in birds of prey was attributed to organochlorine pesticides through a series of field and mechanistic studies that together produced a body of evidence that was incontrovertible. The presence in the environment of synthetic oestrogens is much more difficult to link to decreased sperm counts in men due to the inherent variability of the data and the different interpretations that are possible.

Test systems and study types for ecotoxicology

Test systems for assessment of ecotoxicology have been chosen on pragmatic grounds in helpless acknowledgement that assessment in every relevant species would be impossible. The following descriptions of test species and study types has been put together with reference to the Organization for Economic Cooperation and Development (OECD) guidelines (www.oecd.org) and to *Principles of Ecotoxicology* by CH Walker *et al.* (see Bibliography). The intention is to give a flavour of the test species and studies conducted, rather than to attempt a definitive description. Furthermore, the various tests on algal growth and bacterial degradation are not considered here.

In many single species studies the objective is to determine the LC_{50} and a no effect concentration (NOEC). The LC_{50} – the median lethal concentration – is equivalent to the LD_{50}, seeking to determine the concentration at which 50 per cent of the test system is killed. The concentration concerned may be that in water or in a diet and the values for these measures, particularly with tests conducted in water, are greatly influenced by the conditions under which the experiments are conducted. There seems to be a lack of standardisation of some aspects of these tests – for instance algae used as feed or in the characterisation of important test components such as artificial soils. These may lead to deficiencies in trace elements or to other test parameters that have an unsuspected influence on the test data. It is probable that this situation will improve over time with development of knowledge in these areas but, in the mean time, it is as well to be aware of the possibility of these problems and the difficulty caused in data interpretation, particularly when comparing data between laboratories. The majority of tests are single-species experiments, conducted in isolation; there is a brief discussion on mesocosm studies at the end of this section. Study designs are given in the appropriate guidelines.

Invertebrates

Daphnia magna are tested to assess effects on mobility and reproduction. In the immobilisation test the percentage of *Daphnia* that are not swimming after 24 or

48 hours is assessed for each concentration of test chemical. For the reproductive test, young *Daphnia*, less than 24 hours old, are used and the total
number of offspring produced by each animal that survives the test is assessed
against the controls. The clone of *Daphnia* that is used is important as there are
differences in sensitivity, which make comparison between experiments difficult.
The algae used to feed the *Daphnia* can have an important effect on the test
results and, in the absence of standardisation, it may be difficult to compare
results between laboratories.

Earthworms are studied by exposure to test chemicals in containers of artificial soil, with an assessment of mortality 7 and 14 days after application; at
least two concentrations – one with mortality and one without – are examined,
with appropriate controls. Experiments may include an assessment of reproduction, which has been found to be a more sensitive marker of effect in some cases.
Another experimental procedure exposes the worms to the test material on
moist filter paper.

Bees (used for agrochemicals only) are subject to acute oral and contact tests.
Oral toxicity is assessed by feeding the bees with different concentrations of the
test chemical, with mortality checks up to 48 hours. Contact toxicity is assessed
by direct application to the thorax, which can also be used with other insects.
Other invertebrates that can be used in test programmes include woodlice,
springtails and marine arthropods from sediments, such as those found in
estuaries and other areas with high pollution loading.

Vertebrates

Various species of fish are used, including rainbow trout, fathead minnow,
zebrafish and bluegill sunfish (for the US EPA). Tests may be static (where the
water is unchanged for the duration of the test), semi-static (the water is
changed at intervals) or flow through where the water is changed constantly.
The duration of exposure is generally for up to 14 days, although shorter
exposures are used to determine the LC_{50}.

Birds such as quail, mallard duck, pheasant or partridge are used in a variety
of tests, including dietary tests, which may use five test diets with increasing test
substance concentration over a 5-day period. A 3-day off-treatment period
follows.

The majority of these test systems are used in single-species studies in which
the classic toxicological design of controls and several treatment groups are
examined, usually with the added dimension of time as a factor.

Mesocosms and field tests and studies

Single-species testing is, in some ways, analogous to *in vitro* toxicity test systems
in that only a part of the ecosystem or animal is being examined and
interrelationships between species or organs cannot be easily predicted. The

problem of single-species testing can be partially circumvented by the use of mesocosms or field tests. Whereas a mesocosm is an artificial ecosystem of a manageable and controllable size, field tests use pre-existing areas in the environment for studies with chemicals such as pesticides or to determine the causes of observed environmental effects. The latter is analogous to an epidemiological study in humans. As always with toxicological investigation, size and complexity are associated with significant cost and these experiments or investigations are inevitably expensive and time consuming.

Mesocosms are large-scale experiments that attempt to reproduce a section of the ecoytem in miniature, usually including a pond or water system such as an artificial stream. The use of 'miniature' in this context is deceptive, however, because these may have a volume of 50 m^3 or greater, with a surface area of up to 25 m^2. The advantage of both these test types is that they have a number of different species, which can interact in a way similar to that in the real world.

A mesocosm is constructed, in an appropriate container, according to the experimental duration and objective; longer experiments need larger systems. The components of the system and their origins and quantities are defined in guidelines (e.g. those from the OECD). All components, such as the sediment (with indigenous fauna and flora), fish species, plankton and plants, are carefully characterised and sourced so as to be free from confounding contaminants. Before addition of the test chemical, the system is allowed to equilibrate and mature, the duration of this being proportional to the size of system. Experimental duration is influenced by the type of chemical being tested, persistent chemicals requiring longer examination that those that are readily eliminated by biotransformation or degradation. Several mesocosms may be set up to examine different doses of the test chemical, in which case the reproducibility of the system becomes critical to interpretation of the data.

By definition, field tests do not use 'constructed' locations but the experimental parameters are still carefully defined before the test is undertaken. The areas covered by field tests may be substantially larger than with mesocosm experiments and are typically performed for pesticides, which may be applied at doses expected to be toxic. Measurements made are dependent on the chemical class, habitat, type of agricultural system and application method. They include determination of persistence of the chemical in soils, water and in the flora and fauna, including an estimation of any bioaccumulation risk. Study of population change in response to the application is an important aspect of these trials.

Changes in population that are noted independently of field tests are the trigger for field studies. The difference between a study and a test being that no chemical is deliberately applied in a study. As with an epidemiological study, the object is to determine the cause of an observed difference from expectation. Such studies depend on the initial observation – development of male sex organs in female dog whelks or declining reproductive performance in seals – and the painstaking investigations that follow. These include precise definition of the problem and analysis to determine the presence or not of abnormal chemical residues such as organic tin compounds or polychlorinated biphenyls, either in the affected species or in their environment. The relationship between the effect and the proposed cause is usually only accepted on provision of a credible toxicological mechanism of effect or an incontrovertible association that is not present in other locations. Frequently, as in many other walks of life, a strong or circumstantial association between a chemical and an effect is not enough to offer 'proof' to authorities, especially if money is involved in rectification, either directly in clean-up costs or in increased costs for a profitable industry.

There is evidence that morphological change, resulting from pollution, may be counteracted by natural selective forces. Thus, populations of the peppered moth, *Biston betularia* responded to carbon deposits on trees by increased proportions of a darker variant, the incidence of which has declined with declining carbon-based pollution. Similarly there has been evidence that the development of male sex organs in female dog whelks (imposex, which hinders reproduction) is being circumvented through selective pressures. These population responses are apparently based on existing genetic diversity in the normal population and it seems unlikely that this type of adaptive response to morphological change would be readily duplicated in the case of biochemical effects on basic molecular function.

An important aspect of field studies is the use of biochemical or morphological markers of effect to assess exposure. These may be easy to assess, as in the presence of imposex in female dog whelks exposed to organic tin compounds, or more challenging as in the analysis of carcases for chemical residues. Classic markers have included the thinning of eggshells in peregrine falcons, which was the mechanistic response to exposure to DDT and its major metabolite DDE. The routine monitoring of marker species can also be used in the assessment or development of local pollution. Increased metabolic capacity in the livers of river trout may imply exposure to excess concentrations of xenobiotics. Such hypotheses may be confirmed by analysis and this could be extended to the carcases of predatory birds or mammals such as herons or seals. These are markers of effect and the distinction must be drawn between the presence of a chemical and its effects on individual species and its impact on the ecosystem as whole. To determine the impact of a chemical it is necessary to carry out detailed population studies. Crucially, it is important to know what the population distribution was *before* the pollution occurred or to know the situation in an *identical* area in which no pollution has (yet) taken place.

Pitfalls in environmental toxicology

The principal problem of ecotoxicology is the simplicity of the test systems relative to the complexity of the ecosystems and the multi-factorial nature of many of the possible adverse variations that may occur. Although the test systems may be good models for individual components of the ecosystem, the specific tests may not be predictive for ecological effects in the target species or groups when they are removed from the relative simplicity of a laboratory environment. Furthermore it is extremely difficult to assess the significance of change seen in a laboratory environment and to predict effects in the whole ecosystem.

The most complex ecotoxicological experiments attempt to reproduce entire ecosystems in miniature and to examine the reactions of components of this artificial system to the controlled introduction of the chemical. The principal difficulty with this type of test, apart from the eye-watering expense, is that with increasing experimental complexity it becomes much more difficult to control the many variables. Although an artificial stream is probably a good reproduction of an ecosystem in miniature, it cannot reproduce the wider picture of the whole ecosystem.

A further factor is the likelihood of effects that are attributable to unconsidered relationships, for example the effect of ivermectin on the degradation of dung from treated cattle. Although this type of effect might be predicted by lateral thinking, rigidly regulated testing and data assessment does not readily lend itself to such thought processes. The interrelationships and co-dependencies inherent in the ecosystem are not easily assessed a priori but, with the benefits of hindsight, become painfully predictable when the effects are first noticed. Extrapolating laboratory change – will an effect on one species significantly affect the whole ecosystem? – is fraught with difficulty.

Epidemiology – a brief review

Epidemiology, the study of factors in human disease, can act as a starting point to a programme of toxicological investigation or as the final phase of surveillance that follows marketing of a new drug. Classically it is associated with linking cause and effect in human disease. The science has a long history, from the eighteenth-century observations of Percival Potts on scrotal cancer in former chimney sweeps to the association of thalidomide with phocomelia and vinyl chloride with haemangiosarcoma. It is not the intention here to go into a detailed examination of epidemiological technique or study type, but simply to review the field briefly and to look at some of the pitfalls that may be encountered.

In contrast to laboratory toxicology, epidemiological study is conducted in the field with a diverse population in which the exposure is often poorly defined and outcome is often compromised by other factors such as smoking or alcohol. Good epidemiology is dependent on rigorous control of variables and of confounding factors that may invalidate the conclusions if not fully appreciated and allowed for. Thus, in a study of respiratory disease due to an occupational hazard, smoking could be expected to influence the results and is therefore a confounding factor. Because the natural variability amongst humans is so large, it is difficult to detect minor deviations from controls without using vast numbers of subjects. Epidemiology is therefore good for detecting clear effects that may be associated with exposure to a specific substance. Clarity of effect may be due to rarity of the observed disease or to numbers affected. Thus, cause and effect linkage of vinyl chloride with hepatic haemangiosarcoma was made easier by the rarity of the tumour and the distinct population in which it was seen. The importance of numbers is illustrated by the association of smoking and lung cancer, which has been taken further to show that smoking exacerbates respiratory disease in occupational exposure to asbestos or in uranium mining. For 'normal' diseases such as leukaemia, variation from normality is more difficult to define, especially as the human population tends to be naturally inhomogeneous. The result of this inhomogeneity is the presence of clusters of diseases in particular areas, for example a high incidence of meningitis in some villages or the presence of leukaemia clusters around a nuclear plant. The normal presence of a disease in a population makes it extremely difficult to separate low-level effect, which might be due to exposure to a chemical, from normal variation. One product of this uncertainty is often a succession of studies, each seeming more authoritative than the last and each with a different conclusion. For many years it has been considered that all alcohol should be avoided in pregnancy because alcohol in large amounts has been clearly associated with fetal alcohol syndrome; recently it was suggested that small amounts might be beneficial. Equally, it has long been suggested that saturated fats should be avoided in favour of polyunsaturates; then it has been counter-suggested that too much polyunsaturated fat is not good. Although it would seem sensible to take all the data from all the studies and pool it to establish the cause of the effect or correctness of attribution, this is usually made difficult or impossible by variations in experimental technique, population differences, differing criteria for differential diagnosis, etc.

Establishment of a relationship between cause and effect by epidemiology is dependent on comparison of an exposed population or one showing the effect with a control that is unaffected or unexposed to the chemical or agent of interest. Correct choice of controls is crucial as they are the 'normal' population against which the test group will be compared. If you are looking at minor differences between individuals or study groups the definition of normality is very important. Move the normality goalposts and the conclusions will change.

Studies may be conducted prospectively on living people by following them until the object of the study is achieved or retrospectively on case histories where previous history is associated with current disease. The collection and long-term retention of occupational health monitoring data under the Control of Substances Hazardous to Health (COSHH) will facilitate epidemiological study, although the sheer volume of data collected and potential doubts about the method and accuracy of recording and collection may make this difficult.

Where the condition investigated in epidemiological studies is associated with a naturally existing background incidence or with a wide range of values it is quite possible to have different studies indicating different and opposite effects. The influence of interest groups is also a factor to consider. The information that red wine is good prophylaxis against cardiovascular disease was good news for the red wine producers of Bordeaux but less wonderful for white wine sales. Within a relatively short time a study emerged showing the benefits of white wine. The toxicological overview might be that a sensible amount of alcohol accompanied by appropriate antioxidants is a good combination for avoidance of cardiac complications.

Another example of contradictory epidemiological study results is provided by examination of the relationship between electromagnetic radiation from power lines and leukaemia in children. In this work the definition of the exposed population varied between studies, some including houses up to 100 m either side of the power lines while others used a smaller distance. Lack of comparability between study protocols made an overall assessment of the data impossible, leaving little scientific proof but a lingering public perception that they had been misinformed or led astray. The absence of any mechanism by which the leukaemia could be induced was also a crucial weakness. In the final analysis no amount of epidemiological research into a fuzzy problem will overcome public perception.

Chapter 9

Interpretation

Introduction

The intention of this chapter is to give guidelines on the interpretation of toxicological data and to indicate an overall philosophy to this sometimes seemingly black art. Interpretation is distinct from prediction, for example in attribution of cause/effect before versus after the event: 'She smokes a lot, so she may get lung cancer' versus the finding that she has lung cancer. Did she smoke? Yes, 20 a day. We have a probable cause for this cancer.

The most basic object of interpretation is to assess the significance of difference, once it has been established that there is a difference to explain. The questions to be asked include 'Is there a difference?' and if there is, how has it arisen. Does an observed difference mean toxicity? Equally, if no difference is discernible, where one was expected, why has it not been detected? Were the methods used sensitive enough to show difference? Has exposure been achieved or is the lack of effect due to true lack of toxicity? Is the lack of toxicity relevant to other species? When the data are clear in showing an effect of exposure there is usually little debate about the results and, with appropriate supporting studies, the mechanism is also generally accepted. However, as is often the case, the differences – especially in epidemiological studies – are often small, confined to one group or species and have no clear origin or mechanism. In these circumstances it is quite possible for conflicting interpretations to be put forward for the same set of data. Furthermore, additional studies may serve simply to produce contradictory results and are often performed to protocols that are not directly comparable with earlier work. The net result is that the data from the various studies cannot simply be combined to give a larger population size (and so more statistical power). The outcome is a body of data that is almost impossible to negotiate without falling foul of one group or another and conclusions are left hanging.

The interpretation challenge

The main challenges for toxicological interpretation, which are of clear relevance to the public (the ultimate customer of toxicological investigation), include the causes of cancer (threat to the individual), reproductive effects (threat to the children) and general disease and debilitation which can result in loss of quality of life or shortened lifespan. The public perception of risk and its assessment are dealt with in chapter 11, but it is clear that public interest can put enormous pressure on the process of interpretation and may exert an undue influence on the end result. This is a particular problem when any degree of urgency exists, especially if more studies have to be conducted; it is all too easy in these circumstances to arrive at a conclusion, based on insufficient data, which is at best misleading or simply wrong.

Frequently the task of interpretation is made more difficult by the lack of clarity of cause and effect. For any finding that has a significant normal incidence in the general population, asthma for example, attribution of a set of cases to a specific cause can be tenuous. Unequivocal demonstration of cause and effect is possible only if there is a clear relationship between exposure to an agent and a condition present at a significantly higher incidence than normal. For this reason, minor increases in conditions that may be due to toxicity are extremely difficult to ascribe with certainty to individual chemicals or classes of chemicals. This leads to contradictory epidemiological studies that cause opinion to veer from one side to the other, in a manner that does nothing to help scientific credibility.

The scope of interpretation

Data presented for toxicological interpretation ranges from the results of individual toxicity tests or whole data packages or large epidemiological investigations to a single data point from an occupational monitoring scheme. The complexity of interpretation increases as the number of measurements and the amount of data increase. One of the interpretative tricks with large multi-endpoint data sets is to group the data together into easily definable sets so that the conclusions can be better focused on the mechanism in operation. The complexity of a full clinical pathology data set for an individual in a health screen (perhaps 20 to 30 parameters) may be contrasted with the same type of data for a study in animals where there may be 40 to 50 parameters for 30 or more animals. With both sets of data it is not sensible to try to interpret each parameter separately because links between functional groups of analytes or haematological cell counts may be lost in the maze of increases and decreases and uncertain abnormalities. In these circumstances one data point that is seen to be abnormal may be supported by other abnormalities or may be dismissed because there are no other supporting variations from normality. Equally, the changes seen at various exposure levels may be contrasted with those seen in other groups or in other members of the same group.

Interpretation as a dynamic process

Interpretation is not a static process and it is quite likely that new data will at least influence previous perceptions, if only to confirm them. As a toxicological programme of testing or research develops it should be possible to build up a picture from individual studies and to define extra studies to be undertaken in the light of these data. From the conclusions of the individual studies the wider picture of the effects and mechanisms emerges, allowing overall conclusions on the activity, mechanism and hazard posed by the test chemical. This in turn facilitates assessment of workplace risk, clinical dosing information, clinical treatment of overdose, acceptable daily intakes or harvesting intervals (time to harvest from last spraying or treatment). Appropriate interpretation may also suggest better practice, for example improvements in food storage in the light of Balkan endemic nephropathy, in which the presence of ochratoxins, produced by moulds in poorly stored food, was implicated in progressive renal toxicity and failure.

There is often pressure to attempt interpretation of part data sets, for instance part way through a long study or in the middle of an ongoing programme of investigation. This should be performed with caution and in the clear understanding that data that follow on may invalidate the interim assessment. It is in this type of circumstance that interpretation of environmental disasters often comes adrift, leading initially to the wrong conclusions or inappropriate investigative studies.

Steps in interpretation

It is not sensible to set hard and fast rules for interpretation, as these are too readily disproved by exceptions, however, as the chapter develops the general principles that should be applied to interpretation will emerge. These include the following, whatever the size of the data set:

- Validate the data
- Look at all the validated evidence
- Define the controls or baselines
- Decide what evidence of exposure is available
- Examine the mechanism proposed as support of the attribution.

When these have been adequately addressed it may be possible to draw a conclusion as to cause and effect. Failing this, it should be possible to define further studies that should be conducted to elucidate the effects seen.

Study design

The first step is to assess the study design to ensure consistency with the study objectives and good practice. Part of this should be to look for procedural oddities (or deviations from protocol) that might influence the data. For instance, food consumption can be distorted by difficulties in recording discarded food or the practice of giving supplements, which may not be recorded quantitatively. From this base, the credibility of the data has to be assessed by review of the methods for factors such as sampling error, faulty procedure or design. One such bias is found when more samples are assessed from treated groups in comparison with the controls, leading to an apparent treatment-related difference that is purely a product of sampling frequency.

A critical aspect of study design is the choice of dose or inclusion levels, as overload may lead to unrepresentative toxicity. This is particularly true in studies where the chemical is mixed with the diet, as high inclusion levels will have an effect on the nutritional value of the food offered. The comparators used also need to be examined as use of the wrong ones will invalidate the study. Thus, when trying to demonstrate similarity, old should not be compared with young, smokers with non-smokers, uranium miners with office workers, etc.

Controls and expectation

One of the precepts of toxicology is the detection of adverse change from normality and the controls in any experiment give a baseline of experimental normality against which all the treated groups or individual experimental units are assessed. It is critical, therefore to be assured that the controls are, in fact, normal. Given that the numbers in any toxicity study will be merely a sample of a much larger population, it is inevitable that there will be a degree of normal biological variation between control groups in different experiments. Some of this variation will be extreme and this can lead to apparent difference that is not biologically real.

When confronted with an apparent treatment-related difference from controls the assessment should seek to indicate if the treated group values are simply higher than the controls or have they been increased as a direct influence of the test substance. Box 9.1 summarises the questions that need to be asked.

Box 9.1 Confirmation of the validity of the control data

The validity of the data from the controls in any experiment should be critically examined to confirm that they represent expectation or normality. Invalid controls call the whole experiment into question. The following should be considered:

- Were the controls experimentally appropriate and within the limits of expectation?
- If there is more than one control group, are the data consistent between controls or positive controls and treated groups?
- Have the data been distorted by procedurally related stress or, in animals, by the presence of an observer?
- Is only one parameter affected?
- How large is the difference?
- Is the difference reproducible or consistently present in other data or studies?
- Has the difference arisen through the way the data has been processed?
- When the validity of control data is checked against historical controls, is the comparison valid?

The presence of a dose response is a particularly important criterion in assigning a difference to treatment, while the presence of differences in associated parameters also lends weight to the argument for causal relationship with the test substance. To a degree, the size of a difference determines its reproducibility, as small differences seen in small studies are notoriously difficult to reproduce. The presence of the effect in similar studies or mechanistic evidence from related data would also support a relationship to treatment. The influence of data treatment procedures on the perception of difference cannot be ignored, especially when the only difference is statistical; appropriate data treatment may eliminate difference.

The critical question relates to the appropriateness of the controls and whether they were within expectation for the parameter under analysis; in other words were they normal? Choice of appropriate controls is particularly critical in epidemiological studies where confounding factors or poor differential diagnosis can invalidate a study. In toxicological studies the choice of controls is easier as the experimental population is usually supplied as a uniform set of individuals that can be randomly separated into control and treated groups. In this case you can be confident that the controls and treated groups have similar starting baselines. However, due to the presence of normal biological variation, especially with small group sizes, differences between the groups can be reasonably expected before treatment starts. At this point it becomes useful, essential in some cases, to have historical control data to hand to assess where the control and treatment group values lie in relation to expectation.

Use of background data in interpretation

There will come a point in the examination of toxicological data when it must be decided whether an unexpected observation is natural or when an unexpected difference is a change from normality. The contemporary study control should always be the first and chief comparator in any toxicity study. However, as indicated above, there is a role to be played in interpretation of toxicological data by focused use of historical control data. These data should be used to indicate if the controls have strayed from expectation and to back up the concept of normality; they should not replace the contemporary control. Only when the intention of an experiment, often an early or sighting study, is to look for gross differences from normal should historical data be used to indicate normality in the absence of study controls.

Provided the controls are selected from the same population as the treated groups it is possible to be confident that they are truly comparable with them. With historical control data, care has to be exercised that this is true. The greater the similarity of the historical control individuals with those in the study with which they are being compared, the greater will be the confidence that can be placed in using them to support interpretation. The criteria that should be checked before historical control data are used in a particular study include:

- Strain
- Route of exposure
- Age of test system
- Media or vehicle
- Supplier
- Contemporaneous data
- Husbandry or storage
- Study procedure

(See chapter 2 for more discussion of these points.)

The greater the deviation of the historical control parameters from the study test system, the less relevant they will be to the interpretation of that experiment. Inappropriate use of historical control data is one of the easiest errors to make – especially if there appears to be no reasonable alternative. In fact, if there are no comparable historical control data it is probably better to avoid their use entirely. It may be possible to use historical data from other laboratories but this carries risks, which should not be ignored. Although the strain and age may be similar, the care of the test system and other factors such as environment, instrument settings and so on may be sufficiently different to produce data that are not directly comparable. Such data may be used as a guide in the initial setting-up of an assay but are of dubious use thereafter. This is illustrated by historical tumour incidences in rodents, which are available from suppliers. The problem here is that the data are compiled from studies conducted in different laboratories under undefined husbandry conditions. Differences in diagnosis and nomenclature used by the individual pathologists are also a confounding factor. It is therefore not possible to place much confidence in these data but they are better than nothing and may be useful in discussing the incidences of rare tumours. In general, the less reproducible the test conditions, the less useful will be the historical control data from other laboratories.

Statistics and significance in toxicology

Statistical analysis is routine in sufficiently sized toxicity studies and the results can be slavishly reported to the general detriment of credibility. It is important, however, to remember that statistics is a fallible tool. A useful analogy is comparison of the use of statistics by toxicologists to the use of a lamppost by a drunk; they should be a source of illumination not of support. It is easy to misuse them and to draw incorrect conclusions based solely on the presence of statistically significant differences.

In simplistic terms there are three levels of significance that are important in toxicology, namely statistical, biological and toxicological or clinical, in increasing order of importance. Data should be analysed with these significance levels in mind, taking into consideration any dose response (or its absence), the inherent variability or variance of the data being examined and the sample size. Variance is a function of the range of the values (minimum to maximum) and of the deviation of the individual values from the mean and indicates the extent to which the values are distributed about the mean. Variance increases when the data includes outliers, data points that are radically different from the majority of the group.

Statistical significance means simply that the test group is different from controls in a numerical sense and that the difference in means is large enough for the effects of variance to be overcome. This can be numerically ridiculous and a disaster in presentation terms; computer programs often work on unrounded figures but report to one or two decimal places. This means that it is possible for a table to contain four group means for one parameter from different treatment groups, all of 1.1 but with significant differences flagged for one or more; this is also often a reflection of the differences in variance in the data for each group. Equally, it must be pointed out that a difference that is not statistically significant may still be of biological significance.

Likewise a statistically significant difference is not always of biological significance, which relates to a change that may be important for the animal but that is not necessarily adverse and that is probably reversible. Examples of this would include normal hepatic adaptation to treatment, possibly seen as a minimal hepatocellular hypertrophy or an increase in urine volume due to increased water intake after administration of a foul-tasting substance. Transient diuresis of pharmacological origin without other change would also be included, if it was not seen to excess. Cessation of treatment or exposure is associated with a speedy return to normality. Biological significance does not equate to toxicological significance, especially as most data are representative of a single time point and do not analyse a continuum, which might show an increasing difference attributable to treatment. However, it should be noted that if a biological difference is allowed to persist, it may result in toxicity.

Toxicological significance denotes change which, if allowed to persist, may impact the survival or well-being of the exposed population or test system. Although reversibility may mean that an adverse change is not of toxicological significance, the degree of change is important, for example administration of carbon tetrachloride to rats can result in extensive liver damage which is clearly the result of toxicity. This damage is clearly evident in the first few days following treatment but, due to the liver's powers of recuperation, there may be no difference from normality after 14 days.

Tumour data provide examples of the distinction between these levels of significance. A doubling of the incidence of a rare tumour over control incidences, if seen at the highest dose level, may not be statistically significant but would probably be considered to be of biological significance, if not of toxicological significance, depending on context. Equally, a 25 per cent difference from control in testicular tumour count in some strains of rat may be flagged as statistically significant but is unlikely to be of biological or toxicological significance, especially if significant difference is established against only one control group or at the low or intermediate dose level. Toxicologists seem to be fond of an overall threshold of significance set arbitrarily at 10 per cent; a difference of less than 10 per cent relative to controls is not significant, a sort of numerical comfort blanket, which has the benefit that it is well accepted but with little scientific basis. A 10 per cent increase in plasma activity for an aminotransferase is unlikely to be of any biological significance, whereas a 10 per cent difference in plasma sodium concentration could be seriously unwelcome. This distinction is due to the low physiological impact of variability in enzyme activities versus the more precise requirement for electrolyte concentrations.

This might cause closer examination of the statement, frequently used in toxicology reports, that 'as the difference from controls was less than 10 per cent, it was not considered to be of toxicological significance'. Having raised that caution, it should be said also that the 10 per cent level is a useful, if arbitrary threshold and that larger values should be used with care.

At the simplest level, the use of statistics merely examines the differences between control and treated groups and gives a probability that the two groups represent different populations. In other words they test the null hypothesis that there is no difference between control and the treated group(s). The results of statistical analysis can therefore be used to answer the question 'Is the difference from controls caused by treatment or exposure to the suspected factor?' Note that it generally only *indicates* the answer and does not provide it unequivocally in every case. All too often a single statistically significant difference will not be enough to prove the wider hypothesis, particularly if the sample size is small or there is wide variation between the individual data points. The smaller the sample size and the greater the variance in the data the more unreliable will be the statistical values that result from any analysis. For sample sizes of less than 10 or where the variance is large, a statistical significance is only a pointer to a difference that may be of biological or toxicological significance. It is the responsibility of the toxicologist to interpret the data to indicate the real significance of the difference, in biological or toxicological terms.

Statistical process

In analysing data, it is important to use the statistical tests that are appropriate to the data type being examined, whether it is for a continuous variable or presence/absence data. The following is intended to show the approach normally taken in analysis of these data types and is intended simply as a guide to statistical method. For more technical explanation one of the texts in the bibliography should be consulted but, having said that, it is extremely difficult to find an explanation of statistical method that is accessible to the mathematically challenged.

For a continuous variable, the first line of examination is at the level of group means and, usually, the standard deviation which, in conjunction with the number of data points, n, gives a first indication of the variance of the data. Table 9.1 illustrates the effects of variability on the summary statistics (mean

Table 9.1 The effect of variability in data on summary statistics

Data point	'Normal' data	Variable data	With an outlier
1	31	36	31
2	29	24	29
3	27	25	27
4	34	36	34
5	32	42	32
6	29	19	63
7	28	36	28
8	31	23	31
9	33	33	33
10	30	30	30
Mean	30	30	34
SD	2.2	7.4	10.5

Note: SD, standard deviation.

and standard deviation) for a representative set of data. The 'normal' set has been constructed to represent typical values for an enzyme such as alanine aminotransferase. The second – variable – set is a reworking of the first to introduce greater variability, while the third set illustrates the effect of a single outlying value.

The summary data give a first, crude indication of difference, assessed from the control and test group means and the overlap of their standard deviations. This has been described as the 'very obvious test'; it has a pleasing simplicity, which is a bonus to many but may be frowned on by professional statisticians. There are two approaches to the analysis of continuously variable data, namely parametric and non-parametric methods, the latter generally having less power than the former. Parametric analysis is the method of choice but for this the data should be normally distributed and have homogeneous variance.

The first step in statistical analysis of a data set is to confirm that the variance is homogeneous and, if so, to proceed to analysis of variance and other parametric methods. If the variance is possibly affected by the presence of outlying data points it may be useful to perform the analysis with and without these values. Analysis of variance uses the data from all groups and seeks to establish that the null hypothesis is true – that there are no differences between the groups – or that one or more groups are different. Although much used in the past, Student's t-test is now acknowledged to be unsuitable where there is more than one group.

Where it has been decided that parametric analysis is not appropriate, non-parametric methods offer an alternative, although they are not easily applicable to complex data sets. They are mostly based on ranking the data and are particularly good when there is obvious deviation from the normal distribution but become more difficult when there are a number of tied values. The Wilcoxon rank sum or Mann–Whitney test is the simplest of these methods and is based on assessment of the ranks of the individual values, not on the original data themselves. The Kruskal-Wallis test is the equivalent of analysis of variance, used when there are more than two groups for comparison. This process is summarised in Figure 9.1.

Data that describe presence or absence are generally assessed using chi-squared or Fisher's exact test with more complex analysis being undertaken with tests for positive trend. The chi-squared test is appropriate for high-frequency findings and compares the observed with the expected frequencies, the latter being derived from all the data for the groups being tested. For data with lower

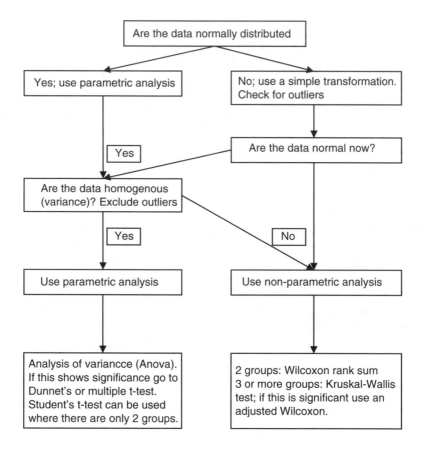

Figure 9.1 Statistical process for continuous data.
Source: Adapted and simplified from Dickens, A and Robinson, J. 'Statistical approaches'. In Evans, GO (ed.) *Animal Clinical Chemistry – a primer for toxicologists*. London: Taylor & Francis, 1996.

incidences, Fisher's exact test is normally used, comparing the numbers of animals in each group with the lesion and those without it. In carcinogenicity bioassays, where analysis of tumour incidence is a vital component of the interpretation of the results, tests for positive trend are used. Cancer is more prevalent in older animals and, as a result of early death due to toxicity, the animals at the high dose will not have the opportunity to express the same numbers of tumours as the controls. Where treatment causes an increased incidence of a tumour in animals that survive to old age this will not be apparent if there is a significant early mortality. Analysis is therefore conducted using the data from all the dose groups and takes account of the numbers of animals that die during the study. In addition the tumours are categorised for each animal as fatal, probably fatal, probably incidental or incidental; an additional category of uncertain may be added.

Data treatment and transformation

In analysing data it is often useful to treat it in various ways in order to make differences easier to discern. One approach to this is to examine change rather than the original value. The classic example is analysis of bodyweight gain rather than the simple group mean data for the absolute weights. This can also be applied to parameters such as alkaline phosphatase which should decrease with age; the absence of decrease may indicate treatment-related effect. In young rodents, food consumption may be readily correlated with growth by the calculation of food conversion ratios – in effect the amount of body mass produced for each gram of food consumed. This figure declines as the growth phase is completed and becomes meaningless after that as food consumption is maintained at the same values without significant gain in bodyweight.

For parametric analysis it is necessary to have normally distributed data. With skewed data it may be possible to achieve this by transforming the data, for instance by using the log of each data point, which can also be used where variability increases with the mean; the square root of the data may also be used. More esoteric procedures, such as use of reciprocals or trigonometric functions start to show a degree of numerical desperation, indicating that the use of non-parametric methods would probably be better.

Assessing exposure

Toxicological effect is always related, directly or indirectly, to exposure to an active molecule or to an agent such as radiation. Assessment of exposure is therefore essential to interpretation of toxicological data because, although the presence of an effect indicates exposure, exposure cannot be assumed in the absence of effect. In addition, the presence of an effect does not necessarily mean that it can be attributed to the chemical under investigation. Box 9.2 looks at some of the factors to be considered in assessing exposure.

Box 9.2 Questions in assessment of exposure

Exposure, and its significance, should be assessed via the following considerations:

- Was the test system exposed to the test material or a metabolite? A particulate material may not be available to cells *in vitro* and an oral dose may not be absorbed.
- Was toxicity due to a metabolite or an indirect effect (e.g. hormonal imbalance)?
- Did this exposure extend to the target tissue?
- Was the target tissue exposed to greater concentrations than elsewhere in the test system?
- In a life of mixtures, if there was exposure, was this the cause of the effect?
- Was the observed exposure sufficient to cause the observed effects? 'Sufficient' may be defined from no effect levels in previous studies; also consider any inter-species differences. 'Sufficient' includes duration of exposure (area under the curve as well as treatment period).
- In absence of toxicity, was the exposure medium or vehicle appropriate to achieve exposure of the test system?
- Is the analytical method sufficiently sensitive and specific to detect the test substance or its derivatives?
- Was there any cross-contamination of the controls that might invalidate the data?

The normal sequence of known chemical exposure resulting in an effect may be turned on its head when an effect is observed without an obvious explanation. In this case the interpretation effort relies on finding common exposure factors and confirming that these are consistent with the observations. There have been many incidents or findings that have provoked such epidemiological study, including scrotal cancer in chimney sweeps due to soot, lung cancer and smoking and more recent cases such as the Spanish toxic oil syndrome (TOS) and eosinophilia-myalgia syndrome (EMS). The last two, which had clinical features in common, related to contamination of rapeseed oil (canola) and tryptophan, respectively. Both were associated with widespread malaise amongst the exposed populations and with a number of deaths. In the case of TOS, the effects were traced to rapeseed oil contaminated with aniline to make it unsuitable for human use. The investigation of the incident was partly hampered by the policy of giving money for returned oil, which resulted in the handing in of numerous spurious samples. EMS was eventually associated with the ingestion of products containing contaminated tryptophan, the contamination resulting from changes in production, including a new production bacteria and reduced filtration steps. The causative agents for these incidents have not been definitively identified, although candidate molecules and mechanisms have been proposed.

Evidence of exposure to the test substance is almost always achieved by analysis of samples taken from the medium *in vitro* or of blood or urine samples taken from animals. Occasionally, it is possible to point to effects seen and conclude that the test system must have been exposed but this does not characterise the concentrations associated with the effect or if the parent molecule was present. Toxicokinetic analyses of blood samples gives an indication of basic kinetic parameters including half-life and area under the concentration curve (AUC).

Integration of exposure information

For the reasons given above, integration of exposure data into toxicological assessments is essential for a meaningful interpretation of the results. In assessing the likelihood of exposure, the physicochemical properties of the molecule should be considered, including partition coefficient, solubility and ADME (Table 9.2), as these will have a profound influence on the extent of exposure. The speed and extent of absorption and subsequent distribution into the test system are also critical. These factors determine the maximum concentration of the test chemical at the site where toxicity may be expressed, whether that is a protein or cellular organelle in a cell culture or in a tissue in a whole animal. Toxicity is usually seen once a threshold concentration or level of exposure has been exceeded. Systemically, this threshold is indicated by C_{max} (maximum plasma concentration) or AUC (area under the concentration curve). With some toxicities, especially those relating to transient excess pharmacological action, it is possible to relate the onset, duration and severity of effect to C_{max}. Where there is a long half-life of elimination, such that significant concentrations remain at the time of the next dose administration, it is likely that the chemical or its metabolites will accumulate. This can result in the appearance of toxicity at a late stage in the evaluation programme, due to accumulation of effect. For instance a four-week study may show no effects, whereas the same dose levels in a 13-week study may be associated with minimal onset of toxicity just outside normal biological limits. In longer studies this may progress to the extent that development must be stopped.

Although systemic concentrations of a parent compound are useful as a general indicator of exposure, they do not necessarily equate to concentration of the active molecule at the site of action. Brief excursions into toxic concentrations may only be associated with transient effects, such as those associated with excess or undesirable pharmacological action. The expression of chronic or persistent change is probably due to accumulation of effect (or deficient repair) following brief toxic concentrations or to sustained exposure to a concentration at which adverse change becomes apparent more slowly. This type of toxicity

Table 9.2 Selected ADME factors and their impact on toxicity

Long half-life	Longer systemic exposure and possibility of accumulation with repeated dosing
Short half-life	Transient peaks of high concentration that may not elicit chronic toxicity
Area under the curve (AUC)	A measure of systemic exposure related to half-life and concentration. Increasing the AUC, e.g. through formulation changes, may result in greater toxicity
High binding to plasma proteins	Low free concentration of active substance in plasma. Small changes in binding site availability may lead to large percentage changes in free chemical and so to toxicity; e.g. warfarin
Tissue binding	Sequestration into a tissue compartment, such as bone or lipid, reduces the amount of chemical available to express toxicity. Sudden release later on may have serious consequences
Metabolism	Can increase or decrease toxicity. Inhibition or induction of the enzymes or metabolism can have a marked effect on the toxicity of chemicals; simultaneous exposure to two or more chemicals may therefore have a much greater effect than an equivalent dose of either chemical alone
First pass effect	Significant metabolism of a chemical as it passes through the liver for the first time after absorption from the gut results in low systemic availability reducing toxicity in more distant tissues
Enterohepatic recirculation	Break down in the gut of conjugate metabolites excreted in the bile can lead to reabsorption, effectively increasing half-life and area under the curve
Excretion failure or decline	Age-related decline in renal or hepatic function can lead to increased systemic exposure and hence to toxicity, e.g. benoxaprofen in elderly patients
Concentration in tissues of elimination	Concentrations of chemicals in tissues responsible for their excretion can result in local toxicity, seen particularly in the distal tube of the renal nephron and in the bladder

was apparent with the retinal effects associated with chloroquine, which has a high affinity for melanin in the retina. These irreversible effects are dependent not only on daily dose and duration of treatment but also on the total dose taken; toxicity may be expressed after withdrawal of the drug as the drug persists long after therapy has ceased.

However, toxic effect is not always directly attributable to the chemical that was added to the culture or given to the animals. Following administration, and simultaneously with absorption and distribution, the processes of elimination begin. These encompass metabolism and excretion, which are generally expected to result in the removal of toxic entities but which can increase toxicity. One route of removal from the plasma, that is properly part of distribution, is the sequestering of chemicals into tissues where they are retained, effectively inactive, until released. For instance, highly lipophilic compounds, such as DDT and DDE, accumulate in adipose tissue from which they may be released to produce toxicity long after exposure has ceased. This can be a problem in pregnancy when significant lipid mobilisation occurs during the third trimester. Another example is the binding of heavy metals, like cadmium, to metalloproteins and the subsequent toxicity when a storage threshold is exceeded.

Although, having demonstrated exposure of the test system, it is relatively simple to correlate change with the presence of the chemical or a metabolite or an indirect effect, the absence of effect needs considerable care in interpretation. Before a chemical can be truly said to be non-toxic, it is necessary to show that it was available to the test system and that significant concentrations at potential target sites were achieved. Incubation at high concentrations or oral administration of large doses does not mean that exposure was achieved. Poor absorption following oral administration (low bioavailability) is a frequent finding, resulting in low systemic concentrations; as a result the toxicity of a parenterally administered chemical may be much greater than expected when effects are extrapolated from an oral dose. Poor availability may be due simply to the medium or vehicle in which the chemical was offered to the test system, and a change in this can result in significantly greater toxicity.

The assessment of exposure is dependent on the sensitivity and specificity of the methods used to detect the test substance. For small molecules this is usually not a problem; for larger molecules such as peptides or proteins, the analytical challenges become more exacting, especially if the half-life is short or the concentrations very low. This leaves the problem of how to interpret the presence of effect in the absence of measurable exposure. There are a number of possible explanations for this, including analytical methods that are not sufficiently sensitive. Another possibility might be that the correct matrix is not being analysed and that the correct place of analysis is the target site of activity. There is also the possibility that the pharmacological effect persists for longer than indicated by plasma concentrations due to persistent binding at a receptor.

Although it might be assumed that parenteral administration, in humans or animals, would result in rapid exposure to 100 per cent of the given dose, this may not always be the case. Intravenous administration of an inappropriate formulation may lead to temporary deposition near the site of injection, perhaps as a result of local irritation or other damage. Equally, intramuscular dosing of a poorly isotonic formulation may result in slow release from the site of administration. These uncertainties pale into insignificance when the dynamics of oral dosing are considered. Before the compound can get into the systemic circulation, it has to cross the gut wall and pass through the liver without significant metabolism taking place in a 'first pass' effect. Excretion of conjugated metabolites in the bile can be associated with enterohepatic recirculation where the conjugate is broken down in the gut and the active molecule is reabsorbed. This is the mechanism that makes dogs so sensitive to non-steroidal anti-inflammatory drugs.

Although the processes of ADME are clearly important in animals, it should be borne in mind that their absence *in vitro* may have an adverse effect on the results, leading to false negatives or positives. Although this criticism is met to a certain extent by the use of S-9 mix, it may be necessary to use a preparation from a relevant tissue, such as the kidney. The toxicity of S-9 to cell cultures is well known and should also be considered.

The reality of difference – the interpretation of small differences

Toxicology for regulatory purposes is largely about the desire to demonstrate the presence or (preferably) absence of difference from 'normality' and all interpretational effort is directed at this deceptively simple objective. It is relatively easy to spot differences so large that they are barndoor obvious – a 10-fold increase in colony count or enzyme activity or an unusual pathological lesion. Differences of medium size are also relatively simple – they are consistent or outside the normal limits or there is a clear dose response. The real challenge is provided by the small differences, often at the lowest dose level.

One of the reasons for looking for difference is the perceived obligation to show toxicity at one dose and thereby imply safety at a lower one. This leads to pressures to assign significance or otherwise to trivial differences; we *must* show toxicity so this *is* a significant toxicological change. Or we *must* show a no observed effect level (NOEL), so this small difference at the bottom end of the dose-response curve is irrelevant. Although it has been pointed out that, to demonstrate a NOEL there must be effects at higher doses, this edges towards irrelevance when the doses are vastly higher than those expected in humans. Where there is a small difference at the lowest dose level, which is supported by increasing differences at higher doses, it cannot be escaped that treatment has probably had an effect (or an 'influence') at the lowest dose. The significance of this difference is where interpretation becomes more complex. The no adverse effect level (NOAEL) is a useful concept because it acknowledges the presence of treatment-related change while putting it into perspective. The problem is that difference from controls – which is inevitable when using biological systems – is open to misinterpretation unless it is barndoor obvious, as shown by the very obvious test referred to above. For small differences it is difficult to assign significance.

Having noted a difference from controls, the first question to ask is whether there is a dose response. For example, if treated animals are different from controls, is this within background data ranges? It is noticeable that increases or decreases are often present in treated animals and are dismissed as being 'within normal ranges'. It is quite possible to have an effect of treatment that falls inside normal ranges; this becomes more obvious if the controls fall at the lower end of normality while the treated group fall at the top end.

A degree of difference is inevitable as a result of normal biological variation within the limits of normality defined by contemporary controls or similar, independent studies. Any pressure to downgrade a difference by defining limits after the event should be resisted. Although differences due to normal variation are expected, it is reasonable to expect some change in the test system when administering pharmacologically active chemicals at relatively high doses. It is quite possible for a 5 per cent difference in a biochemical parameter to fall inside normal limits and still be treatment-induced, especially if it comes at the bottom of a dose–response curve where the parameter is progressively and clearly affected at higher doses. Such differences show an influence by treatment but are often not biologically significant at the time of observation.

Where there is a classic dose–response curve, interpretation is relatively simple. With U-shaped dose responses it is not so easy; the first problem being to demonstrate that the curve is in fact abnormal, with maximal or minimal effect at intermediate doses rather than at the extremes; vitamin A shows such a curve. Having said that, where there is a difference from controls that is not obviously on a dose–response curve, it is usually easy to dismiss it as being due to chance variation within normal limits. Other reasons for dismissing a difference are that it is present in only one sex (although in rodents this is often not sensible due to metabolic differences), or within background data or inconsistent between examinations. The statement that it is of 'equivocal significance' simply means that it may be related to treatment but not understood. Sometimes the significance of minor differences seen in early studies becomes apparent with prolonged treatment, when lack of biological significance can be replaced by clear toxicological effect. A 10 per cent deficit or increase may not be significant at four weeks but may become fatal if age-related decline in function is accelerated during prolonged treatment.

Differences become impossible to interpret satisfactorily when the data, or the mechanism which generates them, are not understood completely. There is, apparently, a touching, unstated, belief, that more data on more parameters will mean better safety evaluation; this is a fallacy. A single difference from controls does not necessarily mean that the function of the tissue or organ system is impaired in proportion to the difference, as compensating mechanisms exist that cope with change in one direction by regulating in another. The overall goal of evaluating a range of parameters is to look at function, which is the product of many processes that work together. Thus, liver and kidney function are examined in a range of tests in the course of routine toxicity studies and changes in individual parameters are assessed against the data for related measures of organ toxicity. With increasing severity of effect on, say the liver, the number of parameters affected and the size of difference from controls increases, usually with dose. At the low end of the dose–response curve, at or near the NOAEL or NOEL, increasing the number of parameters to be examined may actually confuse the situation because normal biological variation will ensure a selection of differences in both directions, making secure interpretation nearly impossible.

There is a hint of this in the increasing emphasis on immunotoxicology in pharmaceutical development and the enthusiasm for technically demanding methods that generate numbers in the absence of clear understanding of their biological significance. As an example of a single parameter test, sister chromatid exchange went through a phase of popularity. It was agreed that there was a clear correlation between positive results and mutagenicity, as indicated by other tests, but the mechanism and significance of the effect were not understood and it did not become a standard test for regulatory purposes. As a single endpoint it was never interpreted in isolation from other genotoxicity data. There is also a tendency to react to human toxicity with new test requirements. One example of this is the severe cardiac events linked to QT interval prolongation in people taking drugs such as cisapride. Once again the question must be asked where the threshold of difference for rejection lies. A more general, philosophical question could ask if a one-size-fits-all approach to this type of problem is scientifically valid.

The reproducibility of difference

Ultimately there is only one way of confirming the significance of a small difference and that is to see if it is reproducible, either in a second experiment (as for *in vitro* tests) or in the next, usually longer, toxicity study. Furthermore, if the second experiment is performed using slightly different methods, the reproducibility or otherwise of the difference becomes much more significant. For experiments that are inherently weak statistically – those with small group sizes or with incomplete data sets – it is not unknown for a second test to show up a different set of statistically significant differences from controls. In this case it is easy to write off the differences as being due to normal biological variation; this illustrates neatly the importance of considering statistical versus biological or toxicological significance. Small group sizes, combined with measurement of parameters that have large inherent variances, will tend to throw up statistically significant differences that disappear on repetition.

While it is easy to live with non-reproducibility in small differences, it more complex when larger, apparently toxic differences are not reproduced in successive studies. The potential reasons for this include those listed on page 156 and in Box 3.2, to which should be added any changes in study design that may have taken place. Another consideration is that toxicity may be expressed early in a study but, due to development of tolerance or adaptation to treatment, will not be evident later on.

Interpretation of different data types

The following sections give an overview of the types of toxicological data and attempt a basic guide on how to approach each type.

Individual data sets

The simplest type of data that may be considered to be toxicological relates to a single parameter for one individual, such as a marker for occupational exposure. This may be presented as a single time point or a series of time points, which give a chronological profile of exposure. With this type of data it is important to be sure that the marker is either a direct marker of exposure or a surrogate marker such as an easily measured effect. In general the more remote the analyte or effect from the parent compound or the greater the natural background incidence or concentration, the more difficult it is to draw supportable conclusions from the data unless they are clearly at the extremities of or outside the normal range. The best marker of exposure is the parent compound, a known metabolite or by-product. However, this is often not possible and an indirect marker of effect such as inhibition of cholinesterase activity in the plasma following exposure to organo-phosphate insecticides can be used. Although it is possible to analyse urine or plasma for DNA adducts, these are not necessarily specific and may reflect lifestyle or other exposures. A more general approach is to look at clinical pathology data, which rarely looks at a single parameter in isolation, as a guide to abnormality that may be work-related. With any such data set, which is unlikely to have contemporary controls unless part of a full epidemiological study, it is important to have access to robust, trustworthy historical data ranges. If there is any sample analysis for the individual from before the start of exposure, this is clearly a significant advantage, although the date and circumstances in which the sample was taken should be considered. It is also probable that such data will be available for other workers and can be combined to give an overview of the exposed population. Within this data set it may also be possible to identify subsets of individuals who have been subject to greater or lesser exposure depending on their work station.

For chemicals that are accumulated into tissues and released slowly, assessment of exposure may be difficult during the early stages, as the effects only become apparent when a concentration threshold is crossed. For instance cadmium has a half-life measured in decades and accumulates in the kidney until a critical concentration of around 200 $\mu g/g$ is reached. At this point cadmium toxicity becomes apparent through increased urinary excretion of proteins and the cadmium concentration in the urine rises as a late herald of renal toxicity.

General toxicology

In some ways general toxicology is the least precisely defined and the broadest of all the branches of toxicological investigation, due to the number and variety of endpoints examined. A typical programme of toxicity studies includes studies from single dose up to 12 months in length. This breadth of investigation poses a number of challenges in interpretation, which are best approached by taking an overview of the data, rather than trying to interpret change in each parameter in isolation from the others. In many ways, the presence of different parameters acting as markers of change in different organ or tissues gives greater security of interpretation, as change in one parameter may be supported by change or lack of change in another. In addition, the findings in one study should be reproducible in succeeding studies, giving confidence that marginal effects are treatment-related or spurious. Thus, there are classic associations that are useful to remember in everyday situations, particularly in liver and kidney toxicity, which are the most frequent target organs; some of these are listed in Table 9.3.

From this it may be seen that changes in a number of parameters can often be tied in to pinpoint change in a particular tissue or organ system. Some of the associations are unexpected. Thyroid change may be associated with a marginal anaemia due to variations in the plasma concentrations of thyroid hormones. Antibiotic administration in rats is associated with greatly increased caecum size, but also with a decrease in the peripheral neutrophil count, both as a result of a decrease in the intestinal burden of bacteria. Perhaps the most difficult changes to interpret are those that have a multitude of different causes. Reduced growth and food consumption may be due to sedation, true appetite suppression, abdominal discomfort or other less specific and less easily identified causes. Reduced growth in the absence of reduced food consumption may indicate an effect on the GI tract or, in some cases, an effect on basal metabolic rate, as seen with decoupling of respiration. Pituitary tumours in rats are linked with a range of clinical signs such as hunched posture and torticollis

Table 9.3 Classic associations in toxicology

Liver toxicity	Renal toxicity
Increased plasma activity of liver marker enzymes: e.g. alanine and aspartate aminotransferases	Increased water consumption and urine volume. Urine parameters may change, e.g. enzymes and cellular debris
Decreased plasma total protein concentration	Increased plasma concentrations of urea and creatinine. Proteinuria
Increased coagulation times due to decreased synthesis of coagulation factors	Severe renal toxicity may lead to decreased erythrocyte parameters due to effects on erythropoietin synthesis
Increased liver weight due to enzyme induction or accumulation of lipid or glycogen	Increased kidney weight
Change in colour or size at necropsy.	Change in colour or size at necropsy
Histological findings such as necrosis or centrilobular hypertrophy due to enzyme induction.	Histological change, e.g. basophilic tubules or necrosis, papillary necrosis, or glomerular changes

but are particularly seen with weight loss and lowered food consumption. Table 9.4 shows some of the problems encountered in general toxicology studies and suggested reasons.

One of the factors to be aware of in toxicity of any type is stress and the adventitious effects that it may generate in any type of test system. In general toxicology, stress may be associated with decreased thymus and increased adrenal weight. This effect may be induced indirectly or directly. However, it is important to remember that indications of immunotoxicity may be masked by this and it is sensible to check other indicators of immune function before ascribing change in the thymus to stress.

A feature of general toxicity studies is the presence of specialist investigations, such as ophthalmoscopy, neurological examinations and electrocardiography. In particular, electrocardiography poses a number of difficulties in interpretation because the method and conditions of collection are critical in defining the value of the data. In an unanaesthetised animal, the stress of examination will tend to increase heart rate and blood pressure, perhaps masking treatment-related effects that are present in the resting animal. To circumvent these problems, there is increasing emphasis on separate study of cardiovascular effects using animals with telemetry implants to monitor cardiac parameters such as heart rate, blood pressure and electrocardiogram at regular intervals during the day. For the particular problem of QT interval prolongation, which was seen with drugs such as cisapride, there are *in vitro* studies that can give a reliable prediction of the presence or absence of this effect.

Table 9.4 Troubleshooting in general toxicology

Unexpected toxicity, compared with prior tests	Change in formulation or batch of test chemical. Poor predictivity of dose range finder studies due to factors such as differences in animal age, supplier or husbandry
Variation in individual response	Metabolic polymorphism or other genetic factor, social factors in group housing, e.g. nutrition status
Low systemic concentration or area under the curve (AUC)	Poor absorption or poor formulation; isotonicity is important in parenteral formulations. Extensive first pass effect. Short half-life
Low toxicity	Low availability; inappropriate route of administration or dose selection
Interspecies differences	Different ADME; different mechanism of effect; species specific mechanisms such as peroxisome proliferation; entero-hepatic recirculation. Different expression of or affinity for pharmacological receptors.
Different response in males and females	Especially in rodents; due to different activities of metabolism enzymes in liver particularly but also physiological differences such as alpha2-microglobulin excretion in males

Two critical areas of investigation in general toxicity studies are clinical pathology and morphological (post-mortem) pathology. Although both are capable of separate interpretation, their power is much greater when the data from both are combined. In this way, the presence of change in the blood or urine without associated change in morphological pathology can be put into perspective in terms of toxicological significance (Table 9.3). These investigations are useful during longer studies as they can indicate the target organ ahead of the terminal investigations and can lead to the use of specialist techniques for autopsy and microscopic examination. Generally, minor change in a single parameter, without any other correlative change, is unlikely to be of toxicological significance – especially if the values are within expectation (always assuming that there are enough historical data to give confidence).

Haematology

The critical groupings are indicated on page 86. The normal lifespan of an erythrocyte in the blood is around 100 days depending on species, and as they age they become less able to cope with oxidative stress. Aged or prematurely aged erythrocytes are removed by the spleen and if this process is accelerated anaemia can result. If the bone marrow is healthy there should be a compensatory increase in the immature forms of erythrocytes, particularly reticulocytes. Anaemia can also be induced by cell lysis in the peripheral circulation. Increased turnover of erythrocytes may be reflected in the presence of the pigment haemosiderin in the liver. Changes in the leucocyte counts – total and differential – can indicate immunotoxicity or effects in the bone marrow. Changes in coagulation parameters are infrequent but can indicate liver change as the coagulation factors are synthesised there.

Clinical chemistry and urinalysis

Changes in the plasma activity of enzymes can indicate the target organ for toxicity. Thus, increase in both alanine and aspartate aminotransferases (ALT and AST) is a good indicator for hepatic toxicity. An increase in the plasma activity of AST alone suggests a different target tissue, for instance muscle; this could be supported by increases in muscle enzymes such as creatine kinase or lactate dehydrogenase. Within the liver alkaline phosphatase (ALP) is found on the biliary side of the hepatocytes and increase suggests an effect on the biliary tree such as cholestasis. Increases in the plasma activity of aminotransferases may be due simply to increased permeability of the hepatocyte membrane and this may not be associated with microscopic change. Where the enzymes are mitochondrial in origin, as with glutamate dehydrogenase or, in the rat, ALT, increased presence in the plasma may be indicative of necrosis, which should be evident microscopically. The presence of isoenzymes can complicate interpretation. ALP has isoenzymes that are specific for the liver (see above), bone and gut. The bone isoenzyme decreases as growth slows and the gut isoenzyme varies diurnally according to the feeding cycle. There is also an isoenzyme of ALP in the kidney in the brush border of the proximal tubule lumen and the increased presence of this in the urine indicates renal toxicity.

In the plasma, renal effects are indicated by increases in the concentration of urea and creatinine together. Increase in one of these alone is not usually indicative of renal change, especially urea which may be increased due to inappetence and consequent nitrogen imbalance. Other indicators of renal toxicity are urinary volume and specific gravity or osmolality, total electrolyte output and the presence of various other analytes including proteins, blood pigments and cellular debris. Although urinary enzymes such as ALP and N-acetyl glucosaminidase are good indicators of renal effects they are not widely used in routine studies. The procedures used in urine collection should not be ignored in interpretation, including the duration of collection. Where the animals are placed in urine collection cages immediately after dosing, it is possible that the urine volumes and specific gravity will not reflect high water consumption recorded at other times of the study when free access to water is available. In this instance, in the absence of other evidence of renal change, the increased water consumption is probably a response to the dosing procedure rather than to any direct effect on the kidney.

A factor to consider in interpretation of enzyme activities is the variability of the values between animals and between examinations. For example, creatine kinase is very variable and the levels can be affected by exercise and other factors, such as restraint. Lactate dehydrogenase, another enzyme with well-known isoenzymes, is also highly variable and is now less often examined. In studies in non-human primates, ALP is often considered to be too variable for meaningful interpretation and is replaced by leucine aminopeptidase.

During longer studies, where several examinations of blood and urine are undertaken, change with continuing treatment (or reversal of change following cessation of treatment) can indicate the progress of toxicity or the development of tolerance to the effects of the test compound. At the end of the study these changes may be correlated with the presence of changes in the target organs when they are examined at necropsy, weighed and then processed histologically for microscopic examination.

Morphological pathology

Interpretation in pathology is a specialist area very much dependent on the experience of the pathologist performing the examination. Toxicological pathologists are famous for the variability of their opinions and it must be realised that an unwelcome conclusion will not be removed simply by getting another pathologist's viewpoint. What you then have is two opinions that are often slightly different and sometimes conflicting. The key to pathological confidence is to ensure that the peer review, which is undertaken before finalisation of the pathology report, is scrupulous, fully recorded and agreed. In examining differences in lesions, especially tumours, it is vital to ensure that the same number of sections have been examined from all the treated groups. Where macroscopic abnormalities are seen at necropsy in the highest dose group, more sections will be prepared and examined than in the controls. This can easily increase the recorded incidence of routine background findings, thus giving a false impression of treatment-related effect. Non-neoplastic findings are usually graded from minimal to severe or marked and it is possible to see effects as increases in severity with increasing dose or as increases in incidence and severity. It is important that the interpretation takes this into account. In general it is not practicable to provide historical control data for non-neoplastic pathology because the data collection is to a degree subjective, for instance in assigning grades. However, if there is an increase in incidence of a normal finding over the expected incidence in controls, it should be possible to offer an opinion on its significance. Considerations in this assessment include any increase in severity over expectation with increasing dose and the location and type of change.

In simplistic terms, the tissue, type, extent and reversibility of the findings determine the significance of pathological change. A minimal, centrilobular hepatocytic hypertrophy, with a slight increase in liver weight but without associated clinical pathology change, is likely to be of low toxicological significance if it is shown to be readily reversible. This type of effect is seen typically with minor induction of hepatic metabolism. Where the mechanism for an effect is known, as for haemosiderin deposition in the liver in haemolytic anaemia, the finding is also unlikely to be of toxicological significance, if the cause itself was not so great as to be of concern. Pigment deposits are unlikely to be quickly reversible, as the pigments tend to be slowly metabolised and therefore more persistent than easily repaired changes in tissues such as the liver or kidney. Changes in tissues that do not repair readily, such as the nervous system, are of much greater concern. These have to be considered in terms of no effect dose levels and the difference between toxic levels and those seen or expected in human populations. The levels of endocrine hormones are frequently not investigated in routine toxicity studies, in part because of the effects that stress can have on their plasma concentrations. However, examination of endocrine glands, or tissues under hormonal control, can indicate the presence of hormonal change and point to potential problems that may be seen in longer studies. This is due to the large influence that hormonal levels have on non-genotoxic carcinogenesis.

Reproductive toxicology

In general toxicology, the principal time-dependent change is growth, with increasing maturity and metabolic capability, which occur over the lifetime of the animal. In contrast, reproductive toxicology adds extra layers of complication, because of its sensitivity to disturbance and the added dimension of transient, time-specific processes, which themselves have considerable complexity. The final outcome – offspring that can reproduce in their turn – is influenced by effects on processes that start with male spermatogenesis and function, continue with mating behaviour in both sexes and gestation, culminating in parturition and post-natal care and development. To this can be added, in rare cases, transplacental carcinogenesis, as expressed by diethylstilbestrol.

Reproductive toxicology is an area in which *in vitro* screening has been adopted in order to speed the selection of compounds for further development or for chemicals already on the market, which have not been examined previously. These tests, although reasonably predictive of effects *in vivo*, are not infallible and it has to be asked whether the experiment has produced a result that is relevant to humans. Where the compound has been marketed for a significant time without problem and comes from a class of chemical which is not known for reproductive toxicity, it is probably reasonable to dismiss the *in vitro* data as not relevant – although it would be sensible to say why. Taking whole embryo culture as an example, the major differences from the situation in life are the absence of a placental barrier and of maternal metabolism, both of which can have a protective effect for the fetus.

Although it may be relatively simple to conclude, from basic data, that a chemical reduces fertility or that it causes a reduction in post-natal survival, the root cause may not be obvious. In considering the results of fertility studies it is useful to refer to the data from general toxicity studies for effects on reproductive organs or for data which might imply any hormonal effects. Depending on these data, and the existing knowledge of the compound's class and expected actions, it is important to confirm that the males were treated for long enough before mating to show any effects. Maternal toxicity is also a factor to consider. In general, guidelines require that the high dose be chosen so as to show toxicity but excessive maternal toxicity can result in delayed development in the uterus, which may imply effects that are not immediately relevant to humans at low exposure levels. Typical of these are retarded ossification and reduced fetal weights.

Much of the sensitivity of reproduction arises from the interdependence of factors such as hormonal balance, nutrition, behaviour, physiology, maintenance of the placental barrier and the complex balance in the embryo between growth, programmed cell death (apoptosis) and essential processes such as angiogenesis. Table 9.5 shows some of the problems that may be encountered in reproductive toxicity studies; it is by no means exhaustive. The conclusion is that interpretation of reproductive toxicity studies must be undertaken only when a full data set is available, including data for ADME. The data relating to fetal exposure and to excretion in the milk are particularly important in this and these tests should be undertaken if there is any question that these factors may be relevant to the results in the routine testing programme.

Genotoxicity

This is the one area of toxicological testing in which *in vitro* tests have been accepted by regulatory authorities, largely due to the relatively easy definition of

Table 9.5 Troubleshooting in reproductive toxicology

Reduced fertility – male	Spermatogenesis or other testicular change (see histopathology); epidydimal function changed; change in sperm quality (CASA results); behavioural change; stress
Reduced fertility – female	Lower implantation rate, increased post-implantation loss – possibly due to excessive maternal toxicity; behavioural change; stress
Wavy or extra ribs	Variant that is generally not thought to be significant
Unexpected toxicity in rabbits	Inappropriate vehicle – oils or other vehicles which affect gastrointestinal function are not suitable in rabbits. Stress can also be a factor in this species
Prolonged or abnormal parturition	Hormonal imbalance
Poor survival of pups post partum	Defective lactation or maternal care; excretion of test chemical or metabolites in milk

Note: The factors listed in Table 9.4 should also be considered.

the endpoint, which is essentially that of DNA damage either at the level of the gene or the chromosome (Tables 9.6 and 9.7). For secure conclusions to be drawn, all the genotoxicity studies need to be considered together. In contrast to other branches of toxicology, strength of response is not generally taken to be a prime factor in interpretation, as even a weak genotoxic response indicates mutagenic potential. Extrapolation from effective concentrations *in vitro* to those seen or expected *in vivo* is not sensible without caution and, as a consequence, no threshold is accepted for mutagenicity *in vitro*.

Having said that, interpreting the results as positive requires some care. A positive result is indicated by a clear dose–response curve; if there is a sudden increase in effect at high concentrations, this may be due to physical effects or toxicity and be irrelevant biologically. In addition the difference from controls should be statistically significant. The weakness of the statistical approach, as for many of these tests, is that as *n* is only 3 the statistical method is inevitably not especially powerful; use of larger numbers of negative controls (e.g. 6) helps this situation. Finally the results of the test for controls and positive controls should be compared with historical control data to confirm that they are within expectation. Positive results are sometimes found when testing early research batches of the chemical, due to the presence of impurities. These can also be introduced (or eliminated) by changes in production methods.

As with all toxicology, exposure must be demonstrated; this is generally not a problem *in vitro*, where even precipitates have been associated with geno-toxicity. Physicochemical properties that prevent the substance crossing the cell membrane and solubility in aqueous media may become limiting factors. Proof of exposure of the target cells is a particular problem in the *in vivo* micronucleus

Table 9.6 Guide to genotoxicity interpretation

Negative result	No dose–response curve or statistically significant increase in effect compared with the negative controls, providing the positive controls have performed as expected. *In vitro* this is confirmed in a second experiment, sometimes with different harvest times
Positive results	There should be a statistically significant increase with dose response. A two or three-fold increase over control values has been used
Micronucleus test	Mean micronucleus count in controls and positive controls must be sufficient for the study to be acceptable; indicative values are 4 and 10 micronuclei per 2000 polychromatic erythrocytes per animal respectively. There should be a dose–response curve with at least one point with a statistically significant increase in aberrations over the vehicle control
AMES tes	There should be a dose-related statistically significant increase in numbers of revertant colonies in two separate experiments. The strains indicate the following: TA1535, TA100 → Base substitution. TA1538, TA98 → frameshift. TA1537, TA97 → single frameshift
Cytogenetics – CHO cells	Clastogenic effect is indicated by a dose–response curve with at least one point having a statistically significant increase in aberrations over the solvent control. Reduced damage scored at higher dose levels may result from complex interactions between cell cycle and induced damage and the dose–response curve may not be a simple increase in damage with dose
Mouse lymphoma assay	Small colony size may indicate slow growth due to DNA damage, while large size indicates point mutation
UDS	Increase in nuclear grain count indicates a positive result. Autoradiography allows correction of grain counts for cytoplasmic synthesis of nucleic acids

test, especially with a negative result. In some cases, excessive toxicology or pharmacology limits the doses that can be achieved leading to inadequate exposure of the bone marrow. In these circumstances a negative result *in vivo* cannot offset a positive *in vitro* result.

The initial response to a positive result should be to ask if it is biologically relevant and how it has arisen. Before a positive result can be dismissed it is important to understand the underlying mechanism. Thresholds of response are a factor in assigning a negative result to a test. These may be due to interaction with non-DNA targets for instance through conjugation or lack of availability to DNA at low concentrations. This is seen with paracetamol, where the active metabolite is conjugated at low concentrations. There may also be metabolites that are not formed *in vivo* or in humans. Pharmacological activity, such as spindle inhibition, can also produce positive results.

Table 9.7 Troubleshooting in genotoxicity

General problems

Lack of toxicity or negative result	Possibly due to poor exposure. Mouse micronucleus test – limit dose 2000 mg/kg orally → no effect → has it been absorbed? Try parenteral dosing. (Negative result may be due to excessive toxicity)
No response in postive controls	Has the test system been correctly characterised?
Different results for different batches	Test substance purity. Manufacturing process changes
Cytotoxicity	Excessive cytotoxicity may give a positive result in chromosome aberration studies. In the mouse lymphoma assay positive responses at >90% cytotoxicity are not considered biologically relevant BUT need a close dose range to demonstrate reliable negative results
Positive *in vitro* not verifiable *in vivo*	Exposure *in vitro* cannot be replicated *in vivo* at target tissue. Can be due to poor absorption or excess pharmacology or different metabolism. If the positive result was with S-9 mix, does this mimic metabolism *in vivo* or in test species or in humans. Perform new *in vivo* test (UDS) or *in vivo* mutation
Positive result	Review of all data and assessment of cost/benefits. Choose additional assays that will help explain the result rather than simply add to the data set.

Troubleshooting in specific tests

Ames test	Lower colony counts at high concentrations may be due to toxicity which can conceal a positive result
In vitro mammalian cytogenetics or micronucleus	Chromosome damage at high concentrations in mammalian cells *in vitro* may indicate that the harvest times were inappropriate; different harvest times in the second experiment may help to clarify effects seen. Threshold effect or lack of dose response at high concentration may be without biological relevance, due to physical effects or toxicity or presence of metabolites at high concentration (in presence of S-9 mix)
In vivo micronucleus	Excess pharmacology or toxicity or poor absorption. First pass metabolism → poor systemic exposure to parent. Different active molecule at target tissue compared with *in vitro*. Excess stress may lead to a small increase in micronuclei
UDS	*Ex vivo* preferred over *in vitro*; autoradiography preferred over liquid scintillation counting

It is routine in genotoxicity testing *in vitro* to confirm the results of a first experiment in a second, preferably with slightly different conditions or harvest times. Because the assays are relatively inexpensive, it is easy to react to positive data by repeating assays or performing new tests. Amongst these, due to normal biological and statistical variation, there will be a proportion of results that are also positive. In these cases, as the data set grows, an overall interpretation becomes much more difficult.

Carcinogenicity

Data relevant to potential carcinogenicity are contained in several different study types, including the classic rodent lifespan bioassay. As with genotoxicity studies, which are a critical part of carcinogenicity assessment, the data package should be viewed as a whole. Data relevant to carcinogenicity can also be derived from routine toxicity studies and these can give valuable indicators for potential non-genotoxic carcinogenesis. Effects such as enzyme induction or the presence of hepatic foci with different staining characteristics may be associated with a later positive result in the carcinogenicity bioassays. As already said elsewhere, the genotoxic carcinogens are relatively easy to detect before getting to the stage of long-term studies, the chemicals that are carcinogenic indirectly are much more of a challenge. Classifications of carcinogens, for instance by IARC (International Agency for Research on Cancer) (Table 9.8) give useful background to interpretation in this often contentious area.

The mainstay of carcinogenicity assessment is still the two-year bioassay in rodents, although transgenic models are becoming more important, especially in the USA. The basic intention is to demonstrate the presence or absence of an increase in tumour incidence or burden in treated groups compared with appro-

Table 9.8 Carcinogen classification

Good epidemiological evidence in humans; about 30 compounds	Known human carcinogens, e.g. arsenic, benzene, vinyl chloride, aflatoxin	International Agency for Research on Cancer (IARC) group I
Limited epidemiological evidence, sufficient evidence in animals	Probable carcinogen; e.g. polychlorinated biphenyls, diethylnitrosamine, phenacetin	IARC group 2A
Insufficient human evidence, reasonable evidence in animals	Possible carcinogen; e.g. TCDD, DDT, diethyl-hexylphthalate	IARC group 2B
Not classifiable	Diazepam	IARC group 3
Not considered to be carcinogenic	Caprolactam	IARC group 4

Note: Compiled from sources in the bibliography.

priate controls. This apparently simple objective becomes increasingly complex as the various supporting or influencing factors are considered. Differences in tumour burden or time of onset (latency), between control and treated groups, may be attributable to a range of factors other than the simple mechanism of action of the test substance. These factors may be additive or negative in effect. Increased growth and bodyweight tend to increase tumour burden and to produce a different tumour distribution compared with animals that grow less and more slowly. This has been the subject of considerable debate in recent years and has resulted in the use of strains that do not eat and grow so much. In some models, the tumour incidence in the controls can approach 100 per cent which effectively reduces the information derivable from the study to an assessment of effect on latent period for tumours; this has been seen in some photocarcinogenicity protocols.

As with reproductive toxicology, carcinogenicity assessment is very dependent on the quality of the historical control database. If that is deficient, the assessment of the significance of rare tumours becomes much more difficult. Although use of a double control group will alleviate some of this, it cannot completely answer the problem. The use of mortality adjustment and statistics can only be of assistance with more common tumours and cannot address the single renal carcinoma that may be found in the high-dose group. In the lower dose groups a single rare tumour may not be a problem, providing there is no evidence of a U-shaped dose–response curve or of excess toxicity at the highest dose.

Other data that are available for assessment of carcinogenicity potential include the routine toxicity studies, genotoxicity, pharmacological actions (including those peripheral to that expected) and the metabolism and pharmacokinetics (Table 9.9). It should be borne in mind that pharmacokinetics and metabolism may differ at high doses from that seen in the lower dose groups and that the pharmacokinetics for the test compound may well change as the animals get older. In particular, renal function declines with age and, if there is any subclinical nephrotoxicity, may be accelerated by treatment. The assessment of toxicokinetics in long-term bioassays may not be available for the later stages of the study, as this is not always a regulatory requirement. This is a significant weakness of current guidelines.

Where a chemical has been shown to produce tumours in both sexes of both species or in several organs, it is a clear indication that this is a carcinogen of probable relevance to humans. Having said that, it has been difficult with some known human carcinogens, such as arsenic, to produce tumours in animals. Where there is an increase in tumour incidence in one sex in a single tissue, it is possible that this may be due to a non-genotoxic mechanism that is unlikely to be of relevance to humans. This requires mechanistic studies for confirmation of lack of relevance. This category contains a large number of chemicals acting through well-established mechanisms, such as peroxisome proliferators and those that act on the α2u globulin. These are associated with significant non-

Table 9.9 Guide to carcinogenicity interpretation

Tumour increases in both sexes, both species	Clear carcinogen with probable relevance to humans. Review genotoxicity data
Tumour increase in one sex in both species	Equivocal result; mechanistic studies may resolve this issue. Review genotoxicity and ADME data and all non-neoplastic pathology
Negative genotoxicity data, with tumour increase in one tissue, possibly in one sex	Possible non-genotoxic, species specific mechanism. Mechanistic studies should demonstrate (non)-relevance to humans. Results of routine toxicity studies may show evidence of early change in the affected tissue. Tumour increase is often associated with non-neoplastic change predisposing to tumour formation. Possible class effect. Established classes of chemical and effect, e.g. peroxisome proliferation
Low toxicity	MTD may not be achieved leading to doubtful regulatory acceptance; a 10% decrease in bodyweight gain due to reduced food consumption is not evidence of MTD unless backed up by pharmacokinetics and/or metabolism. Presence of excessive pharmacology at higher doses may be a factor
Lower food consumption in treated groups	Leads to lower tumour burden and increased lifespan through dietary restriction. Possibly due to poor palatability of diet if test substance offered with feed
Higher food consumption	Increased tumour burden and reduced survival
Increased survival in treated groups	Longer exposure may lead to different tumour burden of routine tumours in comparison with controls
Decreased survival	Tumour rates must be adjusted for mortality to account for lower numbers of animals exposed for full test duration. If this is confined to high dose this may be due to differential toxicity expressed only at high doses. Survival below 50% or 25 animals at completion of the study may invalidate the results for regulatory authorities
Increased incidence of tumour and associated non-neoplastic changes not seen with other compounds of same class	Compare pharmacokinetics of other compounds from same class; achieving similar levels of exposure may show similar histopathological changes indicating a class effect. Differential metabolism may be a factor
Increase in rare tumour.	Is the tumour in the high dose only? Is there a mechanistic explanation that is not applicable to humans? How recent and extensive is the background data at the test facility? Was this seen with other compounds of the same type? How frequent is this tumour in other historical control databases?
Increase in common tumour	Is the incidence within the historical control range? Is there a shorter or longer time to onset or is there a difference in survival between the groups? Dose response?
Increase in tumours in mouse liver	May not be relevant to humans as the mouse liver is sensitive to non-genotoxic compounds

neoplastic pathology in the affected tissues and are, theoretically, easy to predict from the results of the routine toxicity studies. With this type of data, it may be possible to prepare for interpretation of the carcinogenicity studies in advance by performing appropriate mechanistic studies. Non-genotoxic mechanisms of carcinogenicity are often accompanied by a clear threshold dose below which no effect is seen. Within a class of chemicals, differential absorption of the class members may lead to unexpected differences in effects in the rodent studies. This may be investigated by comparative assessment of toxicokinetics, as was shown for the fibrate family of hypolipidaemics; this is described in the ciprofibrate case study at the end of this chapter.

Environmental toxicology and ecotoxicology

Data for these linked disciplines relate to testing following deliberate (and known) exposure of individual test systems or specified areas (ecotoxicity tests), or investigation of unexpected effects in the environment as a whole (such as eggshell thinning or population changes) (Table 9.10). These data sets are distinct and set different challenges in interpretation. There is an implicit distinction between environmental events that affect people and those that affect the ecosystem as a whole. The former represents the interface between epidemiology and environmental toxicology and includes episodes that affect human populations. Ecotoxicology, by contrast can be taken to include effects

Table 9.10 Factors to consider in environmental toxicology

Controls	Are the controls correctly chosen and defined? If an area is selected as a control, is this area truly comparable with the study site?
Normality	How is normality or expectation defined and how recently was this definition produced?
Population dynamics	Populations change naturally in the absence of effect from synthetic chemicals and this may mask or enhance ecotoxicological differences. Population balance may be disturbed by factors outside the definition of the study limits.
Measured parameters	Was the correct parameter chosen for measurement – variability, normal levels, ease of measurement and relevance?
Observed differences	Are these direct or indirect? Are they (a) real (b) relevant?
Transient excess mortality	Was the period of record long enough to show effects that may have persisted beyond the study period? What were the effects of concurrent disease and increased susceptibility to subsequent disease? What is the differential mortality between polluted and non-polluted areas?

on other fauna and flora and their environment (the ecosystem), although the studies may well be similar to epidemiology, in that they concentrate on a single species. The presence of effects in humans due to pollution does not rule out effects on the local fauna and flora. In reports of smogs in Los Angeles or London, there are very few references to the effects on the urban wildlife. However, although there may be few reports of wildlife effects, it is counter-intuitive to infer an absence of toxicity when such far reaching human effects were seen.

Experimental ecotoxicology tests – of the type carried out to support registra-tion of chemicals such as pesticides – produce data that follow similar rules of interpretation as for other toxicity studies. With single species studies conducted in laboratory conditions, the data have to be extrapolated to the ecosystem or environment as a whole in much the same way that single-tissue studies *in vitro* have to be extrapolated to the whole organism. Understanding the dynamics of the test environment and study apparatus is an essential for correct inter-pretation and subsequent efforts to predict ecotoxicity. Mesocosm tests based on replicas of ecosystems or parts of ecosystems may give a better insight into effects based on interrelationships between different fauna and flora. In all cases it is important to define exposure and to chart distribution of the test chemical through the environment and then to follow its sequestration or elimination and to link this to the presence or absence of effect. One aspect of mesocosms is that with increasing complexity the greater the inherent variability becomes and, as a result, normality is more difficult to define. It is possible that clear-cut effects seen in the laboratory may be lost in the wider variation possible in a mesocosm experiment. At least with a mesocosm study the source of all the components should have been characterised before they were added to the system. With a field study this is less feasible but characterisation of the components must be as scrupulous, to avoid masking of treatment-related differences which might confound interpretation.

When an unexplained environmental effect is observed, there are similarities with the problems encountered in epidemiological studies. These include poor definition of exposure, difficulty of choice of controls and a multiplicity of interrelationships and dependencies that complicate interpretation. One of the first questions to be answered relates to exposure to synthetic chemicals, which may be previously identified markers of exposure or effect. Analysis of relevant tissues, corpses, soil samples or whatever sample is appropriate or available for chemicals is a specific indicator of exposure. One problem with such specificity is the greatly increased sensitivity of analytical technique. Presence at low levels is not necessarily causative and it must be decided if a chemical is present in sufficient quantity to be responsible for the observed effect. This is not always cut and dried. At one time Americans contained quantities of DDT but this was not linked to significant toxicity in the population as a whole, probably because most was sequestered into adipose tissue. One reason for the absence of human effect is specificity of toxic mechanism; another is the usual epidemiological difficulty of assigning cause and effect in conditions that are widely present in the general population. In predatory birds that showed eggshell thinning in response to accumulation of DDT up the food chain, it was found that a metabolite, DDE, reduced calcium deposition in the eggshell; this has so far not been a significant problem in Americans. Although markers of effect may also be indicative of exposure to a xenobiotic or environmental factor, they are not necessarily specific and the question has to be asked – 'were the markers relevant?' As with epidemiological studies it is important that a proposed cause and effect be linked by a credible toxicological mechanism, otherwise other causes should be considered.

Population decline, which can be a first indication of an ecotoxicological effect, may be due to a variety of causes such as reproductive failure or incapacity, habitat destruction, direct toxicity, amongst others. Accumulation of toxins in the study population in comparison with suitable controls from a similar location is a good indication of cause but it must be considered that such accumulation could be responsible for a different effect than the one being studied. Populations are dynamic and can respond to changes in pollutant levels quite quickly; this can make interpretation of studies carried out in successive breeding years much more complex. Any ecosystem is subject to a range of pressures and changes in species distribution and population are likely to be influenced by more than one simple factor. In the Great Lakes, populations of fish-eating birds have been affected by DDT-induced eggshell thinning, changes in fish populations in terms of numbers and species due to fishing practices and habitat; these various factors have worked together or independently to make year-to-year comparisons more difficult.

Data sets that accumulate following known pollution events such as oil spills or high concentration chemical releases into rivers, pose their own particular challenges. The first of these is that a trustworthy pre-incident characterisation of the local ecosystem is not always available. Spillage into a bay with low tidal exchange of water may mean that the effects will be localised and comparison with nearby or similar sites may be possible. Release into a river can be associated with long-distance transport of pollutants, as has been illustrated in the Rhine on at least two occasions. Interpretation of all such data is dependent on prior knowledge of the affected areas; the discovery of a difference from expectation does not necessarily imply relationship to recent high-profile pollution. Chronic low-level release – leakage from old mining activities or water reservoirs for holding washings from mines – is likely to have as significant effects as sudden release in large amounts. Furthermore, such low-level release may not become evident until long after the pollution started. One challenge is that a pollution incident seldom provokes only one study and that the data from different studies may not be collected in a manner that allows easy comparison of results or pooling of data to enable more powerful analysis. Uncoordinated study can simply lead to a greater database that is not conclusive.

Epidemiology and occupational toxicology

The differences between epidemiological and occupational toxicology, which are in some ways different parts of the same field, are subtle and relate in large part to the size and definition of the population under study. Both involve the study of chemically induced effects in populations, the epidemiological population usually being larger and more diverse than a worker group. This may be summed up by the difference between the workers in a chemical facility and the effects of discharge from the same facility on the surrounding community. The difference is also exemplified by smoking and vinyl chloride. The former investigation involved the population at large and in the latter a small, defined group of chemical workers was examined. The overlap between the two disciplines occurs at the point where a small group becomes a population – a community versus small focused groups of workers in an occupational setting. Epidemiology differs from mainstream toxicology in the methods used and the fact that sometimes it gives different results. It also tends to highlight an effect after it has happened, as was the case with asbestos, rather than indicate its probability beforehand.

In both areas it is important to ensure that the correct comparators are used with avoidance, as far as possible of confounding factors such as the healthy worker effect, where workers tend to be healthier than the general population (Table 9.11). Investigation in a wider context may be complicated by small differences from controls and differences in protocol. In the examination of the influence of the Mediterranean diet on longevity and health there have been suggestions that the genetics of the local population may be a significant factor and that the influence of olive oil and red wine may be less than hoped for by interested parties. Clearly, a lot more research is needed here, conducted locally in appropriately smoke-free bistros.

Epidemiology

The most contentious aspect of epidemiology is the interpretation of small differences from expectation or controls. This is seen with conditions or events that have a significant natural background incidence in populations or environments that are inherently variable and often poorly controlled. This leads to poor reproducibility of results from one study to the next, interpretation of which is made more difficult by differences between protocols and chosen populations. These methodological differences reduce the extent to which data can be pooled for extended analyses of the whole database. It is only when associations are very strong that the results of epidemiological study are accepted with anything resembling speed. The postulated decline in sperm counts in response to environmental oestrogens is a case in point. Interpretation has been hampered by analysis and re-analysis of data with conflicting results, variability in sperm counts due to seasonal factors, donors, health, occupation, counting techniques and sample quality. Although there may be, intuitively, a

Table 9.11 Factors in epidemiology and occupational toxicity

Controls	Healthy worker effect. Population chosen – influence on study outcome
Confounding factors	Alcohol, smoking, occupational exposures. Effects that are synergistic or additive to that of the investigated substance
Faulty or inconsistent differential diagnosis	Poor distinction between conditions having similar symptoms but different aetiology; e.g. bronchitis may be bacterial or viral or associated with smoking, atmospheric pollution or occupational exposure
Questionaire	If questionaires were used for data collection, was the wording structured so as to avoid bias?
Definition of exposure	In epidemiology by history of persons; in occupational toxicology by personal monitoring equipment and by urine and blood collection for analysis
Biological markers	Is the chosen marker specific for the chemical of concern or for the same group, e.g. cholinesterase inhibition. Is it a measure of exposure or effect or susceptibility?
Statistical significance	Spurious significances due to numbers of relationships being examined in some studies – leads inevitably to a number of false positives
Data accessiility	In some data sets there is a temptation to collect and analyse only the more easily accessible data; this can lead to bias
Significant contributing factors not considered	Genetics, lifestyle, intercurrent disease. Recent papers have suggested that the greater survival seen with the Mediterranean diet may be due to genetic factors

toxicological mechanism that can be held responsible, the differences from controls have not been large enough to satisfy epidemiologists of cause and effect. The overriding problem here is the normal variation that is inherent in the population and the consequent inability to produce a sufficiently robust definition of normality.

A crucial task for epidemiological toxicologists is the definition of the extent and duration of exposure to the chemical of concern. Human life is seldom challenged by a single chemical at high doses, but is subject to exposure by a mixture of many chemicals at individually low doses, although the total exposure may be huge when expressed in milligrams per day. In general, mixtures, especially undefined mixtures, are much more difficult to assess due to antagonistic and synergistic interactions of the various components. The effects of oxidative attack by chemicals, present naturally or as contaminants in the environment, can be offset by high levels of dietary antioxidants, absorption of which may itself be compromised by the presence or absence of other dietary components.

Added to this is the problem that disease is seldom an immediate response to exposure, although asthma and other allergies are notable exceptions to this.

The time lapse between exposure and response, especially to long-term (chronic) low-level exposure, makes attribution nearly impossible unless the response is unusual or rare. Therefore, it is generally not possible to ascribe a common tumour such as breast cancer to a specific cause in a patient for whom there is no predisposing exposure defined. In contrast, despite the long latency period, it is relatively straight forward to ascribe mesothelioma to occupational exposure to asbestos because it is rare tumour found in an easily characterised population. One approach is to use the concept of excess mortality. That is, in specific conditions, it may be possible to attribute deaths above the normal rate to those conditions. In smogs in London in 1952 the numbers of excess deaths attributable to the atmospheric conditions was calculated up to December of that year. However, if the excess mortality figures are plotted into the following months, the number of deaths that may have been due to the initial smog increases significantly.[1,2] A challenge for epidemiologists, therefore, is knowing where to draw a line between clear toxic effect and normal background and showing when change in normality is due to toxicity.

Occupational toxicology

While epidemiological data may relate to hundreds of people, the occupational toxicologist may be presented with data from a single individual, for instance DNA adduct analysis in the urine of an employee handling a potentially reactive chemical. Unless the difference from expectation is large, interpretation of a single data point is difficult. Ideally there should be baseline data from the same individual before exposure took place or from unexposed workers in the same plant or area. It should be possible to chart the exposure from baseline and start of work, to abnormal DNA adduct levels during work and then a return to normal when the shift stops. Before any trustworthy assessment is attempted it must be confirmed that the increase in DNA adducts is not only a marker for exposure but also for the adverse effect attributed to the chemical being handled; without this vital linkage being made, valid conclusions cannot be drawn. One of the principal advantages that an occupational toxicologist has over an epidemiologist is the relative strength of definition of exposure that is available in the workplace, in terms of identity and, often, of dose. In either field, the criteria for attribution include definition of exposure, exclusion of confounding factors, a clear significant connection between exposure and condition and a supportable mechanistic explanation. With such data to hand it should become possible to attribute an individual case or group of cases to a particular cause. The confidence with which this can be done becomes critical when there is a legal case to answer, especially in occupational health cases.

When attempting to interpret the relationship between exposure to a particular chemical and effects in the workplace, it is important to consider alternative sources of exposure to the substance of interest. For example formaldehyde, a commonly used chemical, has a wide presence in the home, in carpets, furniture, clothing and home insulation products. Other factors must be considered, for example radon, smoking and other agents such as diesel exhausts may make a synergistic or additive contribution to the incidence of lung cancer in underground miners. When these additional external factors are taken into consideration, it should be possible to draw a conclusion as to whether the cancer is connected with occupational exposure to the chemical. For individual cancers, which are not part of a group or specific to a particular agent, it is highly unlikely that a connection between it and a specific exposure can be drawn.

In contrast to epidemiology, interpretation of effects in the workplace may be facilitated by the relative certainty of what the exposure was, the presence (usually) of a condition in a specific group of workers and the timing of effect in the affected individuals. Thus, response to a chemical in the workplace may be seen at a higher level or incidence towards the end of the working day or at particular times or during particular processes and may resolve at weekends. Ventilation, especially the recirculation of air in new buildings, is an important consideration and can be associated with sick building syndrome.

Biological markers are an essential tool of the occupational toxicologist but, as with all tools, their limitations have to be accounted for in interpretation of their data. The basic contention is that exposure to a chemical is associated with change that may be seen as variations in the concentration, expression or activity of a biological marker. This type of change, which in all probability is subclinical in the early stage of exposure, may lead to organ dysfunction later in life, with associated clinical consequences. If levels of the biological marker are monitored, pre-emptive action may be taken to prevent further exposure. From the data it should be feasible to extrapolate backwards to the exposure and forwards to the prospective clinical outcome. In order to be of use in the investigation of potential effects, biological markers should be as specific as possible to the chemical of concern. In essence they are markers of exposure, effect or susceptibility to effect. The most specific marker available is analysis of blood or urine for the presence of the chemical or its metabolites. Certain markers of effect are specific for particular groups of chemicals, such as inhibition of acetyl cholinesterase due to exposure to organophosphate or carbamate insecticides. Other markers, such as DNA adducts, are produced by a wider range of chemicals and are not peculiar to any single chemical unless specifically identified as such.

Once a biological marker has been validated as being specific or indicative for exposure to a particular chemical or type of exposure, it should be possible to interpret data from individuals. A change in the value for a marker from baseline for that individual (beyond normal variation) or from general expectation indicates excessive exposure and the possibility of subsequent clinical effects if exposure is not minimised or halted. In validating biological markers in animal experiments it should be remembered that the thresholds of toxicity may differ between the experimental animal and humans; this is especially significant if humans are more susceptible than the test animals.

There should be interactive interpretation between toxicology and epidemiology. Increasing use of biological markers should encourage the interaction between the two disciplines through consideration of toxicological sequelae of exposure and the mechanism of effects attributable to chemicals.

Case studies – ciprofibrate and genetically modified potatoes

Ciprofibrate

Ciprofibrate, a derivative of phenoxyisobutyrate, is one of a series of hypolipidaemic compounds (fibrates) which includes clofibrate, bezafibrate and fenofibrate. All have marked hypolipidaemic activity in humans and animals, reducing both plasma cholesterol and triglycerides through effects on low or very low density lipoproteins. The animal toxicity of fibrates has been reviewed by Bonner et al.[3] They are well known as peroxisome proliferators, an effect that is known to be associated with hepatocarcinogenicity in rodents; the class as a whole is non-mutagenic. The safety evaluation programme for ciprofibrate, which was conducted in the light of previous work on earlier members of the series, showed up a number of toxicities in rodents, which required explanation. These consisted primarily of liver changes, with associated effects in the thyroids and the presence of a low incidence of carcinoid tumours in the glandular mucosa of the rat stomach.

Peroxisome proliferation was noted in both rats and mice.[4] together with increased liver size. This was associated with hepatic adenomas and hepatocellular carcinomas, which were seen in the long-term carcinogenicity studies. There were also functional and morphological changes in the thyroid of rats,[5,6] which were associated with decreased plasma concentrations of thyroxine (T4) and with minimal to mild thyroid follicular hyperplasia. The morphological changes were considered to be consistent with increased thyroid activity. Increased metabolism of thryoid hormones as a result of hepatic enzyme induction is often associated with increased plasma concentrations of thyroid-stimulating hormone (TSH) as a result of the absence of the negative feedback provided by normal T4 or T3 levels. Although TSH was shown to be increased over short administration periods this was not demonstrated in longer studies, a situation that is not unusual due to compensatory mechanisms.

To demonstrate the rodent specificity of the hepatic effects, a long-term study in marmosets showed a lack of peroxisome proliferation; although liver changes were seen, these were an order of magnitude lower than in the rat.[7] In view of the long-standing association of peroxisome proliferation with hepatocarcinogenesis and of hepatic enzyme induction with thryoid change, these various effects were not unexpected. They are known to be specific to rodents and to have no relevance to humans, a point underlined by the absence of effect in the marmoset.

Although the liver and thyroid effects were expected and explainable, the presence of carcinoid tumours in the glandular fundus of the stomach of Fischer rats posed a problem that was potentially more serious. The incidence of gastric carcinoid tumours was 5/59 males and 1/60 females seen in animals that survived for the whole study at 10 mg/kg/day in the diet. Marked hyperplasia of fundic neuroendocrine cells was seen in non-tumour-bearing animals of this group with other changes in microscopic gastric morphology. These changes were not seen in the mouse and were not reported with other fibrates. However, this type of carcinoid tumour had also been seen with long-acting gastric antisecretory compounds such as omeprazole. An investigation was mounted to discover whether there was a secondary pharmacological action of ciprofibrate on gastric secretion and to determine the sequence of events in tumour formation. Two other objectives were to look for this effect in other species and to ask if other fibrates had the same effects. The duration of antisecretory activity is proportional to the likelihood of tumour formation. Thus, the long-acting H_2-antagonist loxtidine and proton pump inhibitor omeprazole have both been associated with gastric carcinoid formation. Shorter acting compounds such as cimetidine, in once-daily regimens, are not associated with this change.

Following treatment of rats with ciprofibrate, changes were seen in the acid-secreting oxyntic cells – hypertrophy, with eosinophilia and reduced vacuolation of the cytoplasm, associated with reduced secretory cell organelles. In separate studies ciprofibrate was shown to decrease acid secretion and the volume of gastric juice, an effect that was also shown with other fibrates. However, in a 26-week comparative study with once-daily dosing of bezafibrate in rats, no similar changes were seen. Investigation of the pharmacokinetics of the two compounds[8] showed that the elimination half-life of ciprofibrate was significantly longer than for bezafibrate – 3–4 days and 5 hours respectively. To reproduce the systemic exposure pattern for ciprofibrate, bezafibrate was administered twice daily at 12-hour intervals; this was successful in producing similar changes to those seen with ciprofibrate given once daily. Furthermore, ciprofibrate given at 10 mg/kg every 48 hours gave similar sustained plasma concentrations to those produced by bezafibrate given at 125 mg/kg every 12 hours.

Gastrin stimulates acid secretion, with low gastric pH acting as a negative feedback mechanism. It is also involved in regulation of mucosal growth, exerting a trophic action on neuroendocrine cells. Reduced acid secretion can therefore lead to hypergastrinaemia, which, if sustained may produce neuro-endocrine cell hyperplasia in the gastric mucosa. Ciprofibrate given at 20 mg/kg/day to rats gave a modest but statistically significant hypergastrinaemia over a period of 56 days. Investigation of other fibrates showed that twice-daily administration of bezafibrate at 150 mg/kg also produced increased plasma levels of gastrin after 12 weeks. Clofibrate twice daily at 75 mg/kg was shown to have similar effects. That these changes in gastrin concentration were dependent on pharmacokinetics was illustrated by the finding that ciprofibrate given once every 48 hours at 20 mg/kg produced less hypergastrinaemia than with daily dosing. Morphologically, six to nine months treatment two or three times daily with bezafibrate or clofibrate at up to 150 mg/kg produced similar changes in neuroendocrine cells in the stomach to those seen with ciprofibrate, consistent with prolonged mild hypergastrinaemia.

The species specificity of the changes in gastrin concentrations were examined in mice and marmosets. While mice showed a transient increase in plasma gastrin concentrations, this was not sustained and there was no evidence of change in the morphology of the gastric mucosa. These findings are consistent with the absence of gastric carcinoids from the two-year carcinogenicity study in mice. Similarly, there was no change in plasma gastrin level in the marmoset over a 26-week treatment period. Although there were some minor changes in the oxyntic cells in marmosets after 26 weeks of treatment at 100 mg/kg, there was no evidence of change in the neuroendocrine cells. In addition, hypergastrinaemia was not seen in humans.

A hypothesis was constructed that prolonged antisecretory activity induced by ciprofibrate (in contrast to the transient effect seen with bezafibrate and clofibrate in once-daily dosing regimens) leads to hypergastrinaemia and a persistent trophic stimulus with hyperplasia of the neuroendocrine cells. This latter effect is responsible for the gastric carcinoid tumours seen in rats. Prolonging the antisecretory activity of bezafibrate and clofibrate by twice daily administration leads to similar effects as seen with ciprofibrate.

Overview

From this case study it may be seen that rapid clearance of drugs can mean that toxicity is not manifested and that toxic potential is not predicted adequately. Determination of the duration and consistency of exposure is critical in the interpretation of the data and this should be correlated with the pharmacodynamics of the compound. Persistence of an otherwise easily reversible change, as seen with the fibrates and hypergastrinaemia, may lead to unexpected effects that have significance for the development of the compound. Equally, it is important to look at the species specificity of these changes to assess their relevance to the ultimate target species, which is usually humans. In terms of interpretation, it is clear from this investigation that, at each stage, consideration of the accumulating data and of relevant literature allowed a logical progression of studies and a solidly based interpretation of the findings when the process was complete.

Genetically modified potatoes

Whereas the investigation of ciprofibrate was a carefully conducted evaluation of its safety, with a specific goal in mind, many toxicological data sets do not arise from such carefully coordinated programmes. Instead, knowledge bases on particular compounds or chemical classes tend to accumulate as research in different laboratories continues. The challenge for interpretation is that the various research programmes contributing to the database, may develop at best on parallel lines, making for a heterogeneous data set, within which cross-comparison becomes difficult. There is a considerable temptation to interpret individual studies in isolation and without due consideration of any weaknesses in their design and execution.

This is exemplified by some investigations in animals into the effects of high concentrations of normal components of the human diet (see Box 1.2 also). Many chemicals naturally present in our diet are potentially toxic, in accordance with Paracelsius' dictum that everything can be a poison if the dose is high enough. The problem with the study of these chemicals is encapsulated by the consideration that the most appropriate route of administration is in the diet. However, it is difficult to give the very high doses that are necessary to evoke toxicity, without distorting the dietary composition to the extent where nutritional imbalance becomes a confounding factor. Although gavage administration may facilitate higher dose levels, the formulation is unlikely to be representative of the normal diet, which is a complex mixture that has far reaching effects on the absorption of chemicals. Studies using the drinking water are compromised in a similar manner and are additionally subject to the inherent uncertainty of calculation of achieved dose levels.

Potatoes have been a focus for toxicological interest for many years. They are from the same family of plants as deadly nightshade and contain related alkaloids such as solanine, which is found particularly in the green skin of potatoes that have been exposed to light. A review by Christie,[9] suggested that many cases of schizophrenia may be associated with consumption of potatoes. A selection of the alkaloids present in potatoes was assessed in the Xenopus assay in vitro for teratogenesis[10] and their potential for teratogenicity was confirmed. The general toxicity of solanaceous alkaloids is well known. In other words, potatoes are a typical dietary constituent, in that administration to animals of certain natural components at high dose levels could be expected to be associated with undesirable effects. The addition, by genetic modification, of a new chemical entity to this existing cocktail could be expected to be of toxicological interest, depending on the expression levels and final content in a normal diet.

Genetic modification of food plants has caused a storm of controversy in recent years as debate has raged over their potential effects on human health and the environment. Induced expression of compounds that may increase resistance to insects, and so reduce the amounts of damage caused during growth or storage, has been a particular bone of contention. Accordingly, there was considerable debate about an experiment in rats given diets containing genetically modified (GM) potatoes, which were published and reviewed in the Lancet in 1999.[11-13] This work examined potatoes that had been genetically modified to express a snowdrop lectin (Galanthus nivalis agglutinin) to reduce damage from insects and nematodes.

Lectins are a group of proteins and glycoproteins that can bind specific carbohydrates, such as mannose. They are present in numerous plants and include ricin and the toxic component of uncooked red kidney beans. They have known effects on the morphology of the small intestine and combination of lectins with receptors in the intestine wall may result in inhibition of use of some nutrients. In this contentious experiment, groups of six rats (their age and sex were not specified in the *Lancet* report) were fed non-genetically modified potatoes, raw or boiled GM potatoes, or raw or boiled non-genetically modified potatoes that had been supplemented with the lectin. The composition of the diets was not given, beyond indicating that they contained 6 per cent protein and had the same energy levels. However, low-protein diets are associated with reduced growth and impaired liver metabolism and immune function. The diets were fed to the rats for 10 days, after which they were killed and the gastro-intestinal tracts examined. Changes were seen that were attributed to the presence of the added lectin; however, these were consistent with the known gastrointestinal effects of lectins. Kuiper *et al.*[13] point out that caecal hyper-trophy, seen in this experiment in rats fed raw potatoes, is a common response in rats fed poorly digestible carbohydrates such as potato starch.

Overview

The study was imperfectly controlled as there were no animals in the experiment that received a normal diet and the effects of a low-protein diet in rats of the same strain and age were not examined. Thus, there was no indication of what constituted the normality against which the changes could be assessed. The changes seen, which were assessed principally by crypt length, were of the type that is likely to be readily reversible on cessation of treatment. Because the experiment lasted only 10 days, the chronic effects of such high-level dietary inclusion were not investigated. There was no attempt to define the dose–response relationship and so to assess the presence of no effect levels. Finally, the relevance of feeding raw potato should be questioned as this not representative of normal human dietary practice.

Although it might be possible to say that the inclusion of the lectin or the genetic construct, caused changes in the gastrointestinal tracts of the rats, it was not possible to make a scientific assessment of whether this result was significant for human consumers. To do that, it would be necessary to conduct a properly designed longer study in male and female rats with different levels of treatment. This type of study is always difficult to design and interpret because at abnormally high inclusion levels of any dietary component the response of the animals becomes clouded by the fact that they are receiving an abnormal diet. It is usual to restrict non-nutrient components of experimental diets to 10 per cent or less. This work demonstrates the dangers of making sweeping interpretative conclusions from imperfect information. The study was potentially useful as a preliminary experiment but should in no way be considered definitive. In particular, it is impossible to draw secure conclusions from the data from such an experiment; the toxicological significance of the changes seen could not be assessed in such a design. Interpretation of the findings was not sensible without further work and it is certainly not sensible to draw any conclusions related to the relevance of the findings to humans. The only conclusion that can be drawn from this study is that further work might be of interest.

The fundamentals of interpretation

The following are suggested as a basic set of rules for successful interpretation of toxicological data:

- The whole picture is needed for secure conclusions to be drawn.
- A definition of normality, provided by adequate controls or historical control data is essential.
- The experimental protocol must be sufficiently robust to achieve the stated experimental objectives.
- Confounding factors due to husbandry or experimental technique or procedures must be excluded or accounted for.
- Do not over-interpret or extrapolate from small or poorly controlled data sets.
- In the immediate aftermath of a crisis or incident, it is difficult to achieve correct interpretation as data will continue to emerge as the situation progresses.
- Above all, you cannot interpret the data unless you understand what they mean.

When you know the meaning of the results, it should be possible to interpret them and then to perform an extrapolation to humans. Interpretation is an evolutionary process and is supported by appropriate additional experiments to test developing hypotheses for mechanism of effect and species specificity. From this basis it should be possible to perform a prediction of the compounds toxic potential in humans and this is addressed in the next chapter; needless to say, the bedrock of an accurate prediction is secure interpretation of the full set of toxicity data and all other supporting information.

Chapter 10

Prediction of hazard

Introduction

The previous chapters have covered the background and process of testing, that seeks to show differences from normality which may represent toxicity, and the interpretation of the resulting ocean of data. This chapter sets out to explore the process of hazard prediction that takes place once the results of toxicological investigations have been collated and reported. In the context of this book, it is seen as high-level interpretation of the whole data set that takes place after interpretation of individual studies but before risk assessment and management. The emphasis here is on defensive toxicology, showing lack of relevance to humans or other target species, as that is a major driver for continuing the development of a chemical, particularly new pharmaceuticals. The safety evaluation studies identify hazards, which are then subjected to hazard characterisation, after which it should be possible to predict which hazards are relevant for risk assessment. Inevitably there is substantial overlap between these processes. Risk assessment is carried out on one hazard at a time and so it is important to identify and prioritise human-relevant hazards before embarking on the next stage.

There are a number of settings in which this process of prediction is required, including preparation of applications for field trials with pesticides, for first dose in humans with novel pharmaceuticals and when establishing best work practices with chemicals. Assessment of toxicities as relevant hazards for humans has taken on much greater significance as the cost of chemical development has soared. Rising cost has encouraged investigation of toxicity to show lack of relevance to humans and to recoup the huge costs of development. As *in vitro* methods of investigation have improved, these investigations have become ever more focused. Frequently, these take the form of *in vitro* comparative experiments in which human tissues are used with tissues from the test species. If the effects seen can be shown to be irrelevant to humans, the chemical may still be worth developing, other factors being favourable.

Hazard, risk and human-relevant hazard

It is important to distinguish between hazard and risk. Hazard is the description of the adverse effects of a chemical; it is not quantitative and does not take exposure, dose or form into consideration. Risk is the probability that this hazard will occur; clearly, if there is no hazard there is no risk. Hazards of concern to humans are broadly cancer, reproductive effects, debilitating illness or disease and workplace-related effects that might prevent them working. In addition, any potential progressive, degenerative change that may be due to acceleration of normal age-related decline in function should be considered. Needless to say this type of insidiously progressive change is extremely difficult to predict from toxicological data because the circumstances for each individual at risk are so different, in terms of genetics, exposure, diet and other factors that influence individual responses.

A hazard identified for animals is not necessarily a hazard for humans – for example peroxisome proliferation, which is associated with hepatic carcinogenesis in rodents, is not considered to be a hazard for humans due to differences in hepatic metabolism. The object is to predict which toxicological effects detected in the safety evaluation have significant potential to be expressed in humans and so to identify them as being relevant for the risk assessment process. This indicates the need for accuracy in prediction, as it is important that false positives and negatives are avoided; the former may divert attention from real hazard and the latter may expose people to unacceptable toxicity. Hazard characterisation is reliant on correct overall interpretation of the various studies and this, in turn, is dependent on the interdependent interpretation of studies within each toxicological discipline, taking account of any overlap with other areas. For instance the interpretation of data from reproductive studies may be influenced by findings in general toxicity studies, such as testicular atrophy. It is vital, therefore, that all evidence be considered and that the interpretation of all studies is used to extrapolate a prediction of effect in the target species, which is usually humans.

Circumstances of hazard prediction

In evaluating chemicals, especially new synthetic chemicals, it is important to distinguish between hazards that are specific to the various test systems used during safety evaluation and those that might affect humans or the environment. The objective is to protect humanity, the environment or any specific target from potential adverse effects, that might arise from the use of novel chemicals. This can apply also to natural chemicals that are proposed for use in unnaturally high concentrations or circumstances.

Predictions of hazard are made to support the use of new drugs in clinical trials, especially for first administration to healthy volunteers, for pesticide field trials, workplace exposures during production, environmental effects and for the use of food additives. Differences in target populations may modify hazard assessment or significance; teratogenicity is not a hazard for an exclusively male population, although many teratogens, such as thalidomide and diethylstilbestrol, also have effects on the male reproductive system. The presence of disease may modify the response to a chemical, particularly a drug. Thus, patients may benefit from taking a drug but healthy workers may show an adverse response, usually an unwanted pharmacological effect. Although there are populations for which particular hazards are not relevant, factors that affect the response of the individual do not affect the relevance of the hazard, but they do modify the risk. Uranium miners are all subject to the hazard of lung cancer as a result of their workplace exposures, but for smokers the risk is much greater than for non-smoking miners. Likewise, the toxicities expressed by slow and fast metabolisers of isoniazid may be different but it is sensible to consider that the hazard of both is relevant to both populations of patient; it is simply the risk that is different.

Prediction of hazard to the environment or the ecosystem is more complex than that for human populations as the scope for interactions is much greater. There may be some sense in drawing a distinction between an environmental hazard that affects humans directly, for example release of oestrogenic substances or discharge into drinking water, and those which affect the ecosystem as a whole. The latter will affect humanity indirectly but is likely to be much less emotive to the general population than a perceived direct effect such as cancer.

Principles of prediction

There are two 'simple' stages of hazard prediction, firstly identification of the hazard – usually from the animal and *in vitro* studies that are available – and then assessment of the relevance of the hazard to humans. There have been two approaches to these linked questions. The first (and least discriminating) was that any hazard identified in animals was relevant to humans and that the second question was therefore irrelevant. It was this type of assumption that spawned the Delaney amendment, by which any substance shown to cause cancer in animals should not be allowed as a food additive in the USA. The problem with this is that practically anything can be shown to cause cancer in animals if you are sufficiently dedicated and the dose levels are high enough. Such dedication has shown that a natural constituent of mushrooms, 4-hydrazinobenzoic acid, can cause tumours in mice when administered in the drinking water at high dose levels (Box 1.2). This might become relevant to humans if people start drinking mushroom ketchup in large quantities.

The second approach weighs all the evidence and subjects it to a process of expert judgement to arrive at a conclusion as to the relevance of the changes seen. In particular, the inadequacy or appropriateness of experiments should be taken into account when assessing the data and the credibility of conclusions reached in individual studies. Data from inadequate or poorly conducted studies should carry significantly less weight than those that are clearly robust scientific-ally. The terms 'strength' and 'weight' of evidence have been used to describe assessment approaches to data but it is extremely difficult to find a satisfactory definition of either. In view of the ambiguity possible with the use of such similar words as strength and weight in this context, it is probably best to ignore attempts to name the process by which the data are assessed. The clear essential is that all data should be assessed – for adequacy as well as for scientific content – and that there should be an expert judgement of their relevance to humans.

Identification of hazard is essentially independent of dose and formulation but this must be considered within reasonable limits. Thus, for the case of 4-hydrazinobenzoic acid in mushrooms and its carcinogenicity in mice, the relevance of the hazard needs to be assessed. Given that there was a question of formulation relevance in the various studies (the material was given in the drinking water), the inadequate design of the study, and the large daily intake of whole mushrooms that would be necessary to produce tumours, it is likely that this hazard is not relevant to humans. This conclusion is supported by the absence of any epidemiological evidence of carcinogenic effect of mushrooms in humans. Although folklore cannot be considered to be scientific evidence, much is based on historic experience and it *may* be an indicator of effect; this may become politically embarrassing when there is public belief but no demonstrable mechanism of action.

Toxicities – or hazards – that are revealed in safety evaluation studies are usually placed in areas of effect, such as reproductive or genotoxicity. This is simply a reflection of the fields into which toxicology, particularly regulatory toxicology, has been divided for evaluation of the functions that are considered to be significant to the consuming public. These comfortable divisions tend to ignore the fact that some substances have undesirable activity across the whole toxicological spectrum and, conversely, that some very toxic substances do not have toxicity predicted for them in certain areas. Conventional toxicology teaching tends to address one aspect of a compound's toxicity at a time, for instance emphasising the hepatotoxicity of paracetamol (acetaminophen) while not mentioning its renal effects, which may be seen independently of overdose and particularly in combination therapy with other non-steroidal anti-inflam-matory drugs. TCDD is reported to be a carcinogen, immunotoxic, to be acutely toxic in animals, and to affect male reproductive capacity. In genotoxicity, however, results have been largely negative and evidence suggests that it is not genotoxic. For many compounds there is overlap between findings in general toxicology and those in other areas such as reproductive toxicology or carcino-genicity; effects in one area may indicate potential effect in another. The corollary of this is that although it may appear neater to pigeonhole the various effects into simplistic categories, this may not be the best option from point of view of the hazard prediction.

Having identified a hazard from the safety evaluation data, relevance to humans may be assessed by knowledge of the mechanism by which the effect was achieved. For this to be successful there has to be thorough understanding of the comparative physiology of the test systems and of humans. For instance, the action of hepatic peroxisome proliferators in rodents has been shown to be a rodent-specific effect through comparative studies, including long-term studies in marmosets and *in vitro* studies in human hepatocytes. Similarly, the renal toxicity seen in male rats with compounds that complex with α-2u globulin has no human relevance due to the absence of these proteins in humans. Although an effect seen in animals may be expected to be absent in humans due to differences in pharmacokinetics or quantitative differences in metabolic pathways, this does not necessarily remove it as a potential human hazard. Due to the wide variation in the human population, it is possible that metabolic polymorphisms and other individual differences may be able to reproduce the effect in susceptible individuals. The likelihood of this happening is assessed through risk assessment.

In summary, the overriding principle of hazard prediction is that all the data should be assessed and that a mechanistic explanation sought for any effects seen. If there is a scientifically acceptable explanation for an effect, an assessment may then be made of the relevance for humans. If the specific mechanism of toxicity is absent in humans, it is probably reasonable to conclude that the hazard is not relevant to humans. Where there is no explanation of effect other aspects of the data must be considered, including dose response and comparative ADME.

Steps in the prediction process

The following sections look at the process by which toxicities are examined and predicted to be relevant or otherwise as hazards to humans; although the emphasis is on human-relevant effects, the general remarks should be relevant to other targets, such as other animals or the environment.

Prediction of hazard is an evolving process. Initial predictions made from the data of early studies are tested in further studies and then 'finalised' when the programme has been completed. These predictions may be revised as more data are gathered. Epidemiological study in target populations is often the source of such data and is used to test the earlier predictions made from toxicity studies and any trial data in humans. Because epidemiological studies are initiated after the release of the compound onto the market they are not predictive unless used to support changes in use of the test compound. However, epidemiological studies for similar chemicals may be used to support predictions of safety (or hazard) made for the test chemical.

Basic preliminary questions

Before embarking on the process of hazard prediction (or characterisation) the objective has to be clearly defined by asking the question 'What are you attempting to predict?' The reason for the prediction has to be considered in the light of the intended use of the chemical and, as a result, what is the expected target population. The objective should indicate the type of data that are necessary (or optimal, as they are often not all present) for successful prediction. A further consideration is the level of prediction required. The process is influenced by the specificity required, whether the whole population is concerned, a selected part of that population (e.g. farm workers), a patient group, an individual or the environment and ecosystem. Prediction in the early phases of chemical development may simply relate to test system choice, for instance using data from *in vitro* comparative metabolism studies for species selection.

As described below, prediction may also use computer models or expert systems to predict hazard and a choice has to be made of which should be used. Using one system in isolation is likely to give a skewed perception of the real hazards involved, while using every system in existence will cloud the issue irretrievably. System selection should be carried out in the knowledge of the weaknesses of the available options and the desired endpoints for prediction.

The next question to be asked relates to the available database from which the prediction is to be made. How extensive and how reliable are the data? Are there animal data (pharmacology, toxicology or ADME), human clinical data or results from *in vitro* experiments? Furthermore, were the data derived from studies conducted as part of the basic package required for registration with regulatory authorities or were they performed to explain the results of such studies? This database review should also indicate if any further work is needed to clarify the results of any of the existing studies, for instance through an *in vitro* study of toxic mechanism. From these questions the uncertainties involved may be assessed; for instance is an extrapolation from an *in vitro* experiment to humans being requested. The ease of prediction increases with increasing biological proximity to the target species. In this instance 'biological proximity' includes experimental design as well as taxonomic considerations, although precise targeting of mechanistic studies *in vitro* may mean that this latter concern is less important in some cases.

Databases for prediction – quality and composition

Unsurprisingly, the accuracy of hazard prediction is critically dependent on the quality and extent of the database that is used and on the interpretation and conclusions that have been drawn. The available data set may be large or small and, in some cases, may not relate directly to the chemical of interest but to a member of the same chemical class; this is often the case with workplace-related assessments when few data are available. Although it has been said that the whole data package needs to be taken into account in hazard prediction, it is important that the data be relevant to the question asked. Any safety evaluation study can be said to be predictive and, generally, the security of prediction increases with the increasing database. However, large amounts of inadequate or inappropriate data will not help the process and will simply add unwanted complications.

While it is reasonable to assume that a contemporary safety evaluation programme, conducted to modern standards, is likely to be reliable, this should not be taken as a certainty. In contrast, older studies, especially those performed before the inception of Good Laboratory Practice (GLP) in the late 1970s, should be viewed with some caution. This is not because they are likely to be scientifically inept, but because standards of conduct and examination have improved to such an extent that changes dismissed then as irrelevant may be viewed differently today. Older studies need to be assessed in terms of the group size, data records and reporting, and husbandry and treatment procedures. The presence of audit reports by a Quality Assurance Unit working under GLP will add a degree of reassurance to the exercise. In comparing older studies with more recent ones, possible variation in the quality of the test material should be considered. Changes in quality can occur over a period of years due to evolution of production methods; sudden changes in production can lead to unexpected impurity, sometimes associated with unwelcome toxicity, as seen with trypto-phan. Equally, advances in analytical techniques – generally in the direction of vastly increased sensitivity – can reveal impurities in modern batches that intuition indicates must have been present from the outset, but undetected. The composition of an optimal database is reviewed in Box 10.1.

In addition there should be data on the physical and chemical characteristics of the parent molecule and on the physical form used in the evaluation. Although these are important, they have a greater significance in assessing risk. For instance lead poses a number of hazards which do not change with physical form; however, lead on church roofs carries much less risk to the public than lead in paint or drinking water. There may also be predictions derived from computer-based models and systems, which can cover a number of endpoints. These are useful when there is only a small database to work from but they should be considered to be tools, which can be misused all too easily.

There is a stark contrast between what might be seen as a desirable database, as outlined above, and the type and extent of data that are often available. This is especially the case for workplace assessments of chemicals used as intermediate steps in the synthesis of the final product. In these cases the hazard prediction process has to be conservative and is often based on proximity of the molecule to the final product in the synthesis pathway. For a chemical produced late in the synthesis, it may be possible to relate structure to expected pharmacological effects or toxicity; in these cases, the use of computer models becomes more important. Early in synthetic pathways, it is likely that the compounds used or produced will be commercially known or sufficiently similar to known chemicals to be assessed for hazard by literature searches or similar means. Database deficiencies are also frequently encountered when chemicals that have been in use for years, often decades, are considered. Concerns expressed by new producers or people looking for new uses, are sometimes greeted with indifference – 'We've

---

Box 10.1 Desirable database for prediction of human relevant hazard

For a recently developed chemical the normal – and desirable – database would contain information on the following:

- *General toxicology*   Target organ effects resulting from repeated administration should be highlighted in these studies. They may identify progressive or chronic changes, which can indicate significant hazard. These studies provide data relevant to many areas of effect.
- *Reproductive toxicology*   One of the major hazards to look for; endpoints examined that are of concern include effects on fertility, embryotoxicity and post-natal development.
- *Genotoxicity*   Shows potential for genotoxic effects; any positive results are indicative of hazard, as the experimental conditions often do not reproduce *in vivo* conditions.
- *Carcinogenicity* with indication of mechanism if appropriate.
- *Skin sensitisation and hypersensitivity*   Should show potential for dermal effects that could be of importance in production personnel and which are, of course, critically important for dermal preparations.
- *ADME data and information on pharmaco- and toxicokinetics*   There may be information on the particular P450s that are involved in metabolism and this part of the package will act as an anchor for the *in vivo* data, particularly in interpretation and mechanistic work.
- *Safety and efficacy pharmacology* (where appropriate)   These studies should identify transient, reversible hazards, e.g. cardiovascular or respiratory changes.
- *Human data*   These may relate to clinical experience (with drugs) or (very occasionally) to volunteer studies with pesticides.

---

used it for years without any [recorded] problems' – and it is very difficult in these cases to come up with a rational approach that is based on science rather than comfort factors. The production in tonnes of a chemical may also affect the size of the available database because the amount of testing increases with intended annual production.

Data handling

At first sight this might seem to be an oversimplistic item to be included. However, for a full-scale review of a complete data package, an ordered approach is essential as the amounts of data that are available can be enormous and not all of it is necessarily relevant or useful. Although it has been said earlier that putting studies into areas of investigation may be counterproductive, it is an essential first step when there are large numbers of reports or papers, as it allows you to see what there is and gives an initial indication of any deficiencies. It is useful to decide early which studies are pivotal to the assessment and which provide supporting evidence. The quality of study design and reporting come into consideration at this point; if there are studies that are not as good as others, these may be useful as support rather than being seen as definitive. A definitive study may be defined as one which completes a series, confirms a set of findings or offers a mechanistic explanation and which, crucially, has been conducted to high standards of design and interpretation. As the report is usually the only evidence of this available, it has to be complete and to have all the data and details of personnel responsible for the study conduct and reporting. Further layers of comfort for the reviewer may be provided if the testing facility is well known and independent of the developer, although with current controls exerted through enforcement of Good Laboratory Practices, the latter point is less significant than it used to be, even allowing for regulatory cynicism.

The next step is to identify toxicities in the various study areas covered by the reports and check for potential overlap and interdependencies between the various areas. It is also important to check for consistency. For example, where studies have been repeated, were the effects reproducible and consistent between studies or laboratories and, if not, why not? There is a degree of interpretational variation between toxicologists in both contemporary and historic terms. Historically, interpretation may have been different due to lack of knowledge of the significance of changes seen; effects dismissed at one time may acquire new meaning as research continues. In some cases, interpretation may have been weakened by standards of study design and conduct that were acceptable at the time the study was commissioned but are now outdated. It may be possible at this point in the review process to indicate what extra studies are needed to facilitate the hazard prediction. This may save a fair amount of effort in reviewing essentially useless studies.

Factors for consideration in prediction

In considering toxicity seen in test systems used in safety evaluations, the primary questions relate to the effects seen and the mechanisms by which they occurred. Although it is possible to point out toxicities in humans that are not easily reproduced in animals, it is not safe to say that the reverse is true. Much research grant money has been spent in investigation of the toxicity of TCDD, after experience in the Vietnam war and at Seveso. Although it is clear that it is highly toxic in animals and that guinea pigs are extremely sensitive to it, with lethal doses measured in micrograms, it has been said that the only *proven* effect in humans is chloracne. Having said that, however, no-one is queuing up to say that TCDD is safe.

However, there are a number of toxicities that are seen in animals which are acknowledged to be specific to the species. For example, the α-2u globulin

nephropathy is seen only in male rats; others would include peroxisome proliferation seen in rodents treated with hypolipidaemic compounds such as
ciprofibrate or plasticisers like diethylhexyl phthalate. Although these are
'standard' toxicities, there still needs to be proof that they are responsible for the
changes seen. Once the mechanism of an effect has been established, the
relevance or otherwise to humans may be assessed. However, it should be borne
in mind that these assumptions may be challenged as the research base expands.

In some cases, the test system used in the evaluation may be said to be
irrelevant to humans. Although it is clear that bacteria are phylogenetically
remote from humans, a positive effect in the Ames test should not be ignored as
it shows a potential for genotoxicity that may be reflected in other systems. If
there is a particular mechanism by which this was achieved then the relevance
of the effect may be assessed. Historically, it has been usual to indicate an order
of increasing human relevance with increasing evolutionary complexity. Thus, a
progression from bacteria to *Drosophila*, to mouse, to rat, to dog to non-human
primate might be set up to suggest that data from rats are more relevant to
humans than those from mice. This may be so as a general rule of thumb but it
is no more than that. Although it may be intuitive to assume that non-human
primates will give a better indication of human effect than other species, this is
not necessarily the case. The increasing use of transgenic animals will further
challenge these traditional and falsely comforting beliefs. As an additional
complication, a general prediction of effect in humans is unlikely to be completely applicable to the whole population due to genetic variation between
individuals and their circumstances (lifestyle, disease, etc.).

As has been pointed out above, dose is not a primary factor in hazard
prediction as that is considered in during risk assessment. In the same way, the
form of the chemical does not alter the hazard, merely the risk of expressing that
hazard. However, if the margin of safety is very large – expressed as a multiple of
the expected human exposure needed to reach the no effect level in the most
sensitive species tested – it may be possible to say that the hazard is not
predicted to be relevant to humans and that further risk assessment is not
needed. Furthermore, if there is a clear threshold below which the toxicity is not
expressed, this may be used to determine relevance to humans. A large multiple
between the toxicity threshold and the expected exposure in humans is a
significant driver in this assessment.

Another factor that might appear to reduce the significance of an effect from
the point of view of human relevance is reversibility. In toxicological terms, an
easily reversible effect, such as a mild increase in liver size due to enzyme
induction, is often flagged as being of minor toxicological significance. In any
assessment of the relevance to humans of such change, the type of change and
the speed and extent of reversibility have to be considered. In hazard assessment
terms a transient change in the liver – which has considerable recuperative
powers – will be rated as less significant than a transient change in the central
nervous system, which has poor repair capabilities.

The mechanism by which a systemic toxic effect is produced is, in broad terms, a function of physiology or biochemistry and the disposition and elimination of the chemical (ADME) and interspecies differences in toxicity are often attributable to these factors. The nephrotoxicity of α-2u globulin complexes is attributable to the large amount of this protein that is produced in male rats, in comparison with females. There are various hormonal differences between laboratory animals and humans that can be invoked to explain toxicities in test animals. Overproduction of growth hormone in dogs following progestogen administration resulted in an increased incidence of mammary tumours. In rats, increased prolactin concentrations are also associated with mammary tumours. Neither of these hormonal pathways and mechanisms is present in humans and both are therefore not human-relevant. There are also differences in the hormonal control of reproductive processes, including parturition, between laboratory animals and humans and such differences may mean that effects seen in reproductive toxicity studies are not relevant to humans.

The processes of ADME in the test system should be considered when attempting to relate effects seen to those expected in humans. Differences in toxicities seen between species may be due to inherent differences in metabolism; the task for the toxicologist then is to assess which of the species is more relevant to humans. Acetylaminofluorene is a potent animal carcinogen, which causes tumours in the liver, bladder and kidney through N-hydroxylation followed by production of a sulphate conjugate. However, guinea pigs are resistant to the effects of acetylaminofluorene because they have low activities for N-hydroxylation and sulphation; this resistance is overcome by giving N-hydroxyacetylaminofluorene. Acetylaminofluorene has been variously designated as a suspected, potential or probable human carcinogen.

If the pharmacokinetics in animals are grossly different from those in humans, the effects seen may not be human-relevant but this does not entirely remove the hazard as a risk. Much metabolism of xenobiotics is carried out through the cytochrome P450 family and there are differences in activities between the various laboratory species and humans. It needs to be pointed out that these are usually differences in activity rather than presence or absence and that the toxic metabolites may still be present in humans, albeit at much reduced concentrations compared with those in the test species. This may then be considered in a more formal risk assessment if this is considered appropriate.

If toxicity seen in animals is due to a metabolite that can be shown to be absent in humans, it is unlikely to be human-relevant. Equally, the absence of toxicity in a test system that metabolises the chemical differently to humans – either by prediction or observation – does not indicate that the chemical will be safe in humans. Studies with the major human metabolite should be considered, if it (or they) is not present in normally available laboratory animals. (Although it has been said that toxicity studies should be conducted in a metabolically and pharmacokinetically relevant species, this is usually no more than a holy grail, due to expense and practicality.)

In assessing the significance of the effects of one chemical, knowledge of the properties and toxicity of chemicals from the same class or with the same mode of action is also an invaluable aid. Although such knowledge is useful, it has to be treated with some circumspection as toxicity can vary widely across a group. This is illustrated by the organophosphates which have a very wide range of active dose levels as shown by the three examples given in Table 1.1 (see page 4). When comparing chemicals across groups, knowledge of the structure–activity relationships is also important. In organophosphates, the bond types around the central carbon atom of the phosphate group affect whether the compound will be associated with 'ageing' of the bound enzyme and possible delayed onset neuropathy. Ageing involves *in situ* metabolism of the bound organophosphate molecule with consequently increased binding affinity. The presence of a P–O–C bond between the phosphorus and one of the side groups of the molecule, as in tri-orthocresyl phosphate, is associated with rapid ageing, while a P–C bond makes this impossible.

Some of the more complex hazard prediction situations are provided by *in vitro* data from which an extrapolation to humans is necessary. This is often seen with genotoxicity data, where a single positive in an *in vitro* test, usually (but not always) a chromosome aberration study in Chinese hamster ovary or mouse lymphoma cells, can cause a variety of problems. If this is offset by a negative *in vivo* study in the mouse micronucleus test and a negative Ames test, it used to be that the single positive result would be dismissed. However, a more questioning approach has evolved where the circumstances of the various results are considered very carefully before reaching a conclusion on relevance. Once it has been accepted that the positive result is not associated with a threshold of effect or is due to excessive toxicity, a number of questions can be asked in order to clarify the meaning of the data. These are directed particularly at exposure of the test cells but also at mechanism. Partly this is driven by the difficult question of whether negative data in genotoxicity tests constitutes adequate proof of non-genotoxicity. For chemicals that have low oral bioavailability but that are reasonably soluble in routine parenteral vehicles, it should be possible to achieve adequate exposure of bone marrow by intravenous administration. If the results of this test are negative and it can be shown that the bone marrow was exposed to a greater degree than that achieved *in vitro*, this will add to evidence that the positive result *in vitro* is not relevant *in vivo*.

A poorly soluble compound may still be associated with genotoxicity *in vitro* as it has been demonstrated that precipitates may still give positive results. However, such a compound is often associated with poor absorption from the gastrointestinal tract and is usually very difficult to give intravenously at high enough doses to duplicate the exposures seen *in vitro*. Both these factors mean that exposure of the bone marrow cells in the mice is likely to be less than of the cells *in vitro*. Low bone marrow exposure to an active mutagen may also be seen where there is extensive first pass metabolism following oral administration, especially if this results in a conjugated metabolite that is not dissociated in the target tissue. Although *in vitro* tests use S-9 mix as a metabolic activation system, in standard protocols this is prepared from the livers of rats treated with enzyme-inducing agents, which may not be the most appropriate tissue or system for the test chemical. At this point mechanistic studies looking at the activities of specific enzymes in target tissues may be invoked to determine relevance of the results; if there is significant reversion from conjugate to parent in human tissues the absence of mutagenicity in the various tests may be deceptive.

Another approach is to examine tissues that may be expected to have had maximal exposure to the test substance, whether as a precipitate or as a saturated solution; these would normally be the stomach (in oral administration) and the liver. The comet assay is gaining in popularity in these circumstances as a positive result indicates DNA damage in the target tissue and is a clearer indicator of mutagenic potential. As with any toxicity, an understanding of the mechanism by which the result was produced is essential to overall interpretation of the various studies. Interpretation of genotoxicity data is facilitated by the presence of other data relating to the carcinogenic potential of the test or similar chemicals.

In summary, for secure prediction that a toxic effect seen in safety testing is not human-relevant, there has to be knowledge in the following areas:

* Mechanism of effect and whether this is species specific
* Comparative physiology
* Whether there is a clear threshold of effect below which toxicity is absent
* Comparative ADME; these studies are useful but may not imply absence of risk
* Relevant data from other chemicals of the same class and action.

In final analysis it has to be recognised that it may not be possible to predict that an observed toxicity is not a hazard for humans from the available data, in which case appropriate mechanistic studies should be conducted to demonstrate specificity of effect. In the event that these studies are not conclusive a conservative approach must be taken with a formal risk assessment.

Prediction from minimal databases

All too frequently, as implied by the discussion of what a desirable database should include, the amount of data available is less than completely ideal, as for an untested intermediate used during the synthesis of a final product. With the early parts of a synthetic pathway the chemicals used are sometimes well known and characterised by existing research. The problem becomes more acute in the later stages when the end products of each reaction are themselves novel chemicals. The distinction between these intermediates and the final product is that formal regulatory testing is not required and so the database for the former is small. One exception to this would be when the synthetic process is carried out at more than one location, when the toxicity of the transported chemicals would have to be assessed according to the annual amounts produced. Another setting in which the database may be expected to be small is found at the very early stages of evaluating a new chemical. How to predict the toxicity of an unknown and then extrapolating that prediction to a situation of human exposure. Factors to be considered are summarised in Box 10.2.

If the intermediate is synthetically remote from the final product, other factors have to be considered. These include an assessment for the presence of chemical groups or structures that are associated with known toxicity in other chemicals. Thus, 4-hydrazinobenzoic acid (Figure 10.1), the contentious component of mushrooms, is an aryl hydrazine, a structural configuration that has been associated with mutagenicity, carcinogenicity and skin sensitisation. There are a number of tools available that assist in this process of identifying these structure-activity alerts. These are seen in the various toxicity prediction software systems that are available and in systems that can conduct literature searches based on structure as opposed to keywords.

Ultimately, the decision process is similar to that used for large databases. All the evidence is reviewed and an assessment made as to the probable toxicity and consequent hazard. The inevitable difference is that the conclusions of such an assessment must be conservative until supported by more trustworthy evidence. The use of computer-based expert systems has a great part to play in these processes and as they evolve and become more interlinked their reliability will increase.

Box 10.2 Prediction from minimal databases

The following are amongst the factors that should be considered in maximising the database:

- Physicochemical properties of the molecule – partition coefficient and solubility, molecular weight, pK_a (the pH at which it is 50 per cent ionised), volatility. These properties may be compared with the final molecule.
- Structure-activity relationships known for the final molecule; if structure associated with pharmacology or toxicity in the final product are present in the intermediate, it is sensible to assume similar activities for the intermediate.
- Expected dose levels compared with no observed effect levels for the final product.
- Metabolism of the final product; if there are metabolites that are similar to the intermediate this may point to toxicity.
- Properties of chemicals related by structure or intended action.

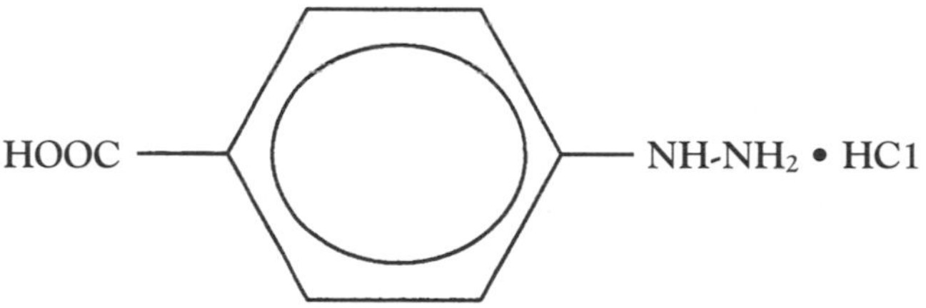

HOOC —⟨benzene ring⟩— NH-NH$_2$ • HC1

Figure 10.1 Structure of 4-hydrazinobenzoic acid.

Computer models for toxicity prediction

The following is based on a combination of personal experience, unpublished presentations and a review of an ECVAM workshop.[1] This gives a detailed review of the systems as they were at the time of the workshop and it is still useful as a guide to the system types and their attributes. However, it is clear that there is considerable continuing development and that a detailed review now of individual systems will be out of date almost as soon as it is written. With this in mind, it is the intention here to give a broad review of the type of system that is available and the weaknesses and strengths of systems in a general sense, without reference to individual systems.

Defining an expert system

Considerable human expertise is available, either from individuals or groups, and there is no doubt that this is a powerful source of knowledge and judgement for use in predictions of toxicity and hazard. However, this knowledge base is best considered as being volatile – due to illness, retirement, resignation or death – and as a result is not always available where and when it is wanted. The intention of an expert system is to bring all such expertise into one place where it may be accessed at any time by anyone. Although such systems need not be computer based, for the purposes of this review, it is assumed that they are. Broadly, they are formal systems that provide predictions on the toxicity of chemical structures which are entered into them by input on a screen. All these systems rely on toxicity data for other chemicals that have been entered into them and on the use of rules that have been devised from or in the light of those data. The rules by which a system works are either based on mathematical calculation, from physicochemical parameters or relationships using regression models, or on existing knowledge – for example the association of a particular chemical group or structure with a specific endpoint such as mutagenicity or sensitisation (a structural alert). While calculation allows a degree of extrapolation into new scientific territory, there cannot be complete confidence that errors made in setting up the rules or in inputting data are not being magnified with repeated recalculation. On the other hand, knowledge-based rules are just that and are dependent on input of that expert knowledge and, to a degree, expert judgement. The mathematical rules and systems are suitable for QSAR (quantitative structure activity relationship) analysis and can produce probabilities that an endpoint will be realised or a value for a dose level such as an LD_{50}. The benefit of such values is that they give a number that can be quoted, in an appropriate context; the downside is that the accuracy of such numbers is often highly questionable and can be little better than chance, especially in the case of dose levels. Another factor is that the process by which such numbers is produced is usually opaque to the user and there is little chance of rationalising the result. In contrast, with knowledge-based systems, there are usually literature references that can be accessed to support a particular conclusion. This may not be as comforting as a number but the results are probably more trustworthy as they do not give a potentially false impression of accuracy for the prediction.

The various endpoints typically covered by these systems are listed in Table 10.1; the fact that some, such as carcinogenicity, are listed with slightly different titles probably reflects the differing confidence (and marketing aspirations) of the people who originated the models.

Criteria for success

In assessing a molecule for potential adverse effects, a human expert looks at it in terms of molecular structure, size, constituent groups and elements, ionisation

Table 10.1 Endpoints predicted by expert systems

Acute inhalation toxicity LC_{50}
Acute oral toxicity LD_{50}
Acute toxicity LC_{50}
Acute toxicity EC_{50}
Ames mutagenicity
Anticholinesterase activity
Carcinogenicity
Chronic lowest observable adverse effect level (LOAEL)
Corrosivity
Developmental toxicity
Irritancy
Lachrymation
log P
Maximum tolerated dose (MTD)
Methaemoglobinaemia
Mutagenicity
Neurotoxicity
Respiratory sensitisation
Rodent carcinogenicity
Skin and eye irritation
Skin sensitisation
Teratogenicity

Note: Compiled from ECVAM report no. 24.[1]

potential and polarity, and probable metabolism. It should also be possible to say if one group will affect the influence of another nearby, for instance by electron withdrawal. The molecular weight gives a rough rule of thumb guide to whether it will be excreted in the bile or urine; the physicochemical data will give some idea of absorption potential and corrosivity. The human expert will assess the three-dimensional structure of the molecule and whether it has any chiral centres of asymmetry. Previous knowledge and experience may be available to the expert to warn of possible effects associated with that class of chemical or with particular structural configurations. This may also be associated with lateral thinking that leads to literature searches for suspected relationships or contributing factors. If allowance is made that lateral thought is unlikely in current software, it is this broad outline that an expert system should be attempting to reproduce.

Although an expert system cannot (yet) replicate the multi-faceted examination and thought processes of a human expert, there are certain aspects that should be considered essential. It should have the following characteristics;

- Allow easy entry of molecular structures
- Recognise structures associated with toxicity or unwanted pharmacology
- Predict interactions between different parts of the molecule, electron-withdrawing characteristics, etc.
- Have some capability of prediction of metabolism and of then assessing the toxicity of those metabolites
- Be transparent as to how or why the prediction results were produced
- Be user trainable, e.g. for specific chemical series
- Accept large molecules
- Allow prediction/calculation of physicochemical properties, such as log P and pK_a or scope for data entry
- Have some appreciation of the three-dimensional structures of molecules and chiral centres
- Be sensitive to the significance of chemically minor changes (such as substitution of S for N) that are toxicologically significant
- Take advantage of the benefits of mathematical and rule-based approaches by judicious combination
- Be easily updated with continuous development by the producers

The ability to enter or calculate the physicochemical properties is an important point when assessing potential absorption or irritancy and corrosivity. Prediction of irritancy/corrosivity can be poor in systems that do not have the ability to calculate physicochemical data. For assessing potential dermal absorption, the ability of a chemical to cross the skin tends to increase with increasing log P (the octanol–water partition coefficient, a measure of lipophilicity), although at very high log P values the permeability starts to decrease again.

The detection of structural alerts is an absolute essential but it is as important to be able to predict interactions between adjacent groups in the molecule.

Given that much toxicity is due to metabolites, the ability of a system to predict metabolism (and other aspects of ADME) is useful and can save time. The range of molecule size that can be assessed should be as large as possible; a limited range may limit the utility of the system. To be successful a system should not be unduly restricted in the type of molecule that it can assess. However, there are certain types of molecule that present particular challenges, such as polymers, and it is probably unreasonable to expect every system available to be able to cope with every class of compound.

Above all else, the strength of the database on which the system or module is based, is absolutely critical for anything approaching success. Ironically, much reliance has been placed on the results from programmes such as the US National Toxicology Program, especially for carcinogenesis prediction, where some of the study designs and interpretation may be open to debate, particularly for the older studies. These are rodent carcinogens and we use a computer to predict rodent carcinogenesis on the basis of sometimes dubious data from old studies, which we must then extrapolate to the human situation. Another factor of debate here is the judgement calls that have to be made when the difference from control was not clear enough to give a clear positive or negative classification. Ironically, for expert systems, use of expert judgements that might be debatable is a weakness – quantitative or black and white data are better. There is no way round this particular challenge; the number of rodent carcinogens is much larger than the number of *proven* human carcinogens and the use of the latter would not give a sufficiently large amount of information for a credible database on its own. A further, inevitable, weakness is that the systems must rely on prior knowledge and this means that for novel toxicities the systems will not be predictive because the mechanism, chemical structure or interactions and properties have not been encountered before. However this could also be said of animal studies. The databases really exemplify the old computer adage of 'garbage in – garbage out'. For this reason it is important to be able to understand how the system has arrived at its prediction and this is where falsely comforting numbers produced by opaque processes are less usable than predictions based on rules with literature references that can be examined for relevance to the molecule under investigation.

Databases are also affected by the tendency to place emphasis on the chemicals that have been shown to have the predicted toxicity, over those that were negative or not toxic. Absence of toxicity is as important as presence in prediction systems. Equally, there is a tendency for the toxic chemicals – the development mistakes – to be buried in company archives in confidential reports that are not allowed into the public domain. Where the data or rule bases are developed by the users in a cooperative manner, there is a corresponding increase in the strength of the system and, inherently, of its credibility and the confidence that can be placed in its predictions.

For the purposes of lead candidate selection, it is particularly useful if the user of the system is able to enter data or rules for the series of chemicals that is being developed – retinoids would be a good example. By this means a database specific to that series can be developed and the effects of additions or subtractions from the molecule may be assessed on the screen without having the expense of synthesising the actual chemicals.

Strengths and weaknesses

In general these largely reflect the achievement or otherwise of the various criteria for success, although each of the systems available has different strengths and weaknesses. This means that care must be taken when choosing a system, especially when a specific type of molecule is going to be assessed on a regular basis. It is probable that any system will have difficulty with one or more types of molecules, although each of these types may well be covered by one or more systems. Many systems are limited in the size or type of molecule that they can deal with. Long-chain polymers can cause trouble, but also chemicals that contain metal atoms and peptides are among the molecular types that cannot be covered by individual systems. More fundamentally, there have been instances when compounds such as organophosphates or polyaromatic hydrocarbons were not assessed correctly due to deficiencies in the database.

The importance of physicochemical properties has been mentioned earlier and it is an advantage if the system is able to calculate these automatically and also to assess stereochemical effects, although the accuracy of the calculations may be somewhat variable. This will, apart from anything else, increase its ability to predict irritancy and corrosivity. Any attempt to increase the three-dimensional recognition of the software is also an advantage.

The software itself is less easy to assess; there is a possibility in some systems that assumptions made in the production of the software may have been wrong, for instance that structures contribute independently to biological activity. The ability to make allowance for such false assumptions is a property of systems in which the database and rule base are available to the user to rationalise individual model predictions, and to define the limitations associated with them. Such transparency indicates why a rule has been invoked; however, this is not possible with all expert systems.

Some systems are more easily adapted to specific user requirements than others, for instance in selection of screen colours and recognition of toxicophores or structural alerts. The ability to build an in-house database for a chemical series for predictions relevant to new members of that series is a big strength of some systems. Although a system may lack this transparency, it may still be possible to do a search to ascertain the similarity of the test molecule to those used in the database; there may be the ability to rank these chemicals for similarity to the test structure.

The overall strength of this type of approach to molecular assessment is that they are generally easy to use and can give results very quickly, making them suitable for high throughput screening and prioritisation of lead candidates.

They can also be used during design of molecules for a particular target; goodness of fit to the intended receptor or predicted activity can be offset by predictions of toxicity. It must be remembered, however, that the absence of predicted adverse effect cannot be assumed to imply safety or that predicted toxicity is inevitable. A significant weakness is that they do not completely replace the need for expert judgement, as a degree of this is desirable to check the predictions for the more obvious inconsistencies. Finally, it may be beneficial to look at the same molecule with more than one system – analogous to the use of several genotoxicity test protocols – in order to assess possible effects. However, due to cost – either in hardware or licence costs – it is not usually feasible to have more than one or occasionally two, in the same place.

Accuracy of predictions

The accuracy of predictions produced by expert systems, and how it is assessed, has been a source of considerable debate. Starting from basics, the accuracy of an individual prediction must be deeply influenced by what is attempted and what data there is to predict from. For a novel molecule, input to the system is simply a chemical structure. On this basis, is it reasonable to expect complex mathematics to provide a supportable prediction of a multi-factorial endpoint, which is influenced by factors external to the molecule, such as physiology? As has been pointed out, the data from which predictions are made – the system's database – is critical to the accuracy of individual predictions; the presence of ill-selected data and faulty assumptions disables the prediction before it gets off the ground.

There are two types of prediction – qualitative and quantitative. Qualitative predictions merely indicate the possibility of the endpoint being realised. They predict molecular events or chemical reactions such as interaction or reaction with DNA for mutagenicity. Where there are well-understood molecular mechanisms and good structure–activity relationships, it may be expected that these predictions should be reasonably 'accurate'. A simple chemical reaction between a molecule and DNA may be relatively simple to predict. In contrast, an endpoint that has many different influences in its realisation – such as reproductive toxicity, which is affected by numerous factors external to the entered structure – is much less easy to predict. From this a first rule of thumb may be raised: the more complex the endpoint, the less inherently trustworthy will be the prediction. A distinction should also be drawn between qualitative predictions that are based on chemical reaction and those that are dependent on interaction with receptors. As the ability to interact with a receptor is sometimes not easily assessed from structure, this type of prediction tends to be less reliable than those for reaction-based interactions.

Quantitative prediction, which is the next stage, is the calculation of a probability for a predicted event or an LD_{50} or MTD, or a physicochemical parameter such as $\log P$. As with qualitative predictions, the values calculated for 'simple' endpoints, such as $\log P$, are likely to be closer to reality than those for parameters that are affected by factors external to the software. Thus, LD_{50}

calculations have been largely a waste of time as the results have shown little difference from what you would expect by chance. The MTD is notoriously difficult to establish *in vivo* and, intuitively, there is no reason to suppose that a computer estimate is going to be any better. In circumstances where data generated *in vivo* for a series of related compounds have been entered into the database, it is possible that computer-generated estimates may be better than those produced for unrelated compounds. In other circumstances, calculated figures for dose levels should be viewed with extreme suspicion.

Performance of computer systems is assessed against pre-existing data or by prediction before testing is carried out. This is a similar process of validation to that carried out for new *in vitro* methods. The correlation of output from a computer system with the results of actual tests is influenced by the clarity of the actual test data and the ease with which they can be interpreted as positive or negative, black or white. For a clear positive or negative there is no problem; for anything debatable there is the problem – given the usually small sets of chemicals used in validation studies – that a single data point will swing the result a disproportionately large percentage in one direction or the other. Other factors that the computer software cannot take account of can also be critical. Impurities in chemicals can have profound influence on toxicity and, while the pure chemical may be correctly predicted to be negative for mutagenicity, the actual production batches may not be.

One aspect of the validation process that takes place using pre-existing data is that, when all the data has been assembled, there is a process of explanation for the discrepancies between the two methods. Thus, for compounds falsely indicated as mutagenic, the toxicophore might have been in a ring structure and not in a side chain, while false negatives may have been associated with weak evidence of mutagenicity in the actual Ames test. By adjusting for this type of factor it is possible to increase the percentage correspondence between the two data sets but it does not remove the fact that the systems were less accurate in the first place. Without conducting a detailed review of all the available systems and models and all the validation studies that have been conducted, the accuracy for most of the predictions for the simpler endpoints does not appear to exceed about 75 per cent, as an upper estimate. Having said that, the performance of systems in particular models may be better than this and there is clear evidence that development and refinement of systems does produce greater accuracy of prediction. This has been seen with rule-based systems and predictions of mutagenicity, which are now accurately predicted by some systems. In fact, if it is considered that a compound may be mutagenic or non-mutagenic and that these form two different positions for prediction, the performance of a system may be better in one respect than in the other.

The problem of validation and how to do it is a constant and the basis for comparisons is changing rapidly as system databases and rule bases are improved and mathematical formulae tweaked. However, there is the continuing problem that prior input of data for old compounds, as a basis for judgement of new ones, will not necessarily mean that the assessments will be accurate, especially where there are novel structural elements or previously unknown intramolecular interactions. No amount of analysis of hit rates, sensitivity analysis or gentle data massage can change this. It is a certainty that accuracy of predictions will improve with system development; it is equally a certainty that some endpoints will always be associated with less accurate prediction due to their complexity, despite the touching optimism of salesmen.

Improving the accuracy of predictions

There is no doubt that continuing development and refinement of individual systems leads to increased reliability and accuracy of prediction – for that system. Such improvement will always be prospective and the promise of accuracy tomorrow is unlikely to be useful in evaluating the problem of the day. In the same way that a single toxicity test is not conducted in isolation, the utility of computer predictions can be improved by using two or more systems. The use of two independent systems gives different angles of view on the same molecule and may give increased confidence in the final decision. Systems or modules can also be used in sequence, using output from one system as input for the next. Thus, metabolism of a molecule can be predicted and the metabolites processed through the toxicity modules of the same system or passed to another for assessment. It should be borne in mind that errors could be increased as the process continues, especially in systems that use calculation in the course of prediction.

Performances figures, whether expressed as percentages or hit rates, are meaningless unless they are considered in the context of what the output will be used for. Opinions on the significance of an accuracy of 75 per cent may well vary. Such figures are produced from comparison of the computer result with those from actual tests, with all their procedural differences or irregularities compounded by debates on the interpretation of the results. These accuracy figures are probably good enough for lead candidate selection or for assessing the possible effects of chemicals for which there is little test data, but they are not yet sufficiently refined to be used in human safety prediction for mainstream marketing applications for chemicals.

If such systems are used as an adjunct to the process of hazard prediction and not as the sole means of assessment, they have considerable utility and cannot be ignored. There are some important caveats, however. The various systems available have significant differences in performance in different areas and some are better with particular molecular classes than others. This means that, for given uses, some systems will be better than others and this must be taken into account when choosing a system.

As implied earlier, it is not sensible to use individual systems in isolation and there are a range of supporting tools that can be used as adjuncts to the prediction process. These include any system used in the design of the molecule, for instance for pharmacological QSAR screening. There are also systems that allow literature searches to be based on molecular structure or on parts of the molecule. It is also probable that physiologically based pharmacokinetic (PBPK) models will become of increasing importance although they have a more traditional role in risk assessment.

Ultimately, in consideration of the performance of computer systems, the cynical view must be remembered, that the toxicity of any novel molecule cannot be accurately predicted until the data for that molecule are entered into the database. Equally, it must be asked at the beginning of the process if you actually need an 'accurate' prediction or whether you simply need to rank compounds in terms of expected toxicity, so that the best candidate can be selected for development. In this case, the consistency and relevance of output will probably be more significant than ultimate accuracy.

Prediction for individuals

The above discussion has focused on the prediction of adverse effects in populations, whether of laboratory animals or of humans. However, the prediction of effect in individuals is becoming more important; although it may be characterised as individual risk assessment, it is covered briefly in this section. Such assessments can cover the likely outcome of overdose to the probable response to treatment with specific drugs and the likelihood of interactions between prescribed drugs. This latter aspect is in its infancy but will become more routine, particularly in respect of clinical trials of new medicines and their subsequent prescription. The results of many clinical trials – which are the ultimate basis for regulatory acceptance for new drugs – are adversely skewed by lack of response of some of the patients entered into the trial. If it can be predicted in advance that a patient will not respond, due to the presence of a metabolic polymorphism or some other phenotypic aspect, there does not seem to be much sense in exposing them needlessly to a drug that may actually harm them. The implication of this is that patient populations for clinical trials can be selected on the basis of their likely responses and that the trial data may be much more favourable as a result. The corollary of this is that the suitability of patients must be assessed by physicians before drugs are prescribed; the time- and money-saving implications of this are considerable as appropriate treatment can be selected immediately and without lengthy experiment. This is the nascent science of pharmacogenomics. The difficulty arises when it is realised that biological situations are rarely black or white and that a patient's phenotype is probably an expression of varying rates of genetic expression and not simply a matter of presence or absence.

As well as phenotype, the reaction of an individual to chemical exposure – intentional or otherwise – is affected by personal circumstance. Thus pregnancy or malnutrition will affect predictions as the relevance of defined toxic hazards. In overdose, additional risk factors to be considered, apart from the dose taken, include the presence of alcoholism, smoking or other drug abuse. The factors relevant in paracetamol overdose are reviewed in Box 10.3.

Box 10.3 Prediction of toxicity in paracetamol overdose[2]

- The lethal dose is about 16 g in a normal 70 kg human; outcome is influenced by hepatic status (e.g. co-administration of enzyme inducers, such as phenobarbital). Dose is always difficult to establish accurately.
- Chronic alcohol ingestion is additive in effect.
- Acute single alcohol ingestion concomitantly is protective.
- Hepatic damage is seen as centrilobular necrosis.
- Hepatic recovery has been noted in biopsies of people who recovered.
- Clinical course – symptoms in first two days do not reflect seriousness of situation. Nausea, vomiting, anorexia and abdominal pain are possible in the first 24 hours and may persist for a week or more. Hepatic damage becomes clinically manifest in 2–4 days; plasma transaminases, bilirubin concentration and prothrombin time are increased.
- Use of the Rumack–Matthew nomogram gives probability of hepatotoxicity from estimation of time of ingestion and plasma concentration of paracetamol; a plasma half life or more than 4 hours is associated with a high probability of hepatotoxicity, which is often fatal.
- Antidote is N-acetylcysteine given before 16 hours post ingestion.

Prediction summary

The following points are given as an overall summary for successful prediction of human relevant hazard:

- Be sure of the parameters for which you are predicting – population group, environmental area, etc.
- What is the purpose for prediction?
- Be sure of your database from which you are predicting hazard.
- Use or consider all data but dismiss those that are not interpretable with any security.
- Today's prediction may look sad tomorrow.

Chapter 11

Background to risk due to toxicity

Introduction

The use of any chemical is associated with risk, whether it is a novel drug, an established pesticide, an intermediate in a synthetic pathway, an industrial by-product or table salt. This chapter examines various aspects of risk, including how it is perceived and described, that are critical in successful communication and subsequent management of risks due to toxicity, either in the workplace or in a wider context. The relevant factors and processes by which the risks associated with the hazards relevant to humans (or another target species) are assessed are then reviewed.

Overview of risk assessment

Risk assessment is, classically, the process of characterising the potential adverse effects of human exposure to a chemical, particularly with regard to carcinogenicity, and assessing the probability that these hazards will be expressed in a target population. Classically, this is a high-level process that uses sophisticated mathematical models and extrapolates from the results of animal testing, usually carcinogenicity bioassays in rodents. Risk assessment is often at the intersection between the science of toxicology and policy – and this is not always a comfortable or smooth relationship. Various definitions of risk assessment and its components have been given, with the more accessible versions usually being from the USA; the Federal government definition is given as 'the characterisation of the potential adverse effects of human exposures to environmental hazards'. It is generally agreed between the various sources that there are four steps in risk assessment, consisting of hazard identification, assessment of toxicity and then of expected exposure, followed by characterisation of the risk. This latter process of risk characterisation was defined by the WHO/FAO in 1995 as the integration of hazard identification, hazard characterisation and exposure assessment into an estimation of the adverse effects likely to occur in a given population, including attendant uncertainties. This includes qualitative and quantitative aspects and is the preliminary to risk management, which is seen as a separate entity.

Although this type of high-level risk assessment is briefly considered in this chapter, the prime intention is to look at what might be termed its everyday use, for example in the workplace and when choosing the first doses to be used in human volunteer studies. This type of assessment considers the possible expression of any of the hazards identified as human-relevant following the overall interpretation of the safety evaluation data (cf. chapter 10), whether these are presence or absence phenomena like cancer or effects such as allergy, reproductive abnormality or other toxicities. The results should allow the setting of parameters such as acceptable daily intakes (ADIs), occupational exposure limits (OELs) and maximum atmospheric concentrations in production facilities. This is a necessary preliminary to risk management.

There has been a long-standing assumption in risk assessment that the results of non-human experiment, whether in animals or in a Petri dish, are relevant to humans. A second assumption is that the effects of high dose or exposure will be seen at lower levels; i.e. that dose response is always linear. These assumptions have weakened risk assessments in the past and resulted in the imposition of unrealistic limits on chemical exposures. Risk assessors have considerable responsibility to get their assessments right, so that the limits of exposure that they propose are reasonable and derived from all the available data, without use of unrealistic assumptions. Setting a limit too high may expose people to toxic concentrations of a chemical with unacceptable effects. Setting them too low may mean loss of any benefit from use of the chemical or impose clean-up processes that are excessively costly in relation to the marginal increase in benefit. In risk assessment it is necessary to apply Occam's razor and to make no more assumptions than are needed to accomplish the declared purpose.

Levels of risk and factors that affect risk

Risk is present at various human levels ranging from personal, through specific populations, such as farm workers, to the general population of an area, to national and international and thence to global. Personal levels of risk are determined by factors such as occupation, lifestyle and home environment. The lifestyle of those about you may also be significant. Smoking is clearly associated with a range of diseases, the most emotive of which is lung cancer. Although there have been epidemiological attempts to correlate the effects of passive smoking with disease, these have generally been unsuccessful. However, to say that there is no quantifiable risk or demonstrated correlation is counter-intuitive. Passive smokers are exposed to sidestream smoke and to exhaled smoke. Although processing smoke through the lungs of the smoker might be expected to remove a large proportion of the chemical and particulates, this will not be totally efficient and, consequently, other people in the vicinity will be exposed to the same toxic mixture, albeit at lower concentrations.

Genetic profile is also important and may determine the individual responses to chemicals both short term and long term. Skin colour and associated sensitivity to UV light is a well-known determinant of susceptibility to skin cancers. Biochemical or physiological factors such as metabolic polymorphisms influence individual responses to drugs and pesticides such as organophosphates. Such individual characteristics may offer an explanation for differences between farmers' long-term responses to occupational exposures, sheep dips being a point of heated discussion in recent years. Box 11.1 looks at cholinesterase inhibition as a toxicological target with specific reference to the use of organophosphates. It is worth noting that the referred paper by Stephens *et al.* provoked two critical commentaries that were published in the same issue of the *Lancet*. The authors' response (also in the same issue) addressed the concerns by reference to

---

Box 11.1 Cholinesterase inhibition: factors in risk determination

Cholinesterase inhibition came to prominence with development of organophosphate (OP) nerve gases and insecticides and of the carbamate insecticides, both of which have been widely used in agricultural and domestic pest control. Latterly, cholinesterase inhibition has been used as a therapeutic objective in Alzheimer's disease, through the action of drugs such as rivastigmine. Cholinesterase inhibition is a property of natural chemicals, such as solanine (see Box 11.4).

- OPs show a wide range of acute toxicities; the nerve gas sarin has a parenteral LD_{50} less than 0.05 mg/kg, while malathion is lethal at around 1000 mg/kg orally (Table 1.1). Carbaryl, a carbamate insecticide, has broadly similar acute toxicity to malathion; carbamates tend to be less toxic than organophosphates due to differences in reactivation rates for the enzyme.
- Organophosphates have been widely used in sheep dips against sheep scab mites and are also used in orchards. Sheep dipping, which was compulsory in the UK between 1976 and 1992, poses significant practical problems in controlling occupational exposure. It is strenuous, dirty work, sheep are inherently uncooperative and, as in all such circumstances, personal protection equipment is difficult to wear with any comfort or, as a result, hope of real benefit. Although the acute effects of OPs are well known, long-term neurological effects have come to prominence as the history of use has increased.
- Epidemiological study of OP-related change in sheep dippers has indicated evidence of neurological effects, especially in those with high exposures over a long period.[1] Another study in 146 sheep farmers indicated deficits in attention and speed of information processing and susceptibility to psychiatric disorder.[2]

- Various papers have examined polymorphisms in paraoxonase, which metabolises OPs in humans; this is present on a genetic level and as different affinities/activities between substrates.[3,4] These papers indicate potential differences in susceptibility to OPs and may explain differences in response seen between farmers. Low paraoxonase activity has also been reported in Gulf war veterans complaining of Gulf War Syndrome, in which OPs were one of the implicated factors.[5]
- Although OPs are clearly acutely toxic and pose significant long-term risk, alternatives are not necessarily better. One possibility is to use synthetic pyrethroids but they have potential environmental problems and resistance by sheep scab mite has been shown in some areas.
- Other factors to consider include run-off from dips into surface water, which has been shown as a significant environmental problem;[6] OP use in salmon farming has also been criticised.
- These various papers refer to OP use in the so-called developed world. Standards of use and acceptance of risk are almost certainly different in other environments.

the full report, neatly illustrating the pitfalls in attempting to draw conclusions from a partly complete account or data set.

Occupation has been always been a factor to consider in personal risk as well as for particular working populations such as miners. Cancers associated with painting radium onto watch faces, working with β-naphthylamine or vinyl chloride are well known and it is fair to say that the incidence of occupational cancers has been much reduced by appropriate application of risk analysis and risk management. There are synergistic factors that affect individual risk, such as the increased cancer risk associated with mining and smoking.

Diet (individual and national) is also a factor of great significance, both in terms of cause and prevention; as a result of this counterbalancing act, it can be difficult to sort out what the significant factors are in a population. High salt intake in Japan was linked to a high incidence of stomach cancer; high intake of rye bread in Finland has been associated with a reduced incidence of gastro-intestinal cancers. Increased intake of antioxidants has been associated with reduced cancer risk. Such factors have clear impact on individuals but, because diet is usually influenced by national traditions and circumstance, the risks associated with it are relevant nationally. While dietary imbalance confers risks in various, sometimes contrary directions – in terms of fibre, fatty acid composition, antioxidants, deficiency or excess of factors such as trace elements – the actual chemical composition of the food is also worth considering. Leaving aside chemicals that are clearly of nutritional benefit there are a host of other chemicals present, some of which are artificial (pesticides or chemicals introduced during cooking) and some of which are endogenous to the food consumed (see Box 11.2). Most plants, such as cabbage, contain their own chemical defences against pest attack – so called natural pesticides – which are present at far higher concentrations than the carefully regulated amounts of synthetic pesticides that may have been sprayed on them.

While individual and national diets are potential sources of adverse effects, they are at least reasonably focused. In contrast, air quality is an international and global concern that has the potential to affect everyone. Poor air quality standards have clear impact in individual cities – Mexico City and Los Angeles being good examples. As airborne pollution can cross international borders, risk becomes a matter of international concern, which requires agreement on standards of emissions from factories and so on. The unintentional export of atmospheric pollution from the UK to countries of northern Europe and the subsequent environmental damage through acid rain has been a bone of often bitter contention.

Risk perception

Understanding how risks are perceived is vital to their management – especially in the workplace, where disregard of risks by employees can rebound on company management in a welter of litigation and financial regret. Lack of risk appreciation, coupled with factors such as uncomfortable personal protection equipment, can have serious consequences for a company and its employees. Before a risk can be managed successfully, it must be understood by the people who are at risk and who need to put the desired measures into practice. If their perception and appreciation of the risk is different from that of the managers, the management process is unlikely to be successful.

Defining risk in terms of the probability of the occurrence of an adverse event is often easier than getting the significance of that possibly remote event accepted and a course of preventative action agreed. The perception of risk, particularly by the public, affects responses to risk reduction initiatives or to new introductions of processes or chemicals and cannot be ignored. This is due to the ways in which risk is perceived by the people involved. Risk that is remote in time or distance is less threatening than immediate risk; a familiar risk is more likely to be accepted than one from an unfamiliar source or one that has been poorly communicated and explained. For an observer or someone else who is not directly affected, even severe risks may not carry personal significance, whereas for the person about to fall off the cliff, the risk is real and immediate. However, if the person is told there is a risk that he or she will fall off the cliff in five years time, there is much less immediacy and so less likelihood of corrective action. In understanding risks of diseases normally present at low incidences, it could be said that any disease is rare – until you get it yourself. If disease is brought into the personal sphere – through a friend or relative or yourself – it immediately assumes much greater significance. Furthermore, if there is no obvious cause, responsibility may be assigned to any local factor or circum-stance, especially if more than one case is present in a small group. Such local incidences may not climb above the levels of normality in a wider context but they may well be perceived as critical.

Risk perception is also influenced by the position or identity of people who are given the task of explaining it. Explanation and assessment from clearly interested parties, generic 'scientists' or – especially – government will tend to be more closely questioned and ignored than that from independent sources. Increasingly fervent dismissal by government of concerns about pesticide residues in food, simply leads to greater levels of disbelief by the public supported by perceptions such as jobs-at-risk or tax losses.

The major health concerns of the public, such as cancer, are driven by personal understanding of risk and knowledge of the mechanisms; the smaller the understanding the greater the concern. While cancer as an aspect of tobacco smoking is well understood it is chiefly of concern to those who do not smoke, as the smokers have accepted the risk, either by acknowledging it or by ignoring it. This acceptance might not prevent a smoker buying organically grown produce in the belief that it has fewer pesticides and carries less risk as a result; there may be a market for organic tobacco. The disparity between the risks associated with smoking and the risks associated with minimal amounts of safety-tested pesticides is not a factor to be considered. One risk (the lethal one) is acceptable while the other is not.

Another difficulty is that risks are often perceived and considered in isola-tion, without considering that risk in one sense may be offset by benefit in another or vice versa; in other words risk is often two sided. Organically grown or stored peanuts may have higher levels of aflatoxins due to the uncontrolled presence of mould, which is usually absent in peanuts treated with pesticides. Aflatoxins are highly potent carcinogens and carry a higher risk than the pesticides. Removing one risk often means promoting another to the same or a higher level. One risk may be enhanced by another; the risk of occupational cancer is often increased in smokers or by excessive alcohol consumption.

Data that appear to indicate differences in risk are another source of false perception. Deaths from cancer may be higher in a poor industrial town than in one that is academic and rich. However, the incidence of cancer could well be the same in the two areas and the apparent difference is due simply to a disparity in health care standards.

Risk perception is one of the factors in the widespread rejection of genetically modified crops and foods and, in this case, poor communication has exacerbated the problem to the extent that any benefit from this technology is likely to be wasted on a wave of public rejection that is – in part at least – ill-informed. Box 11.2 gives a simplistic overview of this contentious area. Normal agricultural development is genetic modification through selection of desirable character-istics via breeding programmes; the critical difference is that normal agricultural development does not involve the insertion of genes from different species. Although genetic modification can produce plants with excessive concentrations of endogenous chemicals or with allergenic proteins (although this has not been proven in any marketed food), these risks could be managed. For foods that are unacceptably hazardous to certain individuals – for instance nuts – genetic modification holds out the possibility for the removal of unwanted genes from foods; non-allergenic peanuts might have considerable attraction to some people.

Box 11.2 Genetically modified foods

- Genetic modification introduces new genetic material, from bacteria or other species, into a plant's genotype to express a characteristic such as longer shelf-life, better flavour, or resistance to pesticides or pests. The action of these inserted genes and their proteins can be very specific, as in the Bt protein expressed by *Bacillus thuringensis* DNA inserted into genetically modified maize to give resistance to corn borer.

- Toxicological risk may be expected in two areas – environment and human health. The former may be seen through effects on wild populations or increased use of pesticides; the latter might be associated with food intolerance, toxicity or factors such as induced resistance to antibiotics.

- Differences from 'traditional' crops are loosely classifiable according to type of chemical expressed – similar or dissimilar to those in normal human metabolism. 'Similar' would include nucleic acids and proteins. 'Dissimilar' would include small molecules such as endogenous alkaloids, which can be present at toxic concentrations in new strains; a new strain of potato was found to have acutely toxic concentrations of solanine and chaconine and was withdrawn.[7] 'Similar' chemicals are likely to be lost safely through natural biochemical pathways; 'dissimilar' chemicals are subject to the normal processes of ADME for small molecules and associated with adverse effects such as the anticholinesterase activity shown by solanine.[7,8]

- Adverse effects on human health are dependent on the composition of the foods and the crops from which they are derived and are most likely to arise from ingestion. However, dermal exposure can also be significant. A new insect-resistant celery was associated with rashes and burns when handling was followed by exposure to sunlight; subsequently, it was found that the new variety contained 7-fold more psoralens than normal celery.[7]

- Genetic modification of food crops might be expected to be associated with allergic reactions. Allergens are mostly proteins and only a small percentage of dietary protein is allergenic. If the protein expressed is similar to a known allergen (e.g. a nut-derived protein) there is a risk that the new food will also be allergenic. As a basic rule, genes should not be transferred from known allergen sources.[9]
- Food has always been associated with certain risks. Genetic modification may also pose risks to the environment, where effects may include gene transfer or toxicity to non-target insects such as butterflies, as a result of excessive expression of proteins such as Bt.
- Pollen from a variety of Bt corn expressing high levels of Bt protein was reported to be toxic to monarch butterfly caterpillars when it fell on the leaves of milkweed plants growing amongst the crop.[10]
- Transfer of genes for herbicide resistance has been reported in sugar beet and in some weeds so that weeds and crops have become resistant to several herbicides.[11,12]
- Narrow spectrum of action of some genetic inserts may mean that use of pesticides is still needed when the crop is attacked by other, unaffected, pests.[13]
- The above should not be taken as evidence for banning genetic modification. Hazards have been identified in terms of food content and environmental effect but risk is determined by local circumstances, such as individual susceptibility and the concentrations of proteins or chemicals expressed in the crop or food, together with local conditions. With appropriate management and some lateral thought the risks can be reduced and managed.

Acceptability of risk

Clearly, risk perception has considerable influence on the acceptability of risk, which may be seen from two angles, that of the public and that of regulators; these are frequently different. The type of hazard and its characteristics define the acceptability of its expression. Increased risk of irreversible change such as birth defects is unacceptable to a greater degree than a minor effect that is seen to be transient. When a transient effect turns out to have long-term consequences, the acceptability of the risk is likely to change. In official terms acceptability of risk is expressed in incidences; one death in 1 million appears to be acceptable although, in practice, this would probably not be detectable.

The relationship between risk and benefit (or cost/benefit ratio) is a critical factor in determining the acceptability of risk due to toxicity. As a broad rule of thumb, acceptability of risk increases with increasing benefit or, for instance, severity of disease. Acceptability is essentially unquantifiable and is influenced by perception of the risk; as such it is a matter of judgement, which tends to be conservative. At the either end of the cost/benefit spectrum this judgement is relatively easy; significant toxicity is acceptable in cancer drugs but is not tolerated in analgesics sold over the counter. In the middle of the spectrum however, the choices can be much harder. For more serious inflammatory conditions such as rheumatoid arthritis, where long-term treatment of a wide range of patients could be expected, a greater degree of risk would probably be allowable but, for example, reproductive effects or human-relevant carcinogenicity would be unacceptable. Although significant toxicity may be acceptable in a cytotoxic cancer drug, as cancer treatments become more targeted in terms of receptor specificity and affinity, it is likely that they too will have to conform to expectations of low toxicity. According to indication, some toxicities may be more acceptable than others; diabetes is associated with a number of clinical effects and any toxicity that might act to enhance these effects or accelerate the progress of the disease would not be acceptable.

Comparative risk

Risk usually has a comparative element that needs to be considered in any assessment, most simply as a cost/benefit analysis. When considering a chemical that has been developed for a particular purpose, the advantages of its use should be considered as well as the disadvantages. This is also true when looking at chemicals that have been used for many years but then shown to be associated with toxicity. Replacement of a toxic chemical with an essentially unknown substitute is not necessarily better, as long-term experience with the substitute can show different hazards that may also be undesirable. Different forms and concentrations of the same chemical will probably be associated with different levels of risk. Hazards posed by different chemicals may be similar but have different risks attached to them; also, hazard does not necessarily imply significant risk. Comparative risk is valid for single chemicals but should also be considered across different origins, chemical groups or boundaries of use, such as when a pesticide is re-assessed for medicinal use. Risk, therefore, should not be considered in isolation; Box 11.3 looks at elements of comparative risk and seeks to put some perspective on this.

Comparison of risk is also valid across location; a risk that is unacceptable in the USA may be tolerable in a less-developed country due to local circumstances. Use of a carcinogenic pesticide is unlikely to be acceptable in a developed country because lifespan is long enough to allow expression of the cancer; where lifespan is shorter, this risk would possibly be acceptable.[16] Other circumstances may be more important, such as the cost of alternatives, the control of malarial mosquitoes and consequent reduction in disease. The environmental fate of the pesticide and the associated environmental risks may well be similar in both locations.

Box 11.3 Elements of comparative risk

The following list is not exhaustive:

- *Similar hazard, different risk*   This may be seen for single chemicals, between different chemicals or chemical groups and may be a function of relative potency, formulation, place of use, physicochemical characteristics, bioavailability, etc. Comparative risks for lead are seen in paint, car fuel, drinking water, organic or ionic or on church roofs.
- *Origin – endogenous/non-endogenous or natural/synthetic*[14]   Natural chemicals are not less toxic than synthetics; they may act as precursors to safer synthetic chemicals. Synthetic chemicals include pyrethroid insecticides developed from pyrethrum in chrysanthemums; antibiotics developed from penicillin.
- *Location*   Risk that is unacceptable in one environment may be offset by benefits in other places. Ceasing chlorination of the public water supply in Peru, due to perceived risk of cancer, was offset by the major cholera epidemic that resulted[15] (see text). The cost/benefit of pesticide use changes with different circumstances of the environment or country in which it is used.
- *Intended use*   Warfarin is an effective rodenticide but is also used as an antithrombotic drug. Use as a pesticide may be essentially uncontrolled; its use as a drug is controlled but is subject to other factors, such as co-medications, that alter the risk factors for the anticoagulant hazard of its use, e.g. by competing for protein-binding sites and increasing the amount of free warfarin in the plasma.
- *Production*   Organic produce is widely marketed as 'better' than produce grown or treated with pesticides or preservatives. Untreated peanuts may contain unacceptably high levels of aflatoxin due to contamination with the mould *Aspergillus flavus*.
- *Substitutes*   An apparently non-toxic substitute may have unsuspected long-term effects of a different kind to the original. In proposing a substitute there is an onus to ensure that it is less toxic than the original chemical. (See Box 14.6 and associated text on methylene chloride.)
- *Type of exposure*   Risk due to low-level radiation from nuclear plants may be contrasted with the risk of melanoma due to sunbathing.
- It may be concluded that concentrating effort on reducing one risk is pointless if other factors pose similar or different risks that are greater. There comes a point beyond which effort to reduce risk become an expensive waste of time and money.

Differing national standards of water quality have also been a factor in bringing to light unexpected hazard and risk. In the USA it was indicated that chlorine in the drinking water could be associated with a small increase in the risk of bladder cancer. Chlorination of drinking water was found to be associated with the formation of chlorinated organic compounds, some of which were mutagenic in the Ames test. The US EPA concluded that chlorination of the public supply was no longer necessary. This decision was noted in Peru and it was decided that what was good in the USA should also be reflected in local policy and that water should not be chlorinated. This did not take into account the differing microbiological properties of the local public water supplies and, as a result, large numbers of people died in the cholera epidemic that followed.[17]

Risks associated with the differing uses of warfarin have already been mentioned in Box 11.3. Another topical example is the use of cannabis and cannabinol-related compounds in therapeutic applications, as against use as a drug of leisure. As always in risk assessment and management, it is useful to invoke Paracelsius, that the dose makes the poison. Given the pharmacological activity of cannabinoids and evidence of their benefit in a range of disorders, it seems less than sensible not to investigate their use more extensively. In considering the risks associated with use of cannabis, the comparative risks of alcohol and nicotine should also be considered. Once again, it seems that science and politics are, to all intents and purposes, incompatible.

Synthetic versus natural

One of the greatest public debates in comparative risk has been on the merits or otherwise of natural versus synthetic chemicals. Many synthetic chemicals have similar counterparts in nature to which humans have been unwittingly exposed for centuries, without epidemiologically perceptible effect. Although there is a great suspicion – fear even – about synthetic pesticide residues in food, it is seldom remembered that these chemicals are far outweighed by those that are present naturally. This emphasis is disproportionate; the synthetics are present in low, regulated concentrations and have all been thoroughly tested for safety, unlike the vast majority of natural chemicals. Concentrations of synthetic pesticides are further reduced by setting the interval between spraying and harvest. Natural chemicals in foods are essentially unregulated; for the most part, there are no epidemiological data that indicate necessity for regulation and, in any case, the database is not present to allow any sensible limits to be put in place. In fact, when natural chemicals are tested, a potentially alarming number of them are associated with unwelcome toxicity, often with a low margin of safety (Box 11.4).

Given the structural similarities between synthetic and natural chemicals there is no scientific future in trying to draw a toxicological distinction between them; synthetic does not mean toxic, natural is not always beneficial. The structures of some natural chemicals are so complex as to make them very

Box 11.4 Risk and chemicals naturally present in food

In 1999 the American Council on Science and Health published a holiday dinner menu[18] to coincide with the Christmas festivities, to demonstrate just how much of our regular diet is made up of potentially toxic chemicals, that are there naturally and in larger quantities than artificial chemicals such as pesticides.

- Endogenous plant chemicals include an assortment of alcohols, aldehydes, isothiocyanates, heterocyclic amines, carbamates, psoralens, caffeic acid, hallucinogens and large numbers of known rodent carcinogens such as benzo(a)pyrene and ethyl alcohol (which is also a human carcinogen).
- It has been shown repeatedly that high intake of fruit and vegetables protects against cancer, despite the fact that they contain chemicals that have been shown to be rodent carcinogens.
- White bread contains furfural, which is a rodent carcinogen. The carcinogenic dose in rodents was 197 mg/kg/day; the equivalent human dose would be 13.79 g *per day for life*; given that a slice of white bread contains about 167 *micrograms* of furfural, you would have to eat 82,600 slices of bread a day to achieve an equivalent carcinogenic dose.
- Although the emphasis is often placed on carcinogens, 'ordinary poisons' are also present. Potatoes contain the glycoalkaloid solanine which is a cholinesterase inhibitor and teratogen;[19] concentrations are much higher in green potatoes (about 2 mg/g compared with 0.1 mg/g in normal potatoes; the human lethal dose is about 500 mg).[20] Concentrations of such alkaloids can increase after harvesting through exposure to light or damage.[21] There has even been a suggestion that the potato may be the 'environmental culprit' in schizophrenia.[22] The safety margin between normally present concentrations and those that are toxic in humans is not large.
- Severe toxicity is associated with improperly prepared food plants such as cassava root, in which cyanogenic glycosides react with stomach acid to release cyanide. Red kidney beans produce toxicity unless boiled before eating.
- Edible mushrooms contain various hydrazines that have been associated with cancer in mice (Box 1.2).
- Against this background the Delaney amendment for food additives – that no additive found to cause cancer in animals after oral ingestion shall be deemed safe – seems a little redundant.

difficult to synthesise in a laboratory, yet these same comfortingly 'natural' chemicals include some of the most toxic substances known. Batrachotoxin is a structurally complex alkaloid found in the skin of the Columbian frog, *Phyllobates aurotaenia*, which has an LD_{50} in mice that is in single figure micrograms; few chemicals that are exclusively synthetic approach this level of lethal toxicity. Another consideration is that there are many times more natural chemicals than there are synthetic ones, also that many toxic chemicals considered to be artificial, like dioxins, are present in the natural environment through processes such as burning wood.

Use of pesticides or preservatives has two sides in terms of relative risk; that is, risks associated with their use and those associated with not using them. A decision not to use pesticides because they are toxic ignores the natural presence in our diet of vast amounts of naturally present chemicals that have evolved as endogenous defences against insect attack (see Box 11.4). Poor preservation of food – in an effort to maintain organic standards or production or for lack of facilities – can be associated with the growth of moulds. Products from these include aflatoxin (found in peanuts) and ochratoxins, which have been associated with the prevalence of Balkan Endemic Nephropathy.

When considering risks associated with pesticide use it is also worth looking at the increasing consumer enthusiasm for organic food produce, driven by the perception that 'pesticides are bad for you'. This has led to production of increasingly insect-resistant varieties so as to avoid the use of pesticides. This can result in insect-resistant crops that contain higher than normal amounts of endogenous chemical, leading to adverse effects. Thus, organic produce has at least the same amounts of natural chemicals as non-organic food and may have more; the absence of pesticides makes a small difference to the overall chemical burden.[14] In the final analysis, there is no dispute that pesticides are toxic but, as with every other chemical, this is very much a question of dose and the margins of safety between toxic concentrations and those acceptable in foods are regulated. Frequently these regulated margins are larger than for endogenous chemicals, such as solanine.

In conclusion, consideration of comparative risk is an essential in risk assessment of new or existing chemicals; there is no scientific point in setting stringent limits of exposure on a new chemical, if similar levels of hazard and risk are posed by an endogenous chemical present at greater concentrations. Too frequently, the public and politicians are blind to such comparison; I think that it is one of the responsibilities of toxicologists in general to communicate this aspect of risk assessment in a more effective manner.

Risk expression and quantification

Risk is the probability of harm and could, therefore, be expressed as a number between one and zero. In practice risk is expressed in terms of incidence per unit of population or as a percentage. Expression as an incidence – y cases per

100,000 – is useful in terms of the general population, within which the wide range of risk determinants, that affect specific groups or individuals can be accommodated without too much problem. A refinement of this is to compare risk in an exposed population with that in an unexposed population. Expression of relative risk implies some knowledge of normality, i.e. the unexposed population. Normal mortality[23] in Scotland is about 12 per 1000 population, possibly a little higher than in England. The same sources give access to a plethora of normal data for the incidences of disease and resulting mortality.

There may be circumstances in which it is possible to say that a percentage of people exposed to a chemical will probably show a particular adverse effect – as in patients receiving monotherapy with a specified drug – but this tends to be an exception. Although the dose makes the poison, it is the individual who makes the response and doses that leave many people unaffected can leave others severely disabled. It is this breadth of characteristic and potential response that complicates numeric expression of risk in terms of particular groups or individuals. In assessing the risks associated with production of a drug, it is simple to look at the incidence of reported adverse reactions in patients receiving known doses and to extrapolate these data to new patients. However, extrapolating these effects to a group of healthy production workers, who do not have the disease target for the drug and who will be subject (theoretically) to lower than therapeutic systemic exposures, becomes so imprecise that numeric expression is not possible, even if it was legally sensible.

Another sometimes useful, but easily devalued, method of risk expression is to use the doses associated with effect in animal studies and to extrapolate from these to the anticipated human dose. This can lead to seemingly ludicrous similes, such as drinking 400 bottles of cola a day while standing on top of a mountain (see Box 11.4). This method is particularly useful when looking at the risks associated with pesticides or natural chemicals. It is sometimes also useful to consider the factors that might increase the probability of death by one chance in a million. These include living with a cigarette smoker for two months, eating 40 tablespoons of peanut butter or living for 150 years within 20 miles of a nuclear power plant.[17]

Although it is desirable to quantify risk when looking at high-level assessments, for instance in terms of carcinogenicity, for the most part this is not particularly easy or necessary. For a workplace assessment, it is enough to know that there is a hazard to be controlled and that a reasonable estimate of risk can be made in general terms. This is arrived at by consideration of the various factors that contribute to the risk of the hazard being realised.

Summary

- Risk is seen at different levels from individuals to worker groups to national and global populations.
- Risk is increased or decreased by factors that include occupation, diet and lifestyle (smoking or alcohol consumption) and local circumstances.

- Risk of use may be offset by risks associated with non-use.
- Perception of risk, which is critical to successful risk management, is not necessarily subject to logical analysis. Perception is influenced by clarity and perceived honesty of communication and the acceptability of the risk expected.
- Risk may be quantified but this is usually only done for endpoints such as carcinogenicity after extensive mathematical modelling. For general purposes a qualitative assessment is enough.

Chapter 12

Risk assessment in practice and setting exposure limits

Introduction

We are now at the point where the hazards have been predicted to be human-relevant (see chapter 10). The information from these earlier stages is assessed to indicate the probability that the toxicities seen will be expressed in the target population under the anticipated conditions of exposure, which are usually assessed on a worst-case basis. This probability is governed by factors such as safety margins, working practices and form of chemical (see Box 12.1). In essence, in a risk assessment the toxicity of the chemical, related to dose levels in safety tests, is considered in conjunction with anticipated exposure levels for the target population. This should lead to an assessment of the likelihood that toxicity will be expressed in the target population, facilitating decisions on risk and exposure limits. These limits and controls may be re-evaluated in the light of the intended measures to be taken to control exposure in the target population.

Single effect versus general risk assessment

The end goal of risk assessment is an expression of risk in a quantitative or qualitative form. Although all hazards are assessed, risk assessments tend to fall into two overlapping types – broad assessments which look at all the relevant endpoints and those focused on a single effect. The latter may be described as high-level assessments, typically conducted for carcinogenicity and using data from rodent bioassays in conjunction with mathematical modelling to give a numeric estimate of risk for a general population. This focused type of assessment, which is an extension of the broad overview, is discussed briefly here but is not the main focus for this book; they are covered in detail in other texts (see Bibliography). The general multi-endpoint approach forms the basis of all assessments and is more likely to produce a qualitative gradation of risk estimate from likely to unlikely. The output is dependent on expert interpretation and discussion of all the data and this essentially opaque and indefinable process concludes with an overall interpretation that results in proposals for maximum exposure levels. Due to the lack of easy definition of process and decision pathways, it is important that records are kept on how and why the decisions were reached. These records may well become significant in a court of law or in discussion with regulatory authorities such as the UK Health and Safety Executive. They also help in the communication of the decision to those at risk, particularly if the decision is unwelcome in any way.

Although assessments may focus on particular hazards or effects, it is quite usual for a compound to show several different toxicities and these may be differently expressed according to dose or concentration and design and type of the experiment. All may be more or less relevant to humans, although only one may be relevant to the target population for whom the risk assessment is intended.

The above gives an indication of the broad approach to risk assessment, which should give a basic foundation on which to build a set of assessment practices. There is no sense in laying down dogmatic rules for such assessments because the circumstances of each type – whether for agrochemicals, industrial chemicals, drugs or food additives – and for each compound, differ to such an extent that they cannot be covered in detail here.

As stated earlier, the single endpoint assessment is an extension of the general assessment on which it is firmly based. These assessments are conducted typically for carcinogenicity and are often more relevant to the population in general rather than specific groups. They rely on numeric data from carcinogenicity bioassays and extrapolation from the low dose to the exposures that may be allowable in humans. For situations where the general population are already in contact with the chemical – for instance in the diet – these assessments can give an estimate of the existing risks associated with continued use. The weakness of this single endpoint approach is that the other risks associated with the chemical may be forgotten and the data on which they are based and the way in which they are manipulated may be of questionable relevance to humans. They are, however, based on defined mathematical models and produce numbers via a traceable process. While a numeric output may give a degree of comfort to the assessors, regulators and the general public, it does not necessarily mean that the conclusion drawn from these numbers is any more secure or sensible than one arrived at by a more flexible or broader method. Judgement, which is rarely traceable and sometimes difficult to explain, should always play a part in the final conclusion. Various aspects of this approach are covered in a brief discussion of models used (below) and later in a section on risk assessment in carcinogenicity (chapter 14). For those who would like greater detail, there are specific and general texts cited in the Bibliography.

Tools and models in risk assessment

There are a number of data-handling tools and models that can be used to assist with risk assessment. This short section looks briefly at physiologically based pharmacokinetic (PBPK) modelling, allometric pharmacokinetic scaling and at models for carcinogenicity data treatments.

PBPK models and scaling

The principle of PBPK models is relatively simple, although their design, valid-ation and mathematical complexity are not; the following is a very basic account. If the factors known to affect the ADME of a chemical – liver blood flow, partition coefficient, distribution into tissue compartments and the kinetics of metabolism and excretion – are known for one or more species at several doses, it is possible to extrapolate the dynamics from known (tested) doses to higher or lower doses and from one species to another. One of the objectives is to predict the behaviour of small doses in humans from the behaviour of higher doses used in animals. PBPK models can also be used to study the relationship between predicted tissue concentrations and toxic effect. Initially, a model is constructed which consists of a series of compartments that are linked by blood flow, the whole being represented by a diagram (Figure 12.1). Basic rules are applied to the design so that tissues which play a prominent role in the pharm-acokinetics or toxicodynamics of the compound are individually specified in the model. Other tissues can be grouped together as single compartments, dis-tinguishing tissues with high blood flow from those which have low perfusion rates. These are then linked by a series of kinetic expressions describing the movement of the chemical or its metabolites between compartments. Values for parameters such as blood flow through the liver or kidneys or pulmonary characteristics can be obtained from the literature. These are linked to para-meters for the chemical or its metabolites such as partition coefficient and binding affinities for proteins or receptors and to biochemical values for ADME. It should be borne in mind that much toxicity is associated with thresholds and that such thresholds are in turn associated with saturation of a process such as elimination or with exhaustion of a protective agent like glutathione. The presence of thresholds and the consequent drift from linear kinetics complicates the mathematics considerably. The model can then be validated against experi-mental data (or such data could be used in the design stages).

By adjusting parameters such as dose in the model, it is possible to predict concentrations in various tissues either of parent compound or its toxic meta-bolites and so to predict effect. In this way, the effects at doses used in toxicity tests may be used to predict the dynamics at low doses in the same species or by extrapolation to another species.

Extrapolation of pharmacokinetic parameters from animals to humans is a critical part of risk assessment.[1] An adjunct to PBPK modelling is the use of allometric scaling, which takes account of the differences in pharmacokinetics that are seen with increasing bodyweight in animals. Broadly, small animals such as mice tend to have shorter half-lives for chemicals than larger animals such as dogs or sheep. Allometric scaling offers a method of relating bodyweight or surface area to parameters such as blood flow through organs such as the liver and to pharmacokinetic parameters, particularly clearance, volume of distribu-tion and half-life. This allows prediction of these parameters by extrapolation

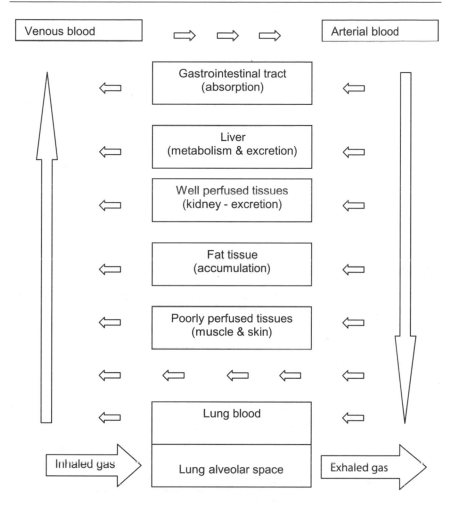

Figure 12.1 A simple physiologically based pharmacokinetic model.

from one species to another. This deceptively tidy and simple concept has encountered a number of problems. Clearance has not been well predicted[2] and the bodyweight model works best for renally excreted compounds.[3] The concept of neoteny – originally meaning the retention of juvenile characteristics in an adult animal – has been invoked to make the process more reliable by taking into account the larger brain weight and longer lifespan of humans. The search for scaling coefficients based on body-derived measurements has been criticised, a search for more mathematically based coefficients being proposed.[4]

This new search tends to demonstrate the ruthless quest of the numerate for greater 'accuracy' of prediction; it must be asked how the resultant 'accuracy' is

to be judged, given that the model can only be set up on one set of characteristics and the target population is composed of thousands of highly variable
individuals. In view of the degree of variation within a normal human
population, 100 per cent accuracy – or even 95 per cent plus or minus 15 per
cent – is a chimaera that cannot be achieved. Furthermore, a drive towards
greater mathematical complexity could mean that the benefits of scaling are lost
to a significant section of the toxicological risk assessment community and the
disadvantages of this outweigh the advantages of any illusory increase in
accuracy. As with all such substitutes for real experimental data, the processes
should be used rationally, with understanding of their weaknesses and with full
explanation of how the conclusions were reached. Used appropriately, allometric scaling is a valuable tool which, as with all other methods in toxicology,
provides useful data that can be used to support the whole database used for
assessment.

Models for rodent bioassay data

Mathematical models for the treatment of data from rodent bioassays for carcinogenicity risk assessments have proliferated over the years (Table 12.1). The
intention of these models is to extrapolate a line or curve from high dose to low
dose, so as to estimate dose levels that are 'safe'. There are a number of such
models, each one adding another layer of mathematical complexity to assessment
of a single endpoint from data that are, in many cases, of questionable relevance
to humans. To the non-numerate the credibility, in terms of relevance and general
application, of many of these models is hidden behind abstruse equations and
figures and assumptions that are not relevant to all data sets. The result of this is
a set of numbers that can prove to be less than perfect, when viewed in the light

Table 12.1 Models for risk assessment

Model	Comments
One hit	Based on the theory of single cell origin for cancer. Simple but producing conservative results
Probit	Assumes a normal distribution of log tolerances. Gives an S-shaped dose–response curve
Multistage	Assumes that carcinogenesis has various stages necessary for the development of cancer and that effects are additive
Multihit	A generalisation of the one hit model
Weibull	Another generalization of the one hit model
Logit	Leads to an S-shaped dose–response curve
Log-probit	Assumes a log normal distribution of individual responses

Source: Compiled from Gad, SC in Salem, H and Olajos, EJ (eds) *Toxicology in Risk Assessment.* London:
Taylor & Francis, 2000.

of subsequent experience. Because of the breadth of the target at which these models are aimed, the assumptions that go into them are necessarily imprecise and tend towards the conservative. They seem to offer a one-size-fits-all approach that, intuitively, is flawed because of the data they are based on (typically single endpoints such as tumours in mice) and the inherent absence of assessment of all the data that is necessary in 'real' toxicology. The end result can be an overestimate of risk leading to an exposure limit that is conservatively low but is not scientifically justifiable. The cost to society of such conservatism is probably considerable, through increased cost of reduction and clean-up programmes. One possible reason for the existence of such models, and their continued use with irrelevant data, is the fact that judgement is essentially unquantifiable and can be disputed – and frequently is. The provision of a conservative number, by a defined route and model with documented assumptions and record of the data used, gives a bulwark behind which some shelter can be found; this may be a poor shield, however, to use in response to litigation.

These models clearly have a valid role to play in the process of risk assessment but that validity is not driven by the elegance of the mathematical gymnastics but by the assumptions and the data that are fed into them. There seems to have been a tacit recognition that the data used were not always especially relevant or uniformly suited to the models available and this has been approached by attempts to make the models more able to cope with them. However, this has not been uniformly successful because the data are the problem not the basic concept of the models themselves. The objective should be to use data that are relevant to the problem under consideration and to have a model that does not rely on unjustifiable (or over conservative) assumptions or fudge factors. The various models used in risk assessment are discussed in detail by SC Gad.[5]

Target population, dose and exposure

In toxicology, risk is largely a function of exposure to the chemical under examination; if there is no exposure there is no risk. For a normal dose–response curve, risk increases with increasing dose, although dose is not necessarily the same as exposure for purposes of expression of toxicity, as a high dose may not be reflected in high exposure systemically or at the site of toxicity. Assessing the expected or actual dose and exposure levels is therefore fundamental to the whole process of risk assessment. There are, theoretically, two basic types of exposure, controlled and uncontrolled. Control may be exerted through the means of maximum allowable concentrations, recommended doses of drugs or pre-set workplace concentrations. In reality there is a sliding scale of control, the highest level being that of a patient who is given a drug and watched while they swallow it and the least during accidents. Control is usually a remote phenomenon and assumptions of regulating authorities may be made meaningless by the practices of the end user or by unpredicted spillage. Exposure can be assessed prospectively or after the event and may be to known or unknown chemicals; in addition it may be voluntary or involuntary. Each case poses its own challenges in assessing exposure – involuntary exposure to unknown chemicals being the most complicated to evaluate.

The expression of toxicity is determined by availability of the parent compound or metabolite at the target (or site of expression), therefore, while the ambient concentrations of the chemical are important, the concentrations achieved internally or at the site of toxicity are also critical. The extent of systemic exposure is dependent on the bioavailability of the chemical for the principal route and circumstances of exposure. To distinguish these, it is probably convenient to think in terms of external exposure (for instance an atmospheric concentration) and internal exposure as shown by maximum systemic concentrations or area under the concentration curve.

For controlled exposure, which is the exception as indicated above, the analytical techniques and matrices – blood or urine usually – are very similar, the main difference being that the dose is known and can be related to the concentration data (exposure) that emerge from the analyses. Methods of assessing exposure are explored briefly in Box 12.1. For purposes of risk assessment, the exposure levels are assessed to answer two questions: what hazards are associated with a measured concentration? and what is the safe concentration of the chemical? The outcome should be a proposed concentration or exposure level that should not be exceeded. The first question may be asked in respect of an existing environmental contaminant or natural chemical. The second question is typically asked about concentrations in production facilities so as to regulate exposure of the workforce or for setting acceptable concentrations of pesticides in foods.

Prediction

Prediction of dose or exposure is necessary when there is no prior knowledge of the chemical, as with a new food additive or on new or excessive release of a known chemical. The process of prediction may need to chart a chemical's progress from release into the environment or situation from which exposure can be experienced to the time it comes into first contact with people and what amounts are available for dermal or systemic exposure. The more steps between release and actual availability to the target population, the more difficult it is to predict exposure accurately. For example, for a chemical carried on or in food, uncertainties such as inconsistent daily intake, absorption effects due to other foods eaten at the same time and preparation losses make the prediction more complex and imprecise.

It is worth briefly revisiting the factors that affect the systemic levels found following external exposure to a chemical, bearing in mind that the duration of exposure may be over several hours each day or irregular and may not perfectly reflect data in safety studies. Following ingestion, the situation is relatively

Box 12.1 Assessment of exposure – basic principles

Uncontrolled exposure may be assessed by prediction or measurement, either direct or indirect. For most purposes of dose calculation a 70-kg person is assumed, although 50 kg is more conservative, especially for female target populations.

Prediction

- By ingestion. Knowing the concentration of the chemical in the diet or water, together with a reasonable daily intake, allows simple calculation of dose level. For example a pesticide present as residues on apples at 1 ppm might result in a daily dose of approximately 2 µg/kg, based on an average apple weight of 150 g, with a pesticide burden of 0.15 mg/apple, eaten at the rate of one a day by a 70-kg person.
- For inhalation exposure, the normal pulmonary tidal volume at rest is approximately 0.5 litre and the respiration rate is between 12 and 20 breaths a minute.[6] For a normal working day of 8 hours at a gentle workrate, a convenient nominal volume of air breathed is 10m^3, based on 20 breaths a minute each of 1 litre. On this basis, a concentration of 3 mg/m^3 translates into a daily dose of approximately 0.4 mg/kg in a 70-kg person. The total daily volume of respired air may need upward adjustment according to the type of work.
- Bioavailability data can then be used to predict systemic exposure from the expected dose.

Measurement

- Direct measurement may be made of the parent compound or its metabolites, usually in blood or urine but occasionally in expired breath, as with ethanol. These data should be specific for the chemical being assessed.
- Indirect measurements use biological markers or biomarkers[7] of effect or response, which include changes in enzyme activity or biochemical parameters such as inhibition of cholinesterase or changes in coagulation times.
- DNA or protein adducts are a useful indication of exposure to reactive chemicals but are produced by numerous chemicals and, unless identified specifically, do not necessarily imply exposure to the study chemical.
- Choice of matrix for analysis should be made according to the chemical under study or the type of marker to be used.

simple compared with dermal or inhalation exposure; systemic exposure (internal dose) is likely to be similar to that achieved in toxicity studies by oral administration. However, it is necessary to make allowance for differences in formulation and duration of exposure (once daily bolus versus probably constant low-level ingestion) but it should be possible to make a reasonable estimate of the amount of chemical that will be absorbed and reach the target site.

For dermal exposure, the local concentration, the duration of contact, local humidity and the extent of any local vasodilation, as well as formulation or form of the chemical should be considered; in addition, the local effects may be more significant than the systemic toxicity. Local concentration may be more important than dose expressed either as a total or in milligrams per kilogram bodyweight and the effects, which may well be local, are likely to be enhanced when high workloads act to increase body heat, peripheral vasodilation and local humidity. The presence of abrasions or skin disease, such as psoriasis, is also likely to enhance absorption across the skin. In some cases it may be necessary to assume a worst case scenario and assume total bioavailability, even if this is unlikely.

When exposure is likely to be by inhalation, the atmospheric concentration may well be constant but dose level will be varied by changes in the breathing rate and volume or air respired, which are normal responses to changes in work-rate or load. For solids or aerosols, the particle size determines the region of the respiratory tract in which the particles or droplets are deposited; the physicochemical or pharmacological properties of the material may also affect dose levels by causing avoidance behaviour in people exposed to it. Clearance of insoluble solids is via the mucociliary escalator, whereas liquids or soluble chemicals are likely to remain in the tract and be absorbed. For purposes of estimating the volume of air breathed in a typical 8-hour working day, 10 m^3 is often used as an arbitrary figure, being about twice the volume anticipated for a person at rest (Box 12.1).

Ultimately, the assessment is likely to produce an exposure level which may not be achieved systemically, due to factors such as genetic polymorphisms or differences in ADME. Once an applied dose has been predicted, use of the bioavailability data for the compound should result in a reasonably accurate estimate of exposure for a given dose.

Measurement

Without doubt, the best method of assessing exposure is directly, by measurement of the parent compound or a metabolite in the blood or urine. This should also be used as a check of predicted exposure levels. Where this is not possible, the use of indirect methods may give good data from which exposure levels may be extrapolated. These measure biological markers or biomarkers of response or effect as indicators of exposure to a chemical. These include inhibition of cholinesterase as an indicator of exposure to organophosphates and increased coagulation due to coumarins. They are usually much less specific than the direct methods; for instance cholinesterase inhibition is produced by all organophosphates and carbamates and, as a result, is an indicator only of exposure to a chemical with this activity, not to a specific agent. This lack of specificity increases as the remoteness of the measurement from the original chemical increases. Normally, however, there is a history of exposure to a particular chemical and it is relatively easy to make the connection between effect and cause. The extent to which the marker is changed from baseline data or from normal, gives a broad indication of the extent of exposure. However, it cannot be used to calculate the dose or plasma concentration of the chemical responsible (if it has been identified) because the severity of response is so much influenced by the individual in terms of genetics and circumstances under which exposure took place. Another factor, working against calculation of dose for unattributed exposures, is the differing potencies seen between members of chemical classes.

Reactive compounds or their metabolites interact with DNA or proteins, giving another method of assessing exposure. The total adduct concentration may be measured which gives an indication of total exposure to reactive chemicals without assigning responsibility to any individual agent. However, where a specific adduct – a nucleotide complexed with an identified additional chemical group – can be demonstrated, this is a clear indication of exposure to the parent compound.

A further group, biomarkers of susceptibility, indicate differing susceptibility to effect, as shown by genetic polymorphisms. A concentration of chemical that is relatively risk-free for the majority of the target population may carry an unacceptable degree of risk for susceptible individuals. This is exemplified by allergic responses to very low concentrations which leave the majority of people unaffected. They do not indicate exposure but are a significant factor in determining individual risk.

Process and factors in risk assessment

Risk is influenced by innumerable factors that act together or against each other in the process of delivering toxic chemicals or metabolites to their site of action. Although it is possible to list these factors, it is probably unwise to do so as this may be unduly restrictive. Risk assessment should not be seen as a box-checking exercise and all the circumstances surrounding the expected use of the chemical must be considered as these may well be unique to the proposed use in the intended location. Some of the factors relevant to risk assessment are reviewed in Box 12.2; these points are expanded in the text that follows.

Physical form and formulation

The physical form of a chemical is significant in determining risk associated with it. A chemical poses the same hazard in whatever form it is present but

---

Box 12.2 Factors to be considered in risk assessment

The following is not in any particular order of importance and should not be seen as complete, as other factors may be relevant to particular chemicals or circumstances of use.

- Physical form. The risks associated with dusty powders, liquids or granulated products are different as the likelihood and type of exposure is different with each. A low-density, easily blown powder offers significantly greater risk than a solid or a viscous, aerosol-free liquid.
- Formulation. In general, diluted formulations pose less risk than concentrated forms; formulation also can have profound effects on absorption and bioavailability.
- Expected exposure, in terms of route, dose and duration.
- General consideration of safety evaluation data for the shape of any dose-response curves and if there are thresholds for toxicity.
- Any human data that exist as a result of controlled experiment or accidental exposure; data from similar compounds may also be useful.
- Type of toxicity or hazard expected.
- Target organ and mechanism for toxicity; reversibility of any effects.
- Species differences in ADME, pharmacological potency and likely impact of any such difference in humans; human or animal polymorphisms in metabolism.
- Safety margins. The relationship between no observed effect level (NOEL), no observed adverse effect level (NOAEL) or lowest observed adverse effect level (LOAEL) and expected levels of exposure in humans. A wider safety margin will be desirable for toxicities such as allergy or carcinogenicity than for other effects such as transient, reversible change.
- Target population for whom the risk assessment is being prepared, in terms of sex, age, disease status, etc.
- Purpose of the proposed risk assessment.

---

different forms carry different risks, as with lead in petrol, paint or on church roofs. As stated above, if the toxic moiety cannot get to its site of action, it cannot cause toxicity at that site. Dermal exposure to a chemical that is not absorbed through the skin will not cause systemic toxicity, although there may be local effects such as irritation. A low probability of exposure is usually associated with a low level of risk. For example, in production facilities a granulated, dust-free product poses less risk than the same chemical in a low-density, easily dispersible form. A liquid form may be less risky to handle, providing aerosols are not generated. Particle or droplet size affects availability through inhalation, micron-sized particles being respirable, while larger ones are trapped in the upper respiratory tract. Physical form is also a consideration in dealing with accidental spillage: a free-flowing volatile chemical goes further when spilled and is more hazardous to clean up than a non-dispersible solid.

Formulation of a chemical with a carrier or excipient also changes risk levels, as this can have significant effects on bioavailability. A solution in a solvent that enhances transdermal absorption is inherently more hazardous than a mixture of the same chemical with a solid excipient such as lactose. A solution combined with a process that allows formation of aerosols is potentially as hazardous as working with a dust. Dilution has the potential to reduce concentrations at the target site and so has benefits in reducing risk.

The expected form, and consequent bioavailability, of the product to which people will be exposed has to be compared with the formulations used in the safety evaluation studies because these are frequently different. A judgement has to be made as to how the form or formulation of the chemical compares with that in the safety data and whether it will be associated with greater systemic exposure levels than those seen in toxicokinetic data.

Route of exposure

The most likely routes and exposure must be considered together with the likely dose levels achieved. Also, the extent of control over the exposure is a significant factor; thus, while it is difficult to control exposure to chemicals present in the environment, much greater control is possible with prescribed drugs (in theory) and in the workplace. This can highlight two populations of exposed people for whom the risks are different. For an orally active drug, patients receive a tablet or capsule of known size at a predetermined frequency; exposure by other routes is expected to be minimal. Workers producing the same chemical, who do not have the disease target for the drug, can expect to be exposed to it dermally and by inhalation. Following inhalation, a degree of gastrointestinal tract exposure can be expected via the mucociliary escalator in the bronchi and, as humans are mouth breathers under exercise, by direct swallowing of deposits left in the mouth. The doses achieved clinically and in the workplace are also likely to be different, as is the duration of exposure. It is possible to have much higher local concentrations of undiluted chemical in a production facility than those encountered in other situations.

Bioavailability

When the likely routes of exposure have been assessed, the bioavailability by the most significant route should be considered. Although risk assessment is often based on dose levels used in the safety data, where possible, the plasma concentrations and systemic exposure should also be considered. Bioavailability is usually considered in connection with systemic exposure but availability for local effects is also important, given that the skin forms a reasonably effective barrier to many chemicals. It should be remembered that the concentration on the skin is likely to be higher than anywhere else and that local concentration on the skin is usually more important than dose expressed in milligrams per kilogram of bodyweight. This principle has relevance wherever the compound comes into contact with the body at high concentrations, including the respiratory tract and eyes, where locally high concentrations can be associated with significant irritation.

Dose response

The relationship, defined by the dose–response curve, between the anticipated exposure levels and the dose levels at which effects were present or absent is absolutely critical to the risk assessment process. The difference between toxic concentrations and the expected dose in the target population gives the safety margin; the steepness of the dose–response curve gives an indication of how quickly the spectrum of effect is likely to change for small increases in dose level. Risk assessment is simplified where there is a large margin of safety between effect and target population exposure levels. This is seen in situations where limited toxicity is seen at very high exposure levels but exposure in the target population is, for example, a factor of 1000 or more lower. Simplistically, large margins of safety are associated with lower risk.

The presence of a concentration or dose above which toxicity becomes evident should not necessarily be taken to mean that the hazard is not relevant, as individual circumstances can act synergistically with the chemical to reduce the threshold. While it may be statistically sensible to take in the 95 per cent of the population who can be expected to fall within two standard deviations of the mean, this does not mean that the other 5 per cent can be ignored.

For drugs, low dose effects may result from the compound's intended activity but these are still likely to be undesirable when expressed in a healthy group of production workers or in the population at large. Where toxicity is expressed only after a threshold level of systemic exposure has been exceeded, this is a clear indication that the effect will probably be absent at the (theoretically) lower levels expected in the target group. This is reinforced if the exposure levels above which the effect is seen are similar in all the test systems in which it is present.

Safety evaluation and human data

Having considered the data that relate to the physicochemical characteristics and form of the chemical and the effect that these and any excipients and concentration factors have on the likely risk, it is time to consider data relating to safety evaluation and human exposure (if any). First consideration should be of any dose–response curve (see above) that has been generated for the effect under consideration and, particularly, if there is a threshold for toxicity below which effects have been shown to be absent.

Although species specificity of response has been cited as a major reason for saying that a hazard is not relevant to humans, a cynical view is that this means simply that the risk of the effect being seen (or detected) in humans is very small. Although the normal approach is to look for differences between species, in some ways a simpler option is to look for uniformity of response. While differences in response can be useful in assessing risks, there is an onus to define these differences mechanistically and this is not always immediately practicable. Lack of definition of mechanism can lead to uncertainty and this must be taken into account in the risk assessment. However, if every test species shows the same effect, it is very likely that humans will show a similar response and this gives a degree of certainty – although this is unlikely to be welcomed.

Expression of the same effect in different species does not mean necessarily that it will be present at the same dose levels or concentrations of exposure. Absorption, distribution, metabolism and elimination will probably be different across the species and possibly between individuals – especially in a genetically diverse population. Much toxicity is due to metabolism by the family of cytochrome P450 enzymes, which show a substantial degree of diversity between species. While a P450 that produces a toxic metabolite in rats may be absent or nearly absent in humans, this does not necessarily mean that the metabolite cannot be produced in humans as the activity needed for the reaction can be expressed by other P450s. Such activity is usually lower than that in the affected species or target tissue.

Where toxicity is expressed through interaction with a receptor, the inter-species differences in affinity for the target need to be taken into account. These differences affect the time of onset of the effect and the speed with which it can be reversed. High-affinity binding can lead to a prolonged effect whereas transient binding to a low proportion of the receptor population is usually associated with transient effect, especially if it is combined with rapid clearance from the target tissue.

In addition to the factors considered above, the safety evaluation studies should also define the hazard in terms of extent, mechanism and reversibility, as well as the factors covered above such as ADME and any differences between species or individuals. One of the most important data points to come from these studies is the level at which no effect has been detected, the NOEL (no observed effect level). If treatment-related effects were seen at every dose level, it may be possible to assign one as a level at which no adverse effects were seen (NOAEL). For this purpose an effect that is not adverse is generally one that is reversible, slight in extent, does not affect the well-being of the organism and is not associated with any permanent consequences. Such slight effects include transient increases in plasma enzymes, reversible increase in liver size due to hepatocyte hypertrophy or transient pharmacological action. Failing this, the lowest observed adverse effect level (LOAEL) may be used but this is not usual.

Each case needs to be considered individually, as an over precise definition of what constitutes 'adverse' may not be helpful. If the hazard for which the risk assessment is being conducted is always adverse, the NOAEL will not be acceptable and a NOEL becomes essential.

Although the acceptability of the risk and the specific hazard under consideration do not affect the numeric process of risk assessment, it is relevant in setting safety margins and acceptable exposure limits. This is influenced by the target organ of toxicity, the extent and type of effect and its reversibility. The last point is a critical aspect of the safety evaluation and has significant impact on the acceptability or otherwise of the risks. Some effects, such as birth defects, cancer or lesions in the central nervous system are not reversible and demand a wider margin of safety than those which do not have any long-term consequences. Some effects, such as allergy, demand wide safety margins as the reaction to even very low concentrations can be life threatening. Allergy is a particularly difficult hazard to deal with because, once established, the concentrations required to provoke a reaction are much lower than those needed for induction. Another factor here is that it is not necessarily easy to predict and can take a long time to develop, as shown by countless animal workers who have become sensitised to animals after years of problem-free work.

Any human data, which may have resulted from clinical exposure, accidental spillage, overdose or even experience gained through working with the chemical, are also an important aspect of any risk assessment. For uncontrolled exposure these data have to be assessed carefully for any estimate of dose achieved and this is not always possible. On top of this the circumstances and adequacy or extent of the data associated with each report have to be considered, as not every exposure is reported with future risk assessments in mind. Where several epidemiological studies are available, care must be taken that the protocols and diagnostic criteria used were consistent (if the data are to be pooled) and that other epidemiological pitfalls have been avoided.

Another source that should not be ignored is information from any similar compounds, either of the same chemical class and toxicological profile or having the same pharmacological action. It should be borne in mind that pesticides can have pharmacological effects (not always welcome) and that this term does not simply relate to drugs. In looking at such data the relative potencies of the chemicals should be taken into account, together with any other toxicities expressed, as similarity of toxicological profile can be used to back up conclusions from the risk assessment of the hazard under consideration.

Purpose and target population

Finally, the purpose of the risk assessment, and the population at which it is aimed, should not be forgotten. The composition of the population that is liable to exposure is relevant as risk factors differ according to age, sex, disease status, occupation and expected circumstances of exposure. Some risks are not relevant to some populations; teratogenicity is not usually a risk factor for all-male working groups, although it may be indicative of other reproductive hazard relevant to males. Dermal exposure and irritation may be a problem in production workers but should not be significant in patients taking a capsule by mouth. Inequality of risk between populations is demonstrated by consideration of diethylhexylphthalate (DEHP). Exposure to DEHP is significantly higher in US patients receiving dialysis (50,000 patients receiving 4500 mg/year intravenously) than in the general adult US population (220 million) who are each exposed to 1.1 mg/year through dietary contamination. Patients who receive irregular blood transfusions, haemophiliacs and young children exposed orally form further subgroups who are exposed to DEHP to different extents.[5]

The composition of the target population for whom the risk assessment is being generated will define the responses that may be expected. The reaction to any chemical is likely to be different between healthy production workers, a group of patients or the general population. Although it may seem sensible to say that teratogenic effects are not of significance if there are no women in the target population, the situations where it is possible to say that women will never be exposed are infrequent and this approach should be used with caution.

Pharmaceuticals offer a number of examples of the way risk assessment works and illustrate the dynamics of the whole process, showing that an assessment for one group is unlikely to suit another. The first contrast can be drawn between patients and production workers; the former have a disease and would be expected to benefit from exposure. Furthermore this exposure is more controlled than for the production workers who do not have the disease and for whom the pharmacological effects may be unwelcome if not actually adverse. Another group who can be expected to be exposed to a new pharmaceutical are the healthy volunteers who, for non-life-threatening diseases, are the first humans to be purposely exposed to the drug. The assessment of risk for this group has to be very conservative because of the significant step that is being taken – from the laboratory animals of the safety evaluation to a first dose in humans. For this reason, first doses in humans are usually conservatively low, with a large margin of safety from the NOEL identified in the most sensitive species. However, for drugs intended for life-threatening conditions such as cancer, it is normal to start human studies in patients rather than volunteers, especially if the drug is toxic, which is frequently the case for cancer therapies. For these patients the risk/benefit ratio is clearly different from other drugs and, as a result, the starting dose is often close to those associated with toxicity in the safety studies. The risk evaluation is complicated in these patients by the general expectation that they are likely to be seriously ill and taking co-medications that are likely to affect responses to the test drug. As the clinical evaluation continues, the risk evaluation of the drug must be continuously revised as the human data accumulate. Thus, a risk evaluation conducted in the final stages of clinical trials is likely to be very different to that carried out for the human volunteers in the first trial.

Setting safety factors and margins

Safety factors are set with the intention that the hazard being assessed will not – with reasonable confidence – be seen (at unacceptable levels in some cases) in the target population. The use of safety factors in risk management has been routine for many years to establish a margin of safety between the doses used in safety evaluation tests (normally in animals) and the levels to which humans will be exposed. Therefore, agreement on safety factors is a basic requirement before exposure limits can be set. The traditional (i.e. questionable) approach has been to use a factor of 100, being a factor of 10 lower to take into account possible differences between species and a further factor of 10 lower to take into account variation amongst the human population. Although this is a simple approach requiring limited numeracy to put into effect, it was based on the fact that there was little knowledge to justify any other method. In reality, therefore, the two factors of 10× are uncertainty factors that have to allow for differences in toxicokinetics and toxicodynamics within the test species and between human individuals. In either case, the traditional approach may not give a large enough safety factor or, equally, may give one that is larger than is warranted by the actual data. With greater understanding of mechanisms of toxicity, differences in ADME and toxicodynamics, a more refined approach is becoming possible.

Box 12.3 summarises the factors that need to be taken into account when deciding safety factors in respect of a particular hazard and target population.

Box 12.3 Choosing safety factors

A safety factor is a desired margin of safety over doses which have shown to be without effect or to show change that is not adverse. When deciding this margin, factors considered should include the following, although each case is different and other factors may well be relevant.

- Database available; increasing study length, statistical power (sample numbers or individuals) and quality increase confidence in the data; small-scale, short studies are a poor basis for extrapolation and so an extra factor should be added.
- Type of effect under consideration – knowledge of mechanism, duration and reversibility. An additional safety factor may be added but apply this to the toxicity of concern not to another lesser effect seen at a lower dose level or in another species.[8]
- Type and use of chemical. The class of compound and its mode of action – toxic or pharmacological – should influence the size of safety factor chosen. Replacement therapies such as hormones or potent pharmacological disruptors of normal physiology (e.g. bisphosphonates), which could have significant adverse effects in a healthy population, need particular care.

- Precedent with chemicals of similar structure, class or mechanism of action. This information, taken with data on relative toxicity in terms of NOEL or NOAEL and knowledge of their effects, should allow more precise choice of desired safety margin.
- Acceptability and perception by the target population of the risk being assessed.
- The traditional method – 10× for species plus 10× for individual variation and a further multiplier to take into account the factors above; e.g. reproductive effects in safety studies might add a further factor of 5×.
- Additional factors may be added for different absorption between test route and exposure route, different ADME and any other clear differences.
- The approach suggested by AG Renwick[9] splits the two factors of 10×. The first (for inter-species variations is split into 4.0× for toxicokinetic and 2.5× for toxicodynamic differences; the second 10× (for extrapolation to humans) may be split in the same way or as two factors of 3.2×[10] (see text). This approach is intended to remove some of the uncertainty in the use of the traditional factors but is dependent on detailed knowledge of the kinetics and toxicodynamics of the material.
- The use of safety factors in respect of chemicals naturally present in food is probably inappropriate.[11]

Hazard weighting and safety factors

The type of toxicity expressed – the hazard – affects the weighting of the subsequent decisions on how the risks are managed. Reproductive effects and frank carcinogenicity are seen as more undesirable than transient effects and so carry more weight in any subsequent risk assessment – and demand larger safety factors in deciding permissible exposure limits. With increasing dose and toxicity it is normal for the number of changes to increase also, producing a range of effect from low to high dose level. The various dose levels associated with change in degree of effect – from NOEL to NOAEL to LOAEL – may be relevant for different populations and, as a result, any targeted risk assessments should take this into account. The result may be to set exposure limits that differ for particular groups and exposure situations, for example production facility workers and consumers.

Safety factor rationale

Looking at the traditional approach of two multiples of 10×, the first is intended to account for potential (probable) differences in response between species. In setting exposure limits, it is normal to use safety evaluation data from the most sensitive species, which may be a non-rodent. Due to the greater variability between individuals of non-rodent species and the smaller data sets in comparison with rodents, a 10× factor to allow for extrapolation between species may not be enough. If there is not much difference in response or sensitivity between the species that have been investigated, a lower factor than 10× may be reasonable. For the second factor of 10×, to account for variability within the human population, there may be huge potential differences in response, a situation that is seen with allergens. It is possible to be exposed over a number of years to an allergen without any evidence of adverse reaction, a situation that is seen repeatedly with animal allergy. The problem for this type of hazard is that the majority of the population will be able to tolerate quite high concentrations whereas a relatively few sensitive individuals – who it may be difficult or impossible to exclude from the target population – could be sensitive to concentrations 100-fold lower. In this case, the only approach is to select a safety factor that should protect everyone, even though this may place costly restraints on the production or containment processes.

To remove some of the uncertainty from the use of the traditional 100-fold safety margin, AG Renwick has argued (see Box 12.3) that the two 10× factors should be split to take account of differences in toxicokinetics and toxicodynamics in the test species and differences in pharmacokinetics and pharmacodynamics in the human population. This method clearly depends on fairly detailed knowledge of the behaviour and fate of the chemical not only in animals but also in humans and on the correct choice of starting dose (see below).

Whatever approach is used, a safety factor must not be derived from an exposure limit chosen simply because it can be achieved. It is not acceptable to say that exposure limits cannot be reduced because (for example) the equipment in use is not capable of greater containment levels or the personal protection equipment is inadequate or wrongly used. The safety factor should be decided first, based on the best data available, and the exposure limit is then derived from the safety evaluation data as described below.

Exposure limits

One of the first hurdles to overcome in this discussion is the plethora of abbreviations that are used for the various types of exposure limit. These can become confusing when all are discussed together; Table 12.2 provides definitions of the more usual limits. These are broadly divisible into those that are relevant in the workplace (OELs and OEBs) and those that are relevant to the human population in general, although there is some overlap. Those that cover the workplace generally assume intermittent exposure, usually for no longer than a typical working day of 8 hours in a 40-hour week and can set average exposure limits (TWAs) or maximum concentrations which are tolerable

Table 12.2 Definitions of exposure limits

OEL	Occupational exposure limit	Average airborne concentrations of a chemical to which workers may be exposed over a defined period
PEL	Permissible exposure limit or permissible dose	The dose that has no adverse effect in a worker. Mostly US term for limits for industrial chemicals that are enforceable by a central authority such as the Occupational Safety and Health Administration.
OEB	Occupational exposure band	An absolute upper limit of exposure based on categories to which compounds with few data are assigned based on hazard
TLV	Threshold limit value	The upper permissible airborne concentration
TLV-C	Threshold limit value – ceiling	An airborne concentration that should not be exceeded at any time
STEL	Short-term exposure limit	The upper airborne concentration that is acceptable for short-term exposure (e.g. not longer than 15 minutes experienced no more than 4 times in a day at intervals of not less than 1 hour) without prolonged or unacceptable adverse effect.
TWA	Time weigted average	The average concentration to which nearly all workers may be exposed repeatedly without adverse effect, during a working day of 8 hours or a 40-hour week
MRL	Maximum residue limit	The maximum acceptable concentration in foods for pesticides or veterinary drugs
ADI	Acceptable daily intake	The daily intake of a chemical that is expected to be without adverse effect when ingested over a lifetime
TDI	Tolerable daily intake	Used in similar contexts to ADI, for residues and food contaminants

Source: Compiled from the Dictionary of Toxicology and reference texts cited in the bibliography.

transiently within the working day, usually for no longer than 15 minutes (TLV-C, STEL). The OEB, as distinct from the OEL, places compounds into four or five bands of acceptable concentrations based on their known or expected toxicity. They are used when there is little information about the chemical, particularly for human effects.

Exposure limits that are applied to the general population cover chemicals such as food additives or pesticides (ADI), although a similar limit, the TDI is used for residues of veterinary drugs and food contaminants (which may be pesticides but may also be other unintended contaminants such as aflatoxins). The MRL is an offshoot of the ADI/TDI and refers to the upper limits of residual drug or pesticide that is allowable in food that reaches the supermarket; in turn this limit influences the interval that is allowed between application or treatment and harvest. These various limits refer to the chemical of concern or, in some cases to metabolites or other degradation products. A further measurement is becoming more common, the biological TLV, in which a biological marker (such as cholinesterase inhibition) is used to define the limit of effect beyond which exposure should cease or be reduced.

Many chemicals are already officially regulated and have set OELs, under European regulations such as Control of Substances Hazardous to Health (COSHH) or the US Occupational Safety and Health Administration (OSHA) and the American Conference of Governmental Industrial Hygienists (ACGIH). If the chemical of concern is not novel, the regulations from these or similar bodies should be checked before setting your own limits that may fall outside (higher than) official ones. Standard texts such as Casarett and Doull have listings of such exposure limits (see Bibliography).

Dose level selection for exposure limit calculation

Dose selection for exposure limit setting is usually carried out by assessing the data from a single species and often one study. If the effect is seen in more than one species the most sensitive species is taken for dose selection, using the longest toxicity study performed. The first step is to ask at which dose level the effect of interest becomes apparent or likely in the test species used in the study being assessed. Usually there are two dose types to look for; the NOEL and the NOAEL. In a typical study of three treatment groups in which progressive liver toxicity is seen with increasing dose, there may be no effect at the low dose (the NOEL), marked hepatotoxicity at the highest dose and minimal change at the mid dose level. If the effects at the mid dose are clearly minimal and reversible, it may be designated as a NOAEL. In this instance use of the NOAEL is sensible because it is a dose that you know to be associated with some effect. In cases where effects at the mid dose are too severe to allow its use, it will be necessary to use the NOEL in the calculation.

There are problems with both these approaches. If the NOEL is used it may be much lower than the next dose up. Although scientifically supportable, dose choice in toxicity studies is often also consistent with numerical convenience, figures such as 3, 10 and 30 mg/kg/day or a similar variation being common; for relatively non-toxic chemicals however, the intervals between doses can be very much larger. The result is that if there is an effect at the mid dose that renders it unsuitable for this use, the low dose may be so much lower as to give little confidence in estimation of the dose at which minimal effects would become apparent (effectively an extrapolated NOAEL, although this is not used routinely). Thus the NOEL may give a lower dose for calculation of exposure limits than is actually justified by the true toxicity of the chemical. Exposure limits on this basis may be more conservative than is desirable, leading to containment or clean-up measures that impose higher than necessary costs on those responsible for managing the risk.

The use of the NOAEL is also flawed in some ways. It does not take sample size into account or variability around the mean that may be due to inhomogeneity in the sample population. Also, because animals tend to tolerate higher doses over short studies than over longer treatment periods the NOAELs in subchronic studies are likely to be higher than those in chronic studies. This is particularly true for toxicities that accumulate with continued treatment; nephrotoxicity may not be seen in four-week studies, may be only minimal after 13 weeks but life-threatening after 26 weeks – even if dose levels for the successive studies are reduced according to the data from the previous study. In addition, the NOAEL takes no account of the shape of the dose-response curve and does not take into account the degree of toxicity at higher doses. However, similar arguments may be levelled at the NOEL.[5,12–15]

In some studies where there is a progressive dose-response curve for an adverse effect, there may be no NOEL. In this case it may be necessary to use the LOAEL or the benchmark dose (BMD). The LOAEL is the lowest dose at which adverse effects were seen and does not refer to a dose at which a defined per cent response is seen – either in terms of numbers of animals affected or in extent of response relative to controls. The BMD seeks to define a dose at which a low response is seen, for example 10 per cent; this may be estimated by extrapolation or calculation from the upper confidence limits of the dose–response curve. It has been seen as a point of departure for the onset of toxicity and replaces the NOEL or LOEL/LOAEL. The drawback of the BMD concept is the need to define a 10 per cent response rate and the statistical weakness of shorter toxicity studies for this purpose. As a result, this is probably best suited to relatively large data sets such as those that result from chronic toxicity or carcinogenicity studies in rodents. If using smaller data sets, as found in shorter rodent studies and those using non-rodents, the uncertainties of this become more significant. The BMD approach used for threshold versus non-threshold effects is also slightly different, the method in the latter being to draw a line from the BMD to the origin of the curve; this is used for genotoxic carcinogens. With the BMD dose it is also necessary to assume an acceptable risk level.

For pharmaceuticals, the minimum therapeutic dose may be used in conjunction with data from clinical trials or adverse reaction reports. However, it is necessary to remember the type of indication the drug is used for, given that toxic treatments are more acceptable for cancer than for non-life-threatening diseases. For non-life-threatening diseases the minimum therapeutic dose may be expected to be relatively non-toxic; for cancer treatments, this cannot be assumed. Examples of these various methods are given in Tables 12.3 and 12.4. Note that because the doses of thalidomide and ethinyl oestradiol are given as the human dose, there is no need to multiply by bodyweight.

For chemicals that have a long history of use or production, it is essential to find out what the existing knowledge base is to indicate currently experienced

Table 12.3 Calculating an OEL for thalidomide using different methods

Data base	Therapeutic dose	Benchmark dose (BMD)
Toxicity seen as birth defects	Assume effect level is 25 mg/day po	25 mg/day assumed as BMD
NOAEL unavailable in animals or humans	$100\times$ factor for extrapolation from effect level to NOAEL	Response at BMD assumed to be 50%. Linear extrapolation to origin
50 mg/day po: 10–50% affected	$10\times$ for human variability	Acceptable risk assumed 1:10,000
25 mg/day po: % response unknown	$2\times$ to adjust for route difference (po instead of inhalation)	$2\times$ to adjust for route difference (po instead of inhalation)
Breathing 10 m³ in an 8-hour workday	OEL=1.25 μg/m³	OEL=0.25 μg/m³

Source: Compiled from a presentation by Ku, Robert H (SafeBridge Consultants Inc) at the American Chemistry Society annual meeting in San Diego 2001.

Table 12.4 OEL calculation for ethinyl oestradiol, a synthetic oestrogen

Method	Calculation
NOAEL and safety factors	Human NOAEL is 3.5 μg/day divided by (safety factor of $10\times$ multiplied by breathing rate at 10 m³/8-hour day) → OEL=0.035 μg/m³. The factor of $10\times$ is for human variability
Therapeutic dose and safety factors ($100\times$)	Lowest therapeutic dose=20 μg/day. Divided by (100x factor multiplied by breathing rate at 10 m³/8-hour day) gives an OEL of 0.02 μg/m³
1% increase over endogenous production	Endogenous production of 17-beta oestradiol in humans=about 70 μg/day. Ethinyl oestradiol is about $2\times$ more potent than 17-beta oestradiol. A 1% increase in activity would be equivalent to a daily exposure to 0.035 μ/m³ if breathing at 10 m³/8-hour day

Source: Compiled from a presentation by Ku, Robert H (SafeBridge Consultants Inc) at the American Chemistry Society annual meeting in San Diego 2001 and Ku, Robert H. 'An overview of setting occupational exposure limits for pharmaceuticals'. *Chemical Health and Safety*, Jan/Feb 2000.

dose levels. This may not be easy when production is being set up in competition with a rival company. If there is a reliable estimate of current exposure levels – for industrial chemicals, food contaminants or endogenous dietary compounds – a margin of exposure (MOE) or safety can be calculated as a ratio by dividing the NOEL, NOAEL or LOEL by the highest dose experienced in the target population. This may indicate that the MOE gives a sufficient safety margin and that no further action is needed; alternatively, it may indicate that additional containment or clean-up measures are needed to reduce exposure.

Setting exposure limits

There are two basic steps in setting an exposure limit; first to take the chosen safety factor relevant to the lead effect that you are guarding against and then apply it to the dose level that you have selected as the basis for your calculations (Box 12.4). Both these steps imply choice and both therefore require a degree of expert judgement. Choice of safety factor has been reviewed above and I have assumed that this far into the process the effect of concern has also been chosen. However, as indicated by AG Renwick,[8] there is little scientific sense in choosing a safety factor for microscopically evident liver toxicity if it is then applied

---

Box 12.4 Setting exposure limits

The first step is the choice of dose level with which to start the process.[5,12] Taking the toxicity or effect of concern, as seen in the longest toxicity study available in the most sensitive species, assess the data to decide which type of dose level is most appropriate, usually selected from the following:

- NOEL, NOAEL or LOAEL – all based on inspection of the data. These do not take account of the shape of the dose-response curve or the risks and effects present at higher dose levels.
- The BMD is the dose at which there is a low response (e.g. 10 per cent), observed or estimated from the upper confidence limits of the dose–response curve. It is probably best suited to larger data sets and requires some estimate of what constitutes an acceptable risk to provide a safety factor.
- For known pharmaceuticals the minimum therapeutic dose may be taken and a safety factor applied to produce an exposure level that can be expected to be without adverse effect or undesired pharmacological consequences.

Then, taking the chosen dose apply the safety factors selected in Box 12.3 and put into the basic formulae as follows:[13]

$$\text{Occupational exposure limit} = \frac{\text{NOAEL (mg/kg/day)} \times 70 \text{ kg (human bodyweight)}}{a \times b \times c \times \text{breathing rate}}$$

$$\text{Acceptable daily intake} = \frac{\text{NOAEL (mg/kg/day)} \times 70 \text{ kg (human bodyweight)}}{a \times b \times c}$$

Where NOAEL represents the dose chosen from the safety data, 70 kg is a standard human (50 kg gives a more conservative figure and may be more appropriate for females), a, b and c are safety factors (a for extrapolation from the test species to humans, b for human variability, c for other considerations such as nature of toxicity, etc.). The breathing rate is usually assumed to be 10 m^3/8-hour working day for a medium workrate). The OEL here is for air-borne particulates and the ADI would be suitable for foods or drinking water. Occupational exposure bands are set for chemicals without official or in-house OELs and for which there are not much data[14,15] (see text). Some basic rules of thumb may be added to this:

- Although it may be politically correct to choose a dose level at which there is absolutely no effect, this may not be relevant to the toxicity of concern if the NOEL/NOAEL for that is higher.
- All activities of the compound should be considered, not simply the toxicities. An undesired effect other than toxicity may indicate a lower ADI.
- Overconservative selection of exposure limits can lead to unnecessary expenditure in clean-up or containment. Setting them too high may mean unacceptable adverse effects.

to a lesser effect such as functional, transient increase in urine volume without pathological correlate.

Occupational exposure bands may be set for chemicals for which there is no official set limit or in-house OEL.[14] These set bands of acceptable air-borne concentration; for dusts these are <0.1 mg/m^3, 0.1–1 mg/m^3 and 1–10 mg/m^3. Gases and vapours are assigned to four bands. There is also a lower, unspecified band for very active substances that cannot be assigned to these bands and for which special arrangements have to be made.

Summary

The following may be seen as the basic steps in risk assessment and the subsequent setting of exposure levels or acceptable intakes:

- The expected exposure of the target population dose in terms of environmental concentration and dose must be predicted or measured; predictions should be confirmed by measurement once the target population comes into contact with the chemical.
- The level of risk posed by a chemical is affected by physical form and formulation, the route(s) of exposure and the bioavailability by that or the most significant route (either in terms of gross absorption or maximal effect).

- The dose response shown by the safety evaluation data should be considered together with the effects expressed. Where there are human data available, these should be examined carefully for utility, given the sometimes imprecise reporting of dose and timing of effect relative to the time of exposure. Good human data are a luxury.

- The purpose and target population of the risk assessment may well influence the final outcome of the assessment. The qualitative factors of perception and acceptability of the risk due to the hazards should also be taken into account; successful management of risk is more likely if the target population is kept informed and in agreement.

- The setting of safety factors and margins is dependent on the weight given to the different effects or hazards, carcinogenicity requiring greater weighting than minor transient effects. Safety factors should be chosen scientifically wherever possible, although the traditional approach may be necessary where appropriate pharmacokinetic and mechanistic data are absent.

- Exposure limits are calculated by using the selected safety factors and the dose level from the selected safety study or studies that indicates a NOEL, NOAEL or LOAEL. Limits should be chosen on the basis of what is necessary rather than what can be achieved.

- This is taken as the basis of workplace risk management, which is considered in the next chapter.

Chapter 13

Risk assessment and management in the workplace

Introduction

The workplace is distinct from other arenas where chemicals may be encountered in terms of the extent and the closer management and control of exposure that is possible within a limited, defined space. The workplace, as a concept, is very diverse and includes offices, farms, shops, and all types of industrial plant, including those producing agrochemicals, pharmaceuticals and industrial chemicals. The conditions of exposure, especially in production facilities, are often very different from those to which an end user is subject. Potentially, in comparison with the end user, the production worker is exposed to high concentrations of the undiluted chemical for long periods in conditions of heat and humidity. This is particularly so for pharmaceuticals where the occupational dose is potentially higher than those needed to achieve the desired therapeutic effect. Furthermore, the ultimate user normally uses the chemical diluted by excipients. However, this does not apply in the case of chemicals used as intermediates in the pharmaceutical or agrochemical industries, which are handled undiluted. However, exposure in the production facility is often better controlled, from the producer's viewpoint, than at the point of use. The following discussion is largely aimed at chemical production facilities such as those in the pharmaceutical and agrochemical industries, but it should be remembered that undesirable occupational exposure can occur in other jobs such as welding, mining, construction and any other place in which chemicals are used or materials worked.

The historical and regulatory background

The causative role of occupation in progressive and debilitating diseases has long been recognised although scientific documentation of the hazards due to particular occupations started comparatively recently. The eighteenth century observation by Percival Potts of the connection between chimney sweeping and cancer of the scrotum, is seen as a milestone in this process. Occupational disease is a roll call of suffering and – in some cases – corporate irresponsibility based on ignorance and lack of understanding. The illnesses with occupational cause include asbestosis, silicosis, farmer's lung, solvent-induced neuropathies, cancer due to agents such as nickel or uranium, sensitisation and allergy including asthma; skin disease in particular is a big problem. Although there may some truth in lamenting that the rising tide of sensitisation and asthma is partly due to the ruthless pursuit of hygiene in childhood and consequent immuno-incompetence, the unpalatable fact is that today's managers have to cope with this and reduce exposures.

One characteristic of occupational disease has been that it tends to develop over many years and may not become apparent until after exposure has ceased, a situation seen with mesothelioma due to asbestos, which has a particularly long period between exposure and onset of the cancer. The corollary of this is that it has often taken a long time for diseases of this type to be associated with their cause, especially where there is an existing normal background. In the latter part of the twentieth century there was a vast increase in chemical production in terms of the number of novel chemicals and increased production of those already existing. A parallel increase in toxicological understanding of the consequences of long-term exposure and better epidemiology resulted in greater appreciation by legislators of the problem, leading to an increasingly stringent set of regulations and guidelines in developed countries.

In the UK, although controls existed before 1974, the Health and Safety at Work Act of that year covered all aspects of workplace safety including exposure to chemicals; this was enforced by inspection. The COSHH (Control of Substances Hazardous to Health) regulations of 1988, which were set up under this act, should be seen in the context of similar legislation in other European countries. In the USA the Occupational Safety and Health Act is administered by the Occupational Safety and Health Administration and occupational exposure limits for many individual chemicals have been set by the American Conference of Governmental and Industrial Hygienists. In Europe these functions are undertaken by organisations such as the UK Health and Safety Executive.

Factors in workplace risk assessment

Risk assessment in the workplace differs in a number of respects from risk assessment in the wider environment.

- The agents to which the workforce is exposed are known and the level of exposure can be controlled by containment of processes or by use of personal protection equipment (PPE).
- The exposure limits can be set centrally by legislation or locally by management but are potentially higher than would be acceptable in other situations. Accidental spillage of undiluted chemical can pose significant hazard
- The workforce is a selected population, whose long-term or day-to-day composition can be controlled by management; susceptible (or potentially

susceptible) individuals can be reassigned or not employed in the first place. Women of child-bearing potential (WCBPs) or who are pregnant may be excluded from certain production processes.

- The use of non-sensitive people does not necessarily mean that higher exposure levels will be acceptable as susceptibility can develop with time in some cases.
- The level of risk is affected not only by the substance but by the process it is subject to. A fully contained milling operation may pose very little risk – no exposure, no risk; however, at the end of this process, if the substance is transferred into polythene bags topped up by someone using a shovel, the risk levels can be significantly greater.
- There is strict control legislation that can result in heavy fines or closure of the plant if appropriate measures are not put in place.

These various factors, with the managerial responsibility of protecting the work-force (and so avoiding prosecution) mean that there is little margin for error. An over-conservative assessment may mean that it is not possible to work on a particular chemical due to cost of unnecessary containment or clean-up. An assessment that is too generous may have serious consequences for worker health.

Workplace risk assessment

The process of risk assessment in the workplace is similar to that in other contexts. The human relevant hazards are predicted from the safety data and information for other compounds is considered as appropriate. These data are then assessed for dose response and mechanism and the likelihood of human toxicity is predicted. In the workplace the physical properties of the compound – particle size, powder density, aerosol formation, etc. – and the process involved are important. For example, milling a compound to produce micronised powder is associated with significant risk as there is greater potential for exposure by inhalation to a respirable form of the chemical, which may also be more easily absorbed by any of the other possible routes of exposure.

Although classic, numerical risk assessment may focus on the most serious hazard, in the workplace all the hazards due to a compound should be considered. If a compound is carcinogenic at high doses in animals but is also associated with significant acute toxicity at lower doses, it is likely that the risk assessment would be based on the latter rather than the potential carcinogenicity, assuming both to be relevant to humans. Each compound assessed poses a different set of problems but, broadly, the most important hazards from a workplace viewpoint are repro-ductive effects including teratogenicity, carcinogenicity, contact sensitisation and hypersensitivity reactions generally and target organ toxicity that is not readily reversible.

The data set available for workplace assessments can be less than the ideal situation outlined in chapter 10. Frequently the route of administration in safety studies is not the same as that expected in the workplace and an adjustment has to be made for differences in absorption and pharmacokinetics between the routes. A further factor is the circumstances of exposure in the workplace. A higher workrate is associated with increased breathing rate and larger inhaled volumes, going beyond the standard figure of 10 m^3 for an 8-hour day. Because humans are mouth breathers at high workrates, the opportunity for ingestion is also increased, either directly or indirectly by clearance from the bronchi via the mucociliary escalator. In addition, these increased workrates will probably be associated with increased temperature, moisture and peripheral vasodilation, which work together to increase local dermal effects and absorption into the systemic circulation. A side effect of these latter factors is that personal protective equipment is likely to be discarded or not worn correctly.

For pharmaceuticals developed for oral use, there is unlikely to be extensive toxicology by inhalation or dermal routes; in addition, any dermal toxicity studies may not have been conducted with the compound as it appears in the workplace. While the finished product will be well characterised in terms of all the data necessary for registration and marketing, any intermediates are often relatively unknown, particularly towards the end of the synthetic pathway, when they are unlikely to be standard off-the-shelf chemicals. In these cases, their similarity or otherwise to the final product has to be considered and it may be necessary to conduct a small set of safety studies. Of course, if the processes in which the intermediate is used are enclosed or adequately contained so as to avoid exposure of the workforce, such studies are unlikely to be necessary.

One aspect of workplace risk assessment that causes a number of problems is the obligatory supply of MSDSs (Material Safety Data Sheets) by chemical suppliers. Frequently the safety database for the more complex chemicals is not complete and, as a result, no definitive statement can be made on various aspects of the compound's toxicity. Thus, an MSDS may indicate that a chemical should be regarded as a potential mutagen and reproductive toxin, even if the studies have not been conducted, in an attempt to avoid litigation if effects are seen later. This leads to a very conservative approach, which is probably wise from the point of view of the supplier but less than useful for the user. In these cases other data sources should be consulted where available and computer-based systems of toxicity prediction can be used. A further limitation of MSDSs is that there is no indication of the quality or extent of the data that are summarised. In conclusion, my opinion is that an MSDS should not be used in isolation unless there really is nothing better available.

Where a facility has been producing a chemical for years with minimal precautions or reported effects, instituting a formal risk assessment may encounter some difficulties, particularly if the safety data indicate an assortment of hazards at exposure levels lower than those actually encountered in the workplace. Although there may have been many years of human exposure, it is quite probable that this has not been quantified or monitored and that any effects cannot be separated from the background by usual epidemiological methods. In these cases, instituting a system of personal exposure and health monitoring over a period of months may well prove useful in defining effects and the precautions to be taken, as indicated by the safety data.

Risk management in the workplace

The endpoint of workplace risk assessment is the setting of OELs (see chapter 12) and the management of the risks that have been identified as significant for the particular worker population and the processes involved. The following sections look at risk management in the workplace, starting with compound hazard categories.

Compound categories for containment

A basic preliminary measure to risk management in facilities that use or produce a range of chemicals is the creation of a series of categories that can be used to define the extent of containment for the chemical and any PPE. This simplifies risk management as it provides a set of basic controls that should work in the majority of cases with minimal modification. There is, however, the possibility that there will be pressure to keep chemicals in as low a category as possible because the higher categories are usually associated with significant containment and clean-up costs.

The system of categorisation in Table 13.1 is based loosely on schemes from several sources; although there are differences between schemes, these are essentially only of detail and the broad outline is the same. Although four categories are often used, I have suggested an entry level 0 for essentially non-toxic chemicals. This system should be workable without significant modification, although minor adjustment may be necessary to take account of local circumstances and preferences.

The criteria for classification given in Table 13.1 are what I consider to be the most relevant but others could be added, such as NOAEL, half-life, structural alerts, percentage protein binding, tissue-specific accumulation, the presence or absence of specific toxicities, or thresholds for specific pharmacological effect; atmospheric concentration may also be relevant. There may also be some utility in including bands of effect on specified markers, e.g. cholinesterase inhibition which could indicate differing potencies for groups such as organophosphates. Another practice is to link the categories to the EU risk phrases that are used to indicate specific hazards, particularly for transport of chemicals.

Although such schemes look very good and undoubtedly have great utility, actually using them is not necessarily straightforward. The central problem is that chemicals do not fall easily into individual categories; they can be category 1 according to one criterion but category 3 for another. The trick is to judge the circumstances and risks of the individual hazards and arrive at a consensus opinion. It may be necessary to categorise one form of a chemical at one level but a more hazardous form at a higher level. In broad terms, the greater the number of

Table 13.1 A basic system of compound categorisation

Category	Criteria for classification
0	Very low acute toxicity; lethal dose >2000 mg/kg. Minimal, transient toxicity due to functional change seen at high doses without pathological findings. No effect on reproductive function. Not mutagenic. No evidence of carcinogenicity by any mechanism. Non-sensitising, non-irritant. Poorly absorbed through skin or by inhalation. Fast elimination without accumulation into any body compartment. No evidence of human effect. NOEL for relevant effect >100 mg/kg/day in animal studies (equivalent to 5000–7000 mg/person/day).
1	Acute lethal dose: 200–2000 mg/kg. Toxicity in single organ system or species seen only at high doses on repeated dosing, without progression of effect with longer dosing, pathological findings no greater than slight or minimal; all effects fully reversible within 4-weeks without treatment. Dose-response curve shows presence of threshold of effect. No effect on reproductive function. Not mutagenic; no evidence of carcinogenicity in animals. Non-sensitising, non-irritant. Transient pharmacological effects present at >5 mg/kg that do not affect ability to work machinery. Pharmacokinetics show no accumulation; short half life. Poor dermal absorption. NOEL shows high margin of safety. NOEL in animal studies 10–100 mg/kg/day.
2	Acute lethal dose 25–200 mg/kg. Reversible, slight toxicity seen at mid to high doses in more than one species or more than one organ system. Not mutagenic. Evidence of carcinogenicity by a clearly non-genotoxic mechanism without human relevance. Minor effects on reproductive function associated with toxicity and not human relevant. Low potential for irritancy or sensitisation. Transient pharmacological effects present between 1–5 mg/kg. Some potential for dermal absorption. Pharmacokinetics show longer half-life with incomplete elimination within 24 hours but without significant accumulation. NOEL 1–10 mg/kg/day in animals.
3	Acute lethal dose 5–25 mg/kg. Potentially moderate to severe human relevant toxicity, with pathological change that is only slowly reversible. Mutagenicity in vitro but not in vivo. Carcinogenicity in more than one animal species. Reproductive effects that may be human relevant, including transient fertility reductions or changes in post-natal care, fetal toxicity without malformation. Pharmacological effects that may be irreversible or debilitating present below 1 mg/kg. Good dermal absorption with or without irritancy; potential for delayed sensitisation; corrosive. Pharmacokinetics indicative of slow elimination and possible accumulation. NOEL 0.1–1 mg/kg/day. Dose response curve with little margin between NOEL and toxicity.
4	Acute lethal dose <5 mg/kg. Potential for severe irreversible toxicity at low doses. Mutagenicity in vitro and in vivo. Evidence for human carcinogenicity. Embryotoxicity seen as malformations in the absence of maternal toxicity; clear effects on fertility. Pharmacological effects present at microgram doses. Severely irritant or sensitising, with potential for anaphylaxis or other severe allergenic reaction. Pharmacokinetics show strong binding in a particular body compartment. NOEL below 0.1 mg/kg/day.

Note: Compiled from several sources.

classification criteria, the greater will be the complexity of applying the scheme to individual chemicals. On balance, where there is uncertainty of relevance or effect, the bias should be towards a higher category rather than a lower one.

The process of risk management in the workplace

The intention is to manage the risks associated with the chemical so as to avoid adverse effects in the workforce or in the wider environment. The theory is that the risks that have been identified are assessed and acceptable levels of exposure agreed against appropriate levels of containment and PPE, remembering that PPE is not the primary means of avoiding exposure. These risks are then managed to prevent expression of the hazards identified, while maintaining awareness of costs and risk benefit ratios.

Assuming that hazards have been identified, the first step is to set OELs, either locally or from central legislation or regulation. Having set an OEL, it is important to know what the processing equipment is capable of in terms of containment. This can be either derived from experience or manufacturer's data sheets or by experiment. There is no point in setting a low limit if the equipment cannot achieve it. Equally, using advanced equipment inappropriately to achieve a much lower limit than is actually required may have unacceptable cost implications.

Look at the processes involved and the characteristics of the compound or the formulation to be used; if the main risk is by inhalation and the material is a liquid without chance of aerosol formation, the level of risk will be lower than for a low-density powder that can be easily blown about. It is normal to work to a worst case scenario and then to manage risks within those limits. Although appropriate measures may be put in place, it may be necessary to institute a regimen of measurement to monitor exposure of the workforce. The first step would be assessment of actual concentrations in the workplace by the use of static and personal air samplers, and assessment of the residue on surfaces, during working and after cleaning. If necessary it may then be useful to analyse urine or blood samples from workers before and after shifts. These analyses can be for the compound itself or a metabolite or for a biological marker of effect.

Throughout the process, the role and impact of local legislation should not be forgotten. In the UK, COSHH plays a central role in workplace risk management and is enforced by the Health and Safety Executive. COSHH assessment of substances takes into account the hazard that they pose and then assesses the processes in which they are used for the risk of that hazard being realised.

When all the above factors have been adequately controlled, the diversity of the workforce should be considered. There will probably be a range of people available for the work, ranging from young to old, from the healthy to those on medication of various kinds. They are likely to have varying susceptibilities to drugs or chemicals, defined by their genetic polymorphisms or lifestyles; alcohol can interact with some chemicals encountered in the workplace and smoking can increase the likelihood of occupational disease. The workforce is likely to contain women of child-bearing potential and the reproductive effects of any chemical should be taken into account before allowing such people to work with it (Box 13.1).

Box 13.1 Risk management in the workplace

The following sets out a basic listing of risk management factors to be considered after hazard identification and agreement on OELs but before starting work with the substance.

- Is the equipment available capable of meeting the OEL or does it require modification or replacement? If performance is known, the correct equipment can be chosen to achieve the OEL. Monitor atmospheres, including personal exposure levels, before and during processing.
- Decide on appropriate containment measures such as local exhaust and the use of isolators or cabinets. Engineering controls and PPE increase in complexity with increasing hazard category.
- Have an appropriate set of standard operating procedures that are relevant to actual practice.
- Decide appropriate levels of PPE bearing in mind the type of work necessary, the efficiency of containment of the equipment and the risks due to substance and process. PPE does not replace containment of the risk and is always a second-line approach.
- Compliance with PPE is often faulty, due to complexity or lack of comfort in the working conditions. Use a what-can-we-achieve approach rather than blind faith in compliance with impractical standards.
- Consider any possible individual susceptibilities to the effects of the substance amongst the workforce.
- Handling – if the process is completely enclosed, there is not so much cause for concern. However, it is useless to enclose everything and then to handle powder manually out of a polythene sack using a hand shovel – even if the operator is wearing vast amounts of PPE.
- Bear in mind that incautious removal of contaminated PPE can lead to greater exposure than the process itself. Cleaning equipment after use can also be hazardous. Contaminated PPE can contaminate other things – personal clothing for instance – and may need to be disposed of rather than cleaned or re-used.
- Consider instituting a scheme of monitoring the workforce for systemic levels of the substance in the blood or urine or for a biological marker of exposure. This will be important if effects are seen.
- At all times remember the impact of local legislation and regulation such as that given by COSHH.

Monitoring for exposure or effect

It should be normal to monitor atmospheric concentrations in the workplace to ensure that the equipment is operating according to expectation and that OELs are not being exceeded. It should be borne in mind that concentrations from one location to another – even in the same room – are likely to be different and that some processes are associated with higher exposure levels than others. This serves also as a check on the original predictions made during the various assessments.

If adverse effects are suspected or expected it may be appropriate to institute a scheme of health monitoring of the workforce. This has been carried out in occupations identified by epidemiological study to be associated with cancer, as with the workers involved in nickel refining (see chapter 14).[1] Evidence of exposure may be indirect (plasma or urinary concentrations of parent compound or a specific metabolite) or indirect as in markers of effect (cholinesterase inhibition or DNA adducts). The further removed the marker is from the actual cause, the less reliable it becomes (see discussion of biological markers in chapter 9, under 'occupational toxicology').

Bear in mind however, that health monitoring is a potential minefield, if there is any doubt about the effect being investigated. This is the case where the effect may be other than that intended for the finished dosage form (for medicines) or is otherwise unexpected. Precursor intermediates may cause different effects than the finished product.

Overview

The workplace is a distinct area in terms of risk assessment and management which is apparently simple (ease of containment, knowledge of chemicals involved, a defined population and known processes) but, on closer acquaintance, has a complexity that can be daunting.

The process of risk assessment in the workplace is similar to that in other areas. However, many of the compounds used are precursor intermediates, which have relatively unknown toxicity in comparison with the final product. As a consequence, data sets directly related to the chemical are often limited; this is a routine situation and requires some ingenuity in obtaining relevant information for a viable risk assessment. The resulting assessment should facilitate risk management through the setting of exposure limits, PPE requirements and containment measures.

Correct choice of exposure limits is critical to successful risk management in a commercial setting. Too high and adverse effects may be seen in the workforce; too low and the costs of containment and engineering measures may make the process too expensive to be financially viable. Where a facility is routinely using many different chemicals, it is useful to categorise chemicals according to the hazards they pose. Bear in mind, however, that there will always be pressure to keep chemicals in the lowest possible category, as expense of production increases with hazard category.

Finally, the complex legislative background must not be forgotten. This is seen in centrally set exposure limits, in requirements for health monitoring, for separate sets of regulations for substances such as lead and for radiation. In putting management controls in place, it should also be remembered that the use of PPE is seen as a last resort in reducing worker exposure, not as the primary method.

Chapter 14

Risk assessment

Carcinogenicity; the environment;
evolution and overview of
risk assessment

Introduction

This chapter looks at the use of risk assessment in carcinogenicity and the
environment (including its international aspects) and moves on to consider the
evolution of risk assessment and offer an overview of the field. The intention is
to look at factors that are relevant to each of these areas rather than write a
standard operating procedure, as dogmatic rules for 'how to do it' are unlikely to
be relevant in every case.

Notes on risk assessment and carcinogenicity

When looking at carcinogenicity as a toxicological endpoint, it is worth
remembering that a very small proportion of cancer in humans is actually
attributable to a specific chemical to which we may be exposed in our diets or at
work. Given that cancer is a high incidence disease of old age with significant
links to the normal human environment (in all its forms), it is very difficult to
partition the risks attributable to individual aspects of that environment and
then pinpoint a cause for a particular cancer in a single individual without clear
evidence of exposure. Risk assessment for carcinogenicity is further complicated
by the natural presence in the environment of well-known human carcinogens
such as arsenic or the products of combustion. In addition, individual chemicals
cannot, for the most part, be classified black or white as carcinogens or non-
carcinogens. The classification of carcinogens drawn up by IARC (see Table
9.8) indicates the gradation of certainty from the clear human carcinogens
through to those that are carcinogenic in one sex of one rodent species, to those
few that are not considered to be carcinogenic.

The risk of cancer is increased by a number of factors, including:

- Diet: eating fruit is risky – not eating it is riskier
- Genotype/phenotype; differential vulnerability of DNA (xeroderma pig-
  mentosum)
- Lifestyle: drinking, smoking, lack of exercise, sunbathing
- Occupation: industrial chemicals, mining, exposure to asbestos
- Reduced immunological competence
- Ignorance of exposure or novelty of mechanism.

These are crudely divisible into those that can be avoided – lifestyle choices such as diet, exercise and smoking – and those that are unavoidable, due to phenotype or to ignorance of their significance. Occupational exposure to carcinogenic chemicals or processes is not necessarily avoidable, due to personal circumstances and other sociological factors. Most occupational cancer has been due to lack of knowledge or understanding or simply ignoring it. In some cases workers learnt to take actions that effectively reduced the risks, such as washing out nasal passages each day after nickel refining to reduce the risk of nasopharyngeal cancer[1-3] (JR Pincott, personal recollections of his grandfather in South Wales).

Inevitably, ignorance has been a significant factor in occupational carcinogenesis, from the scrotal cancer of unwashed chimney sweeps to the more recent exposures to chemicals such as benzene or cyclosporine. These later effects and slow attribution have been due to lack of understanding of carcinogenic mechanisms, poor prediction of effect and the inevitable slowness and imprecision of epidemiological study when there is a low incidence of effect. There is also, apparently, a role for serendipitous observation by professionals; there is a clear tendency to be suspicious of any initiative that comes from the untrained public or which is in any way associated with 'old wives tales'. It follows that these last perceptions are the most difficult to deal with because of the triangle of interest: the *industry* concerned will be seen as wanting to avoid costly clean-up or compensation, the *government* will be keen to avoid expenditure on research or diversion of resources, and the *public* are interested in finding out the cause of effect, apportioning blame and receiving compensation, while maintaining suspicion of the other two sides. In this kind of atmosphere, the necessary growth of knowledge and understanding of all aspects of the case is unlikely to be smooth or progressive.

The following sections look at factors in carcinogenicity and assessment of risk in this contentious field. These include DNA vulnerability and genotype and phenotype, background incidence, data used in carcinogenicity risk assessments, thresholds in carcinogenicity and low dose extrapolation. Finally there is a case study in carcinogenicity risk assessment and an overview of the field.

DNA vulnerability, genotype and phenotype

DNA, and the control of its expression, is central to carcinogenesis, either through direct attack or by changed regulation. Although much is made of genotoxicity due to low levels of synthetic chemicals the level of naturally occurring damage should be considered in any overview of risk due to low levels of synthetic chemicals; this is explored in Box 14.1.

Although change to DNA may be theoretically avoidable, there is no avoidance of genotype and its phenotypic expression – at least until the advent of designer babies. Some aspects of this are readily characterised, such as the DNA repair deficiency that is associated with xeroderma pigmentosum. Many others, however, cannot be defined because of the diversity of influence and effect that

Box 14.1 DNA vulnerability – endogenous damage and repair

DNA is a deceptively simple molecule – composed of only four nucleotides arranged in a regular primary structure – but having great complexity in controls on secondary and tertiary structure, replication, repair, transcription and hence gene expression. It is highly vulnerable to oxidative or other attack or to changes in repair efficiency or gene expression.[4]

- Alkylating agents such as dimethylnitrosamine and cyclophosphamide introduce methyl or ethyl groups into bases, leading to base pair changes or dysfunctional DNA.
- Oxidative attack on DNA bases can lead to base pair changes; UV radiation produces thymidine dimers.
- There are numerous cellular sources of oxygen radicals and hydrogen peroxide, including mitochondria, peroxisomes and some enzymes.
- Fe^{2+} associated with DNA reacts with hydrogen peroxide as follows: $Fe^{2+}+H^++H_2O_2 \rightarrow Fe^{3+}+H_2O+HO^{\cdot}$; the hydroxyl radicals damage DNA and Fe^{2+} can then be regenerated through NADH, making a self-perpetuating cycle of damage.
- Asbestos carcinogenicity has been attributed to generation of hydroxyl radicals in the presence of hydrogen peroxide and Fe^{2+}.
- Daily oxidative damage to DNA has been estimated at 100,000 oxidative hits per cell per day in rats and 10,000 hits/cell/day in humans, assessed by analysis of urine samples for oxidised bases.
- Increased levels of 8-oxo-guanine have been noted in the lymphocyte DNA of smokers.
- Oxidative damage to DNA accumulates with age, associated with a decline in DNA repair.
- Planar molecules (such as oestrogen metabolites) interact with DNA by intercalation into the structure producing disruption to processes such as repair and transcription.
- Infidelity of DNA synthesis and repair leads to abnormalities of gene control or expression.
- Prevention of DNA damage is enhanced by antioxidants such as glutathione, ascorbic acid, tocopherols and enzymes such as superoxide dismutase.
- DNA repair is provided by a range of enzyme systems. Defective DNA repair is seen in the skin cancer, xeroderma pigmentosum where repair of UV damage is deficient.
- Mutation of DNA may be passed on to daughter cells, producing heritable defects in cellular control. For example, the p53 protein arrests cell growth and protects against neoplastic responses; mutation in this gene is relevant to 50 per cent of human tumours.

is possible in an individual. For any individual there is a balance between the processes of absorption, distribution, metabolism and elimination of the chemicals that are naturally present in the diet those taken as medicines or habit (alcohol or nicotine), coupled with any synergistic, additive or inhibitory effects that any of them have on the others. The balance between these factors may result in different exposures to active metabolites or systemic levels between apparently similar people.

Epidemiology and background incidence

The net result of the various risk factors is a background incidence of unattributable cancers above which any new cause has to rise before it can be unequivocally identified by normal epidemiological techniques. Despite the inherent weakness of the epidemiological process, it is still human data that are the most easily accepted basis for risk assessment of human carcinogenicity. Identification is reliant on initial observation, study of incidence in the target population and in an appropriate control group, coupled with evidence of exposure. There may be evidence of a dose–response curve, where dose is indicated by degree or duration of exposure (years worked), bearing in mind that some workers are more heavily exposed than others due to differences in job, for instance between production line and packers. The great value of human data is that it is just that – it is human. However, the likelihood of getting all the foregoing factors in place so as to facilitate a risk assessment based on human data alone is small and decreases as the potency of the carcinogenic effect decreases. The type of effect being modelled is critical in terms of incidence in the target population compared with naturally occurring background. Contrast the relative certainty of vinyl chloride attribution (an unusual cancer in a defined population) versus a chemical causing a range of cancers in the general population with undefined exposures.

The obvious problem here is that humans have to be exposed to the chemical before the assessment can be made. Problems arise when there is a significant background incidence of the cancer, if differential diagnosis is poor and if there are unaccounted confounding factors such as smoking, inter-current disease or prior exposure to other agents. For marginal carcinogens the quality of the data is significant and the vast amount of data required to achieve statistical significance becomes limiting. Many small studies, conducted to different protocols with different assessment criteria, do not form a secure database from which to make an assessment of any precision, as it is usually not possible to combine all the data together to make a statistically sound basis for bulk analysis.

Data used in carcinogenicity risk assessments for novel chemicals

The use of long-term human exposure data is not an option for novel chemicals, although it may be possible to draw analogies with closely related chemicals already present in the market-place or environment. Here, the backbone of carcinogenicity risk assessment is still (currently) the long-term bioassay in rodents, supported by other data derived from general toxicity, genotoxicity and ADME studies.

The data that result from rodent bioassays play a significant role in carcinogenicity risk assessment, particularly for the mathematical models where the statistical power of the large group sizes and any dose–response curve can be taken into account. While these models and statistical power may give a fig leaf of numeric security, this is reduced by the need for judgement to assess the influence of mechanism and other factors such as differences in ADME or pharmacokinetics between humans and rodents. This is quite apart from the fact that the doses in the two species will be radically different and the high doses used in rodent bioassays may unduly influence the carcinogenic response. For proven human carcinogens such as aflatoxins or diethylstilbestrol, there is good agreement between the affected tissues in animals and those that show cancer in humans. The problem is that this is true for *proven* human carcinogens but this cannot be assessed a priori (from a point of epidemiological ignorance) for the vast majority of novel chemicals that are subjected to routine carcinogenicity bioassays followed by risk assessment.

The use of bioassays in two species has been debated for some years, suggestions being made that the use of the mouse could be abandoned or that testing could be reduced by using one sex each from the rat and the mouse. Neither approach has achieved regulatory acceptance. In fact, amongst toxicological pathologists, the use of two species has been seen as an advantage as the results in one could be used to offset the results from the other. Thus, the presence of increased tumour incidence in the livers of male mice could be discounted from human relevance by citing the absence of similar findings in female mice and both sexes of rats. Equally, if a chemical is carcinogenic in two species in a similar manner, it is very likely to have carcinogenic potential in humans at similar dose levels. This clarity decreases as the potency of effect decreases and as the mechanism moves from direct genotoxicity to indirect effect on the control of DNA expression and hence apoptosis and cellular controls. The presence of thresholds in the dose–response curves of many non-genotoxic rodent carcinogens is accepted as evidence that any tumorigenic effect expressed only at high dose levels is unlikely to be relevant to expected human exposure levels. This can be backed up by data from other safety evaluation studies and investigation of mechanism.

Thresholds in carcinogenicity

In non-genotoxic mechanisms, where cellular control is deranged, a threshold indicates a point beyond which the cells can no longer cope with the mechanistic strains imposed upon them, as in the accumulation of protein in α-2u globulin nephropathy in male rats. Such mechanisms are usually tissue specific and often seen in one sex only at high doses. Tumours thus produced in rodents may be dismissed as irrelevant to humans due to lack of an equivalent mechanism, as with tumours in the lungs of mice exposed to methylene chloride (Box 14.3) and hepatic tumours due to peroxisome proliferation.

In rodents, genotoxic carcinogenicity is roughly proportional to general toxicity, is usually associated with a clear dose–response curve and can produce tumours in several tissues in males and females. As, theoretically, a genotoxic event in a single cell can lead to cancer, it has been generally considered that there is no dose threshold for this type of effect. However, biology is very rarely black and white and such assumptions are increasingly challenged, as indicated in Box 14.2. Although damage to DNA may become fixed, no cancer will arise

---

Box 14.2 Thresholds in carcinogenicity

There is widespread agreement that non-genotoxic carcinogenicity is associated with thresholds of exposure below which there is no increase tumour incidence. Equally, there has been a long-standing belief that genotoxic carcinogens are not associated with such thresholds and that even low levels are associated with cancer risk; i.e. that the dose response is linear at low dose levels.

- For a genotoxic chemical, it is theoretically possible for a single molecule act on a relevant part of the DNA, for that change to escape repair and for it to be replicated in cell division and for this to progress to a tumour.
- There is no evidence of threshold for some ionising radiations or diethylnitrosamine.[5]

However, using a promotion protocol with 2-acetylaminofluorence (AAF; 12 weeks treatment with AAF followed by 24 weeks phenobarbital to promote liver tumours) no tumours were seen in the low dose group and one at the mid dose; at the high dose all animals had hepatocellular neoplasia. Non-linearity was also seen for cell proliferation and hepatocellular altered foci.[6] Mechanisms for thresholds in genotoxic carcinogenicity could be:

- Inhibition of DNA repair; effects on cell cycle; interference with apoptosis; meiotic and mitotic recombination; direct interaction with the spindle apparatus; DNA methylation.[6] Low-level DNA damage may delay the cell cycle leading to lower cell turnover.
- Response in some tissues for the same chemical may be linear but non-linear in others. Indirect mechanisms of genotoxicity may result in thresholds.

- A carcinogen may show a J-shaped curve if it increases cell division or oxidative stress at high dose but inhibits them at low doses; this can result in a decrease in tumour incidence at the low dose.[7]
- Modelling on the cell cycle shows the possibility of thresholds for genotoxic carcinogenesis.[8]
- Linearity may be hidden within the background variability.
- Practical or pragmatic thresholds probably exist at background levels below which effects cannot be estimated practically. Saccharin epidemiology is said, by epidemiologists, to be compatible with a small but *undetectable* risk of bladder cancer (despite work showing that rodent metabolism is not relevant to humans).[9]

Conclusion: although thresholds may not exist for all genotoxic carcinogens they do (probably) exist for some and may exist for individual tumour responses.

if the affected cell does not divide and if that process is not continued by further proliferation; mitosis is as important as mutation. To this may be added influences such as apoptosis and immune surveillance. Some carcinogens induce a reduction in cell division at low doses, showing J-shaped dose–response curves. Studies with 2-acetylaminofluorene (AAF), in which treatment with AAF was followed by treatment with the tumour promoter phenobarbital, showed evidence of threshold effects.[7,8]

Where a carcinogen adds progressively to a mechanism that is associated with a background incidence of tumours, a true threshold will probably not exist. When there is no association between background mechanism and tumour incidence, it is likely that there will be a threshold. However, it is likely that there is a practical threshold below which the increase in incidence is indistinguishable from background. In effect this is a no detectable effect level (NDEL) below which cancers caused by the chemical will remain unattributed to that chemical. Arsenic is widely present in the environment at low concentrations and everyone is exposed to it at low dose levels; however, it is clearly associated with carcinogenicity at occupational exposure levels. Although a chemical may be associated with an NDEL, does this mean that its use at low concentrations is acceptable and should we add to the carcinogenic burden that is already present in the environment, even if that is at low levels? Paradoxically, the NDEL would have to be defined by epidemiological study – a science that is inherently not sensitive enough to make such distinctions.

Low dose extrapolation

The basis of carcinogenicity risk assessment, using rodent bioassay data, is the extrapolation of effect from the high dose levels used in the short-lived animal to the much lower doses expected in long life expectancy humans. There are two central problems to this. First, the effects seen at the highest dose level may be a result of pharmacokinetics and metabolism or mechanistic overload that are not present at the two lower dose levels. The significance of this is that the effects at the high dose cannot necessarily be extrapolated from the two lower doses and that the dose–response curve is not linear in the section defined by the data. The second challenge, given lack of linearity in the upper levels, is that linearity at dose levels lower than those tested cannot be assumed. As indicated in Box 14.2, there may be non-linearity in responses to genotoxic carcinogens at low doses and, as a result, the shape of the response curve at low doses cannot be predicted without extensive experiment. The result of this unpredictability is a strong trend to conservatism in risk assessment, as models tend to use the upper confidence limits of the dose–response curve and, as additional cover, a safety factor is added to that. Various models have been used, such as the Mantel-Bryan and Weibull models and derivatives of these have developed into mathematical monsters that try to take everything into account, including time to tumour and spontaneous tumours. The reliability of the final result is inversely proportional to the number of assumptions that are made in producing it. Such mathematical complexity renders these models unsuitable for day-to-day use, returning risk assessment to a point where there is no false security offered by over conservative numbers produced by opaque processes and where expert judgement is essential. The problem is that judgement is open to challenge – scientific and legal. Having said that, a peer reviewed assessment of a full data package which includes comparative ADME and mechanistic data is likely to produce a more realistic assessment of low dose effects and risks.

A case study in carcinogenicity risk assessment

There is a wide range of choice for case studies in carcinogen risk assessment, mostly chemicals with a significant history of use and a large database. These include known human carcinogens such as benzene or arsenic and rodent specific carcinogens such as d-limonene or trimethylpentane from petrol. As a result of commercial sensitivity the number of novel chemicals that enter risk assessment and have the full process published is quite small, although some new drugs may have had their data published for Japanese registration in journals such as *Japanese Pharmacology and Therapeutics*. High-profile examples, such as peroxisome proliferators, offer insight into the factors that need to be taken into account in risk assessment and indicate the type of action that needs to be taken to protect a compound so that it can be registered or its use can be continued.[10]

Methylene chloride has been in use since the 1940s, in industry for decaffeination of coffee and domestically as a paint stripper. The history of methylene chloride risk assessment and regulation is reviewed in Box 14.6 below; its history as a rodent and potential human carcinogen is reviewed in Box 14.3. There is a large body of work published on methylene chloride,

Box 14.3 Methylene chloride and cancer

Methylene chloride has been in use since the 1940s in various industrial applications and as a domestic paint stripper (see Box 14.6); as a result, there is a large amount of human and safety data.

- A US National Toxicology Program study completed in 1986 showed an increase of benign and malignant tumours in mice and benign tumours in rats following inhalation exposure; studies using drinking water exposure or intraperitoneal administration were negative.[11]
- Various epidemiological studies have suggested increased incidence of pancreatic, biliary and liver cancer, while others have refuted these findings.[11]
- Increased mortality from prostate and cervical cancer was reported amongst cellulose-fibre production workers with more than 20 years' exposure. The same study did not confirm earlier findings of increased biliary tract and liver cancer.[12]
- A meta-analysis of data published between 1969 and 1998 indicated weak increases in risk for methylene chloride workers in respect of pancreatic cancer but judged that a strong causal link could not be drawn.[13]
- Two cohorts of photographic film workers were studied, having received exposures averaging 39 ppm (8-hour TWA) for 17 years (1311 men) or 26 ppm for 24 years (1013 men). There was no increase of death from any cause, including cancer and no evidence for effects on target organs identified in animal studies. Combining these results with other studies showed that exposure to methylene chloride does not increase the risk of death from any cause.[14]
- A review of 10 years of work on the mechanism of methylene chloride carcinogenicity in mouse liver and lungs indicated that this is specific to the mouse. In the lung this is probably due to DNA damage in the Clara cells, through interaction with a high-activity glutathione S-transferase unique to the mouse, which is present in the nucleus. DNA damage was not detected in other species, including in human hepatocytes. Therefore, the mouse is not a good model for humans for methylene chloride.[15]
- A critical review of the epidemiology literature concluded that cancer risks associated with methylene chloride exposure are small and limited to rare cancers.[16]

Given the specificity of the mechanism of carcinogenesis in the mouse, its absence in other species and the large body of epidemiological evidence, it is unlikely that methylene chloride exposure is associated with significant human cancer risk at current levels of exposure, which are driven by a significant risk of carboxyhaemoglobin generation[11] rather than cancer.

including human exposure studies, which has allowed a steady evolution of understanding of the hazards and risks associated with its use. The overall conclusion has been that the mechanism of carcinogenicity seen in mice is species specific and that humans are not subject to significant cancer risk. It is instructive to note that the more significant risk is generation of carboxy-haemoglobin and that this has been partly responsible for the reduction in occupational exposure limits over the years.

Overview of carcinogenicity risk assessment

For chemicals already on the market or in the environment, carcinogenic risk assessment is the subject of academic research and debate, conclusions constantly changing as the database grows and understanding of mechanism deepens. For new chemicals the situation is more difficult, especially where there is no human exposure data to assess ADME or actual exposure levels. For these chemicals the main database is the safety evaluation conducted *in vivo* or *in vitro*. There is some official guidance; for example an addendum on dose selection for carcinogenicity studies for the International Conference on Harmonisation (ICH) suggests that a positive result for tumorigenesis in rodents at 25 times the human exposure is probably not relevant as a risk for humans. This type of statement does not mean that such an argument will be accepted by any regulatory authority and it will still be necessary to have evidence of mechanism to back up any marketing application.

In assessing the carcinogenic risk due to a chemical, especially where there is significant environmental exposure or contamination expected, it may be useful to consider how much extra risk (additional cases of cancer) would result if it was introduced into the environment. An acceptable figure appears to be one in a million, although people may ask if they are the individual likely to be affected. (With the advent of proteomics and genomics, individual risk assessment of this type is becoming more possible.) Where the risk of cancer is greater than one in a million there is a moral question to answer; namely should it be accepted that the additional risk – in comparison with that already present naturally in the diet or in the wider environment – is tiny and so can be ignored or that imposing any additional risk, however small, is unacceptable. In any case, given the idea of one in a million cases, how can this be quantified and assessed in the face of the background incidence?

In such cases, comparative risk and cost/benefit analysis become important and subject to judgement that cannot easily be supported scientifically. In Scotland, it is normal for schoolchildren receiving free lunches to be given fruit as an alternative dessert, which almost certainly contains trivial residues of pesticides. There might be argument in favour of organically produced fruit to avoid such residues but the cost could make supply of fruit financially impossible. Quite apart from the endogenous chemicals present at far higher concentrations than the pesticides, the counter risk of reduced cancer prevention through not getting a daily shot of vitamins, trace elements and dietary fibre would hugely outweigh the risk due to synthetic chemicals.

Finally, life is about mixtures and the carcinogenic impact of a single chemical has to be viewed in the context in which it will be used and consumed. No chemical is taken in isolation; even a medicine taken on an empty stomach is subject to the gastric environment and the excipients in the formulation. For chemicals in the diet, the biological matrix in which they are found has far reaching effects on bioavailability and there may well be synergistic or inhibitory effects due to other chemicals. These interactions cannot be incorporated into routine assessments as they are too complex to model or predict; they represent a final layer of uncertainty which may always be present.

Notes on risk assessment and the environment

Environmental risk assessment is a somewhat fraught area, in part due to its high public profile but also due to the complexity of the data and wide range of interactions that must be predicted and taken into account. The usual response to environmental disasters – especially from pressure groups – is invariably pessimistic, although the outcome is often less horrendous than expected. Recovery is possible and can be quite quick, as with the big oil spill recently off the Orkney islands. For prospective assessments, there is the possibility that the risks are understated and that a larger problem may arise as a result. It is extremely difficult to maintain a balance between angry prediction of irreparable harm and a reasoned assessment of data that may indicate safe concentrations of a chemical.

Environmental risk assessment may be divided into retrospective examination of chemicals already present in the environment or prospective prediction of risk for new chemicals, such as agrochemicals. The difference between intentional and non-intentional release into the environment should also be considered. Unintentional release may be from a single point such as an industrial facility or of widespread origin such as traffic pollution, the release of CFCs from consumer goods or the use of contraceptive pharmaceuticals and subsequent environmental release of metabolites or unchanged drug. In theory, intentional release is more controlled or predictable, as with the use of pesticides, but this is not always the case.

There is also a need to differentiate between chemicals present naturally and those that are introduced by human activity. While it is easy to dismiss any artificial chemical as pollution, it is less easy to do so with a compound present in the normal environment. In general the natural chemicals only become a toxicological problem when they are present at concentrations significantly greater than normal. Combustion is a case in point here; naturally induced forest fires are a source of transiently high local concentrations of combustion products, from wood and other organic matter, which include dioxins. It can be argued that similar products produced from burning fossil fuels are not natural and so constitute pollution, especially as these are present at higher than normal concentrations and usually for longer periods. There is, therefore, a concept of excess discharge; using general toxicology as an analogy, there is an exposure level beyond which adverse effects may be expected and below which there will be no significant (or detectable) adverse effects. The environment has the capability to cope with limited release of chemicals in much the same way that an animal deals with a low dose of chemical.

There is the added complication that environmental risk assessment cannot be separated from sociological factors and so it is very much more difficult to bring forward a purely scientific solution that will prove acceptable to the people who feel themselves to be at risk. There is also an element of lack of control in environmental discharges, especially due to non-intentional release from industrial facilities. The concept of pollution avoidance according to the principles of BATNEEC (best available technology not entailing excessive cost) is too easily replaced by the unofficial and unstated concept of CATNAP (cheapest alternative technology narrowly avoiding prosecution). An unexpected aspect of local pollution is that contaminated sites may become wildlife refuges due to restricted human access and that, paradoxically, major clean-up operations may produce more harm ecologically than leaving them alone.

Successful environmental risk assessment is dependent on appreciation of the interrelationship of many factors and the consequent prediction of the outcome. Whereas risk assessment for other purposes may focus on one aspect of a chemical's toxicity, this is not so easy in environmental terms due to the complexity of the ecosystem and the dependency of the whole on its individual components. Although it may be predicted that a pesticide or a genetically introduced chemical resistance may have little effect in a general sense, prediction of effects on single species and through that on the whole ecosystem may well be less easy.

Factors in environmental risk assessment

Much of the difficulty with environmental hazard prediction lies with the simplicity of the test data compared with the complexity of the ecosystem and the difficulties encountered in assessing or predicting exposure. Single species tested in a laboratory environment do not necessarily give a sound basis for hazard characterisation and risk assessment. The use of mesocosm studies may make this process easier but are likely to be undertaken towards the end of the development process due to cost. Certain substance properties make prediction easier, however, such as oestrogenic activity and these can be relatively easily tested for and related to the likely persistence of the chemical in the environment. Persistence is a significant factor in environmental risk, as shown by the relative persistence of TCDD and atrazine in the soil at 10 and 2 years respectively. Where a process of degradation is identifiable, associated with a short half-life, this is an indicator of lower risk than for non-degradable chemicals. This presupposes that the degradation products have been identified, remembering that DDE, a metabolite of DDT, is also very persistent. In a manner analogous to that in protein binding in mammals, sequestration of chemicals into compartments such as clay soils implies potential for long environmental half-life and possible toxicity if there is a sudden release to produce high concentrations. However, high-affinity sequestration may reduce immediate risk levels slightly.

In terms of legislation, in Europe the regulatory framework for environmental risk assessment is based on the risk quotient, which is the ratio of the predicted environmental exposure (PEC) to the predicted environmental no effect concentration (PNEC). Typically, the PEC is modelled using data on expected market volume and use data, together with estimations of diffuse or point source introduction, degradation, distribution and fate. In some cases these predictions are supported by analytical measurement. The PNEC is then estimated by using empirically derived effect or no-effect data from laboratory experiments, applying safety factors of up to 1000 depending on the uncertainties inherent in the test data. A risk characterisation ratio (the PEC divided by the PNEC) of less than 1 indicates low risk while a ratio greater than 1 may indicate a relevant risk. The margins of safety (MOS) are also considered, the risk decreasing with increasing MOS. This process and the reasoning involved is nicely outlined in an environmental risk assessment of methyl tertiary butyl ether (MTBE) carried out by a team from the European Fuel Oxygenates Association (EFOA), NCET (WRc-NSF National Centre for Environmental Toxicology) and ECETOC (European Centre for Ecotoxicology and Toxicology of Chemicals). This assessment is summarised in Box 14.4 and the full report is available on the internet through the referenced websites.

Box 14.4 Environmental risk assessment of MTBE use in Europe

An environmental risk assessment[17] (ERA) was carried out for the use of methyl tertiary butyl ether (MTBE) in Europe, using the European Union System for the Evaluation of Substances (EUSES). MTBE is a highly watersoluble octane enhancer used in petrol, at concentrations up to 14 per cent. Leakage of MTBE into groundwater has caused concern in the USA due to potential contamination of drinking water; it has a pronounced taste and odour. This ERA was performed for three uses of MTBE: as a fuel additive, in production of isobutylene and as a pharmaceutical solvent.

- *Environmental distribution and fate*   Most of the MTBE was expected to end up in the air, with a significant percentage in water but virtually zero in biota with no bioaccumulation. MTBE appeared to be degradable in some circumstances but not in others; expected half-life in air was less than 6 days.

- *Predicted environmental concentrations (PECs)* vary with site and type of use. Background concentrations are <5 μg/l. The annual average local PEC of 172 μg/m^3, for production facilities, was similar to values reported for worker exposure which may be up to 1 mg/m^3. The highest local PEC of 37.7 mg/l was estimated for processing use. The highest reported concentrations in urban air were about 60 μg/m^3 and generally 10 μg/m^3 or less. There were few data for MTBE in soils in Europe.

- *Effects assessment and predicted no effect concentration (PNEC)*   Acute toxicity tests indicated low toxicity to aquatic organisms. The amount of acute data justified the use of a safety factor of 100 (rather than 1000) applied to the lowest EC$_{50}$ value to generate a PNEC. Using the lowest acute EC$_{50}$ value for a freshwater organism (184 mg/l for *Selenastrum capricornutum*), gave a PNEC for the aquatic compartment of 1.84 mg/l. Chronic aquatic toxicity test data showed a 5-day no effect concentration (NOEC) for *Ceriodaphnia dubia* of 202 mg/l; a 21-day IC$_{20}$ value of 42 mg/l for *Daphnia magna*; a chronic NOEC value of 26 mg/l was reported for the marine shrimp *Mysidopsis bahia* and a NOEC for reproduction in *Daphnia* of 51 mg/l. There were also further chronic toxicity data for *Daphnia*, fathead minnow and algae, although not all were completely compliant with OECD test guidelines. In view of the amount of data available, use of a factor of 10 to derive a PNEC from the lowest chronic (NOEC) value was justified for continuous (chronic) release. This gave a PNECaquatic of 2.6 mg/l, in line with the PNEC from acute data, which was used in the EUSES risk assessment modelling. The EC$_{50}$ value for *Mysidopsis bahia* of 136 mg/l was used for intermittent releases, with a safety factor of 10, giving an intermittent PNECaquatic of 13.6 mg MTBE/l.

- *Risk characterisation ratios (RCRs PEC/PNEC) and margins of safety (MOS)*   Except for the sediment and water environmental compartments, all of the RCRs were less than one and all of the MOS values were greater than one. The RCRs that were greater than one were for the use of MTBE as a feedstock for high-purity isobutylene manufacture. From monitoring data for production it was known that the PECs for the aquatic compartments were overestimates and that the true RCRs were probably lower than those calculated by the model.

It was concluded that the environmental risk of using MTBE as a fuel additive, process intermediate or a solvent was low. Where MTBE is released into the environment from production and processing, it was considered that more data and testing were required, including sediment toxicity testing and a sampling and analysis programme to measure concentrations of MTBE in wastewater from sites producing isobutylene.

Environmental risk assessment, in common with other areas of toxicological investigation, should be a dynamic process and is unlikely ever to be static, in view of the continually increasing database. This is particularly true of high-profile chemicals such as MTBE and TCDD. The latter has acquired a dire reputation that has made it into a toxicological icon of all that is chemically evil and synthetic. However, even this is being reassessed in the light of new data and perspectives. Bruce Ames and colleagues have reviewed the effects of TCDD in comparison with those of other natural chemicals, particularly indole carbinole and ethanol, and the indication is that, although TCDD is very toxic, its effects should be seen in perspective with those of other chemicals.[18] TCDD is an example of an environmental contaminant that is present naturally and as a result of human activities. It is characterised by extensive animal toxicity but by few proven effects in humans. The doses humans ingest are, however, far lower than the lowest doses that have been shown to cause cancer and reproductive damage in rodents. The environmental concerns about TCDD have produced stockpiles of this potentially lethal chemical which, if spilled, could have devastating local effects. Any incineration of biological material can produce dioxins, as was complained about in the recent foot-and-mouth outbreak in the UK. This holds true for crematoria as well; should they be closed down?

International management of environmental risks

The environment is global and there is ready potential for transfer of toxic chemicals between countries either intentionally by transport of toxic waste or by natural processes such as river flow or atmospheric pollution and precipitation as acid rain. There have been various attempts to manage toxic risks internationally, with varying success. In general, agreements made with an objective of stopping environmentally bad practice (usually for the benefit of developed countries) are often significantly weakened by the economic or humanitarian need to continue the same bad practices in less-developed countries. Thus, it may be acceptable to ban the use of DDT in the developed world because acceptable substitutes are available (albeit at higher cost). In contrast, in the third world expensive alternatives are not economically available and the environmental risks are seen as less important than the benefits. Likewise, it may appear sensible – from a Western point of view – to ban the transport across borders of toxic material but if the result of this ban is large, ill-managed dumps of toxic waste, the environmental costs may well be greater than the risk of accidental spillage in transit. As a result, this type of agreement is often ineffective due to the influences of interested parties and countries; the wider the proposal, the more difficult it is to reach an agreement that is effective. At this point the mixture of politics with toxicology becomes unstable, to the extent that common sense and science lose out.

Box 14.5 Notes on international management of toxic risks

Management of toxic risks in an international context is fraught with difficulty and frustration; a risk that looks terrible in the West is likely to be acceptable in less-developed countries due to local conditions. Differences in risk perception between countries lead to different approaches and priorities. Toxicology has an initial role in this but then becomes subsumed in politics.[19]

- Toxicology can identify hazard, which will probably vary little for a single form, but risk should be assessed according to local conditions and the use to which the material will be put.
- There is often significant difference between international policy agreement and local implementation.
- International policy can be constructed on inappropriate or incomplete data or flawed premises with little consideration for the side effects of such policy; this can lead to an unbalanced agreement that has undesirable side effects in other, related areas.
- The assumption that all waste is immoral and hazardous is not a sensible starting point for effective policy construction.
- The most successful international agreements are regional, involving few countries, tackle an acknowledged definable pollution problem, have little cost impact on industry and affect rich countries, which can administer them.
- Risk reduction cannot be equated with risk abolition.
- Agreements that are unfocused and have differing standards between developed and developing nations will probably be unsuccessful as the good effects in developed countries will be balanced out by the continuing abuses in the developing nations.

The evolution of risk assessment

The science of risk assessment is dynamic and evolving constantly. For toxicological risks, this has been due to increasing knowledge and understanding of interdependencies in toxicity and mechanisms of action and to increased appreciation that risks should not be viewed and assessed in isolation. Risk is positive or negative, balanced on a host of supporting or dependent factors, to which must be added the perceptions of the people at risk and those who are attempting to manage that risk. Risk assessment results in regulation and management; greater knowledge and understanding should result in better regulation, although this is offset by the inherent (and understandable) conservatism of regulators working in the shadow of the principle that it is almost impossible to prove a negative – that chemical A is safe.

An inescapable factor in risk assessment is the increasing refinement and sensitivity of analytical techniques. When a chemical has been branded toxic and harmful to health, the presence of tiny amounts, revealed by new methods, can result in huge efforts to produce a cleaner environment, even when the chemical is present naturally in greater amounts. John Doull, writing in chapter 1 of *Toxicology in Risk Assessment*[20] points out that we tend to focus 'on the trees of individual effects rather than on the forest of public health. In the final analysis, our mandate is not to use what-if toxicology to produce media headlines and stimulate funding for the investigation of phantom risks but to improve public health, and that should be the most basic principle of toxicology and all science.'

The EPA established a range of 1 in 1 million to 1 in 10,000 for the incremental lifetime risk of cancer associated with possible exposures from contaminated sites, indicating the increased probability above background rate that someone could get cancer following repeated exposure. However, this ignores the risk from naturally present radiation, which is calculated to be 1 in 100. If natural risks are high, what future is there in attempting to manage lower risks from artificially introduced factors?

The evolution of risk assessment for individual chemicals is illustrated by the history of methylene chloride, which shows the changing emphasis in risk assessment and regulation that occurs with over several decades as a database for risk assessment is expanded (Box 14.6). It also highlights differences between different regulatory bodies in the same country.

With increasing knowledge and understanding methylene chloride has been increasingly demonized as harmful. In contrast TCDD, while universally acknowledged as extremely toxic, has become less threatening. During the last 30 years of the twentieth century, one of the greatest advances in risk assessment has been the increased understanding of the toxicity of chemicals present naturally in the environment, whether in the atmosphere, water or diet. Equally, there has been understanding of the balance of nature – that generally the natural percentages of the individual chemicals to which we are exposed are not associated with any detectable epidemiological effect. Where that balance is disturbed and the percentages of certain chemicals increase beyond natural limits, as with increased solanine concentrations in insect-resistant potatoes, toxicity can result. Margins of safety in nature are frequently smaller than those set by regulators. For synthetic chemicals, the Delaney amendment may have looked sensible at one time but is clearly of questionable use now.

Overview of risk assessment

In simple terms, assessment of risk due to toxicity is the process of extrapolation from a limited data set to a wider situation such as the environment or the general population or a specific target group such as a workforce. The data set may contain human data, derived from accidental exposure, clinical or

Box 14.6 Methylene chloride and evolution in risk assessment

Methylene chloride ($MeCL_2$) was first discovered in the nineteenth century. Large-scale production started in the 1940s.[21]

- *1940s* Used as a paint stripper, replacing lye – caustic alkali – with advantages of speed, non-reactivity and safety. In 1946, the American Conference of Governmental Industrial Hygienists (ACGIH) set an 8-hour time weighted average (TWA) of 500 ppm. Safety advice said that employees should keep their hands out of the solvent, because of skin irritation and skin absorption potential.
- *1960s* Approved for preparation of hop extract; residue maximum set at 2.2 per cent. Use in decaffeination of coffee approved with a maximum residue of 10 ppm.
- *1970s* $MeCl_2$ was linked to formation of carboxyhaemoglobin (COHb); the 500 ppm limit was associated with greater levels of COHb than the limit for carbon monoxide. There was evidence that 1000 ppm (allowed as a short-term exposure limit) led to CNS depression. It was also linked to cardiac arrhythmias, which was proved in 1976. In 1974 a limit of 75–100 ppm was proposed and, in 1975, ACGIH indicated a change to 100 ppm as an 8-hour TWA, although 500 ppm was maintained as a limit by the US Occupational Safety and Health Administration (OSHA). The US National Institute for Occupational Safety and Health set a limit of 75 ppm in line with limits set for carbon monoxide.
- *1980s* The ACGIH reduced its limits to 50 ppm. Links to cancer were suggested (Box 14.3).
- *1990s* OSHA proposed a change to a 25 ppm limit. This was the first OSHA assessment to use physiologically based pharmacokinetic modelling. Industrial pressure was mounted for a 50 ppm limit.

Use of $MeCl_2$ as a paint stripper has declined as knowledge of its toxicity has grown, with a return towards alkali based strippers and alternatives. This illustrates the hazards of replacing a supposedly hazardous compound or process with one that is supposedly safer, but unkown.

epidemiological studies, or safety studies in animals and/or *in vitro*. The application of the assessment may be local, national or global. It should be remembered that relevance and utility are likely to decrease as the brief becomes wider because conditions differ from one place or population to another, either in exposure, collateral conditions or, significantly, sociological factors. While it may be possible to arrive at an objective risk assessment for any given (local or regional) situation, application of the conclusions through risk management cannot be separated from local factors such as living standards including income, risk perception and acceptance.

The ultimate use of the risk assessment – which should be based on an objective appraisal of the data and the indicated risks – should take into account any benefits of using the chemical and all the collateral risks and factors. As with chlorination of drinking water in Peru (Box 11.3), the risks of non-use may be greater than those due to use. Ultimately environmental risk must be determined according to local conditions because global assessment is not always appropriate. Environmental risk assessment should take into account the risks that follow any clean-up process; what is the intended fate of the concentrated toxic chemical residues that result? It is better to optimise the production process and prevent the problem in the first place.

Above all, risk assessment has to be communicated to people at risk and to risk managers in an understandable format; it must be user friendly not user hostile, which is not easily demonstrated for some of the more complex models. Depending on the audience, analogies and comparisons can useful, for example something can be said to be equivalent to drinking a small beer once a year for life, or causing as much (or more) of the same toxic effect as a lower concentration of another chemical known and widely acknowledged as seriously toxic.

It is also important that any risk assessment should be honest and not distorted by undue emphasis on one aspect of the problem or by self-interest. An example of this is the 'assessment' of genetically modified foods and organisms. For a food there are two areas of risk – environmental release and ingestion. If the composition of the new food is similar to the existing variety without significant change in concentration, it seems likely that the risk from ingestion will be little different from the risks due to eating the normal strain. The environmental risks are, however, potentially different. The role of environmental pressure groups is very important as they tend to concentrate on one aspect of a problem to the exclusion of all else, thereby devaluing their own arguments. All too frequently risk/benefit and collateral factors are not considered.

It is quite possible to arrive at an objective risk assessment, given a valid set of data and appropriate knowledge of the local situation. The real challenge comes when this assessment is brought into the political and sociological context of its use; science and politics are uneasy companions. At the end of this review of risk due to toxicity and its assessment, the following is suggested as a list of desirables for a successful risk assessment:

- Look at all the data dispassionately.
- Take into account collateral risks and local conditions, including any background presence or incidence of effect.
- Include a cost/benefit analysis where appropriate.
- Make it usable, user friendly and easy to communicate to those at risk.
- Keep it honest, without concentration on a single aspect.

- Combine this with local sociological factors that may increase or decrease the risk of use or how it is perceived and its consequent acceptability to those at risk.
- Produce management proposals that are achievable and are themselves not associated with significant risk.

Chapter 15

The future of toxicity testing

Introduction

All branches of science change and evolve and toxicology should be no different. In contrast to other sciences, however, there is one unchanging aspect of toxicology and that is the responsibility to the general public in terms of chemical safety and the consequent requirement that toxicity studies are conducted ethically and to high standards, whether in industry in support of a new pesticide or in a university as part of a PhD thesis on a chemical naturally present in food. The conduct and results of toxicological study are under public scrutiny, unlike other sciences. As a result there are pressures on how studies are conducted, how they are interpreted and the risks assessed, and how that is translated into risk management. Through all the pressures to change – use fewer animals, ignore that pressure group, keep those jobs, cure my baby, save my crops while not using toxic pesticides – the one thing that does not change is the unattainable public desire for a risk-free existence; the ability to use chemicals without any of the risks.

Current practice

The current approach to safety evaluation has evolved in the light of periodic tragedies such as the thalidomide disaster and is focused by fear of insidious diseases such as cancer. This approach is very much limited to the here and now of toxicological effect and does not take into account any effects (direct or indirect) on future generations beyond our own children. It should be questioned if this self-oriented approach will remain valid or if current practice may endanger future generations, for instance by adverse effects on the gene pool or the environment. Having said that, prediction of such long-term effects is fraught with difficulty as their onset is likely to become clear only with hindsight.

In toxicological terms it is relatively easy to determine the hazards and risks associated with short-term exposure, as the effects are often clearly apparent and easily differentiated from the normality of background data. The real challenge is to detect or predict the potential for insidious long-term effects, especially those which have a normal background incidence. For example, age-related renal and neural degeneration are normal but may be accelerated by exposure to a range of factors such as drugs or excessive occupational exposures. Detection or prediction of such effect can be exceedingly difficult.

For new chemicals, the ultimate purpose of toxicological investigation is to demonstrate safety – the chimaera of negative proof. It is quite possible to demonstrate absence of effect in the constrained circumstances of a laboratory experiment but this should not be equated with safety in a wider context. It is generally acknowledged by toxicologists that there are deficiencies in the individual systems currently used to evaluate chemical safety and that no individual test can offer all the answers. As a result, there is a general desire to move towards a situation where the tests used are individually more predictive so, when they are combined into a cohesive data set, a realistic risk assessment can be conducted.

To further focus this discussion, the broad objective of toxicological testing should be to produce a reliable, reproducible system of evaluation that will allow realistic risk assessment and so minimise any impact of new chemicals on human health. This should be able to answer broad questions, such as 'Is it toxic?' or specific ones such as 'Does it damage DNA?' The process is driven ultimately by economics. Better health means lower health costs. Less expensive test systems and methods and greater precision in targeting testing may result in less expensive drugs or pesticides, which would in turn have economic benefits, especially in the third world. To facilitate this, a toxicity testing paradigm should result in better, faster selection of lead candidates, while remembering that separation of all toxicities from the desired activity or effect is probably unachievable. The drive for non-toxicity will almost certainly mean that some beneficial compounds are discarded without full evaluation.

Current practice is being changed by new techniques used in early development, which are not subject to regulatory guidance or GLPs. These include the use of transgenic animals (knockout mice and rats, humanised mice) and microarray chips for the identification of patterns of gene expression and changes in protein synthesis, together with increasingly sophisticated analytical methods. The amount of data produced is phenomenal and computational techniques are evolving to cope with the flood. The problem is not a paucity of new methods but selection of the technologies that will be useful in the medium to long term. The increase in knowledge and evolution of understanding will always tend to move the goalposts and make previous practice look dubious; there is no easy escape from this.

Current dynamics and pressures

All systems of toxicological evaluation when taken in isolation are fallible and this situation is unlikely to change. The public are more likely to tolerate a false positive than a false negative where predicted safety dissolves into a toxicological disaster such as thalidomide, benoxaprofen or cisapride. There will always be public pressure for better test systems and data and for ethical conduct of safety evaluations. However, because safety cannot be proved but merely inferred, there will always be a possibility of error, whether in a general sense (thalidomide) or in sensitive individuals (cisapride). Complete abolition of animal use in toxicology or complete removal of all restrictions will not produce better safety evaluation. A scientific compromise offers the best way forward but may be difficult to achieve without better communication with the public.

There will always be pressure to reduce the numbers of animals used in toxicity testing, largely driven by animal rights lobbies but also by increasing ethical awareness amongst toxicologists. This has led to better housing and husbandry practices for animals as understanding of the impact of stress on test results has increased. Animals are no longer used in cosmetic testing in Europe, putting pressure on toxicologists to provide viable alternative methods of assessment. The three Rs of Russell and Birch have had great impact on the way animals are used in testing and have resulted in improved study design. In most countries, animal use is strictly regulated by central government and these regulations are always tightening. The use of non-human primates in toxicity testing in the UK now requires far greater scientific justification than previously and is routinely referred to the Home Office. The need for scientific choice of a second species has always been there but it has been easier to say, in past times, that compound supply is tight so a small animal must be used or to make a blanket, unjustified statement that non-human primates are closer to humans than dogs.

The toxicity test most under pressure at the time of writing is the carcinogenicity bioassay in rats and mice. These last more than 30 months from study initiation to reporting and often produce results that are of little or no relevance to humans. Genotoxic carcinogens are readily detected in short-term assays and should not go through 2-year rodent studies. The real challenge is to detect non-genotoxic mechanisms of carcinogenicity that are relevant to humans and the use of a 2-year rodent study is a very imprecise method for achieving this. As a result there are moves to find relevant mechanisms of carcinogenicity by other means, including more intense examinations in shorter rodent studies and by identification of *in vitro* tests that are indicative of human relevant effect, such as intercellular gap junction communication.

Through the whole debate there remains the requirement from regulatory agencies for an adequate margin of comfort before a new test method is accepted, making validation an absolute necessity.

Utility of animal experiments in risk assessment

In looking at the future of toxicity testing the use of animals cannot be ignored. There is much debate about the utility of animal data in risk assessments intended for human use, much of it acrimonious and less than dispassionate.

There have been numerous studies that show either that they are an essential part of the process or are completely useless; the ultimate conclusion must be that if you select your studies or compounds according to your argument and ignore the others, you can prove what you like. Like all the toxicity studies on any chemical, whether *in vitro* or *in vivo*, animal studies are a tool to be used to achieve the objective of a realistic assessment of the compound. As with any tool, they need to be used correctly and appropriately in order to give the most accurate result. During this process their limitations have to be realised and taken into account; this applies just as much to studies conducted in human volunteers or to reports of accidental exposure as to studies in transgenic mice or bacteria. No single study should be taken as the sole basis for a risk assessment; every study is one part of the database that is used and viewed as a whole package and animal experimentation is simply one supporting aspect of this process. Although there may be human data that can carry more weight than other evidence, they may not be definitive for the target population of the risk assessment. Frequently, there are fewer human data than would be considered sufficient for a complete assessment and support from other sources is essential. It is axiomatic that animal studies that have been badly designed and conducted should carry less weight in any risk assessment and their data should be used (if at all) for support rather than definitive conclusion. However, this principle of data quality and integrity applies to any safety evaluation study in any test system, so animal studies are no different in that respect.

In isolation, no testing system is infallible and, with the complexity of the objective, it is likely that no single system will be capable of giving a reliable and reproducible answer – now or in the future. Given the current stage of technological development in toxicity testing and understanding of mechanism, it is clear that animal experiments that have been properly conducted and interpreted are an essential part of risk assessment. This is not to say, however, that the use of animals will not decrease further or that their use cannot be further refined. There is, however, a clear need to move forward and to develop alternative strategies, through the use of new models such as invertebrates or other vertebrates such as fish.

Development of new test methods

In developing new test methods the issue of reproducibility – within laboratories and between laboratories – must be considered. New tests must be robust enough to be transferred readily from one laboratory to another and also be capable of providing reproducible results. It is routine to repeat *in vitro* studies to confirm the results of the first test; at present these tests are performed at the same laboratory. However, there may be an advantage in performing confirmatory studies in a second laboratory, especially where the data indicate a marginal effect, the reproducibility of which is subject to influences by statistical considerations and normal biological variation.

To be successful a new toxicity screen should have the following characteristics:

- *Robust*   The test should be relatively easy in technical terms; complication leads to error and specialist equipment means expense. New animal models should not have over-onerous husbandry requirements.
- *Reproducible*   If not, its utility and relevance may be questioned. Baseline data for individual animals, plates or replicates should not be so variable that change is indistinguishable from historical control data.
- *Predictive*   with good sensitivity and specificity.
- *Quick*   Lengthy experimental phases mean slowed development or lead candidate selection and additional expense.
- *Cost effective*   There is no future for any test if the costs outweigh the value of the results.
- *Multiple endpoints*   This is desirable even if it is addressed through several related models. It is expected that a transgenic mouse would be capable of expressing toxicity other than that shown through the gene of interest. All routine toxicity endpoints could be incorporated into transgenic assays.
- *Dose response*   The new method should be capable of showing a dose response.

Methods using transgenic animals are developing rapidly and the utility and relevance of these models will become clearer during the next few years; however, they may not fulfil the criteria suggested above for ease and speed of technical performance and cost. They have significant potential in mechanistic studies, either for screening for an effect in a chemical class or series or for explanation of effect due to a single compound. There is also the possibility that a transgenic animal could be constructed specially to answer a particular question relating to toxicity.

In vitro toxicology and the future

At the current stage of development, *in vitro* tests are good for mechanistic studies where single (or limited) endpoints are examined. Investigation of a number of mechanistic endpoints, via a battery of tests, could be used to assess the presence of the individual mechanisms or events that lead to a complex conclusion. In terms of the 3Rs the most viable place for this could be assessment of the potential for human-relevant non-genotoxic mechanisms of carcinogenicity. They are also quick to perform and often inexpensive in comparison with traditional methods.

Individually, *in vitro* tests are poor for examining multiple endpoints or toxicities that are multifactorial, such as eye irritation or reproductive effects. In addition, due to the limited viability of the preparations they are also poor for assessing the accumulation of effect that comes with repeated dosing over a long period, for example, the gradual but accelerated decline of functional reserve in non-renewing or non-repairing tissues like the CNS or kidney. Although quick to perform, *in vitro* methods can be technically complex and, as a result, difficult to transfer between laboratories.

For an *in vitro* method to be accepted (especially for regulatory purposes) there must be understanding of the mechanisms and contributing or causative factors in the endpoint studied, plus understanding of how the *in vitro* data relate to the *in vivo* situation. From this position it should be possible to make reliable predictions of human effect. In furthering this process of acceptance, the correlation of the data resulting from new systems *in vitro* with those derived from established methods must be considered, especially where classification is used to rank toxic hazard; but this should not necessarily be allowed to slow acceptance. This process of validation is highly contentious. While it is sensible to prove a concept with the use of chemicals known to target the test system under investigation (e.g. nephrotoxicity and mercuric chloride), use of the new test in parallel with the currently accepted methods is the surest way of achieving validation and acceptance. Using this approach, a percentage concordance with accepted methodology can be produced and the utility of the test or test battery can be assessed objectively. Retrospective testing *in vitro* tends to produce a range of scientific 'excuses' for lack of success in various circumstances and, in my view, this tends to muddy the waters to a point where the utility of the method becomes unclear. To say that a test is 90 per cent successful in predicting neuropathy, providing that certain criteria are met, is the same as saying that the test is handicapped to a greater or lesser extent. A cynic might say that understanding when a test will give a negative result, when a positive result would be counterproductive in your development plans, might unduly influence choice of test and lead to a false indication of safety. There is no satisfactory way round this dilemma, other than careful scrutiny of test choice and results.

Although many people campaign aggressively for the use of animals in toxicity testing to be ended completely, it should be remembered that *in vitro* often means that animals are still used to provide organs, cells or subcellular preparations. This is true for *ex vivo* assays or for the harvesting of tissues for *in vitro* tests in which primary cultures are essential, for instance to retain metabolic capabilities.

In vitro toxicology has a great future for a host of reasons but has significant weaknesses, which mean that complete replacement of animals in toxicity testing is unlikely at the current state of research. They offer potential for use in lead candidate screening assays and in mechanistic research, quite apart from their economic benefits in terms of space and speed of conduct. Organisations such as FRAME, ECVAM (European Centre for Validation of Alternative Methods) and the Centre for Alternatives in Animal Testing at Johns Hopkins University in Baltimore play a significant role in furthering new methods of toxicological testing (their websites are given in the Appendix).

Toxicology *in silico*

The sciences of genomics and proteomics are developing quickly and offer considerable utility in screening for lead candidates; they can be used on animals or on cell cultures. Following a single dose, the number of genes expressed in mouse liver, for example, increases nearly exponentially during the few hours after administration and the pattern of gene expression can be related to the toxicity manifested in the whole animal. The pattern of protein expression can be examined in an analogous way and, when used in conjunction with genomics, offers a powerful tool for assessment of toxicity in the short term. For prediction of long-term toxicity, these short term methods may be limited by the difficulty of differentiating between normality and the slight changes that will result in long-term effects after prolonged exposure *in vivo*.

The future of safety evaluation

It is clear that so-called alternative systems will play a far greater role in the future of safety evaluation. This term is used to describe tests that are not fully validated or currently accepted for regulatory submissions. They have considerable current utility in the selection of lead candidates because they are, on the whole, quick and inexpensive. Although suitable for this type of use, they are currently too little understood to gain acceptance in the more rigorous arena of safety evaluation. However, there is no doubt that further development and refinement of current alternative test approaches will bring them more into the mainstream of regulatory toxicity testing. Their integrated use with current mainstream methods could produce results that are more easily interpreted in the context of their relevance to human toxicity than is currently the case. The biggest opportunity for such advance is offered by refinement of methods of detecting human-relevant non-genotoxic carcinogenicity. This could cut development times and costs.

In *vitro* methods are being developed that use stem cells and expression of genes and proteins in cell cultures and advances are being made regularly in increasing the viability of primary cell cultures and extending their characteristics to cell lines. However, it is not only in *vitro* methods that are improving constantly; there is a continuing development of computer-based prediction systems and these will gain power by becoming more interactive with each other, allowing prediction of metabolism and of the toxicity of the metabolites.

The future approach – not too different from current practice – could be to produce a range of predictions which could be tested in animal models in studies up to 13 weeks for general toxicology. Such an approach could dramatically cut the use of animals and ensure that those that are used are used much more effectively. The use of animals in toxicity testing is likely to continue for the foreseeable future because of the benefits they offer in examining a whole functioning organism over an extended treatment period, with all the interrelationships between tissues, blood supply and ADME that are currently not possible *in vitro*. For these reasons, as well as their multifactorial process controls, endpoints in reproductive toxicity, immunotoxicity and general toxicology will continue to rely on animals. This does not mean, however, that the animal models currently in use cannot be refined and made more relevant to humans by the use of transgenic methods or by the investigation of new species. For instance, the metamorphosis from larval form to adult insect has some similarities to the processes of organogenesis in mammals; strains of *Drosophila sp.* have been developed that have some aspects of human metabolism.

Toxicology is going to come under increasing scrutiny rather than less due to the pressures on us all to make our assessments as safe and as accurately as possible, while maintaining the highest ethical standards in our work. Through all, we should be prepared to change and not be ruled by the 'We have always done it this way' philosophy; tradition is not necessarily science.

Appendix
Useful websites

Regulatory sites

EPA – US Environmental Protection Agency : http://www.epa.gov/

EEA – European Environment Agency (the main European-level provider of environmental information to policy makers and the public): http://www.eea.eu.int/

FDA: Center for drug evaluation and research: http://www.fda.gov/cder/. Center for biologics evaluation and research: http://www.fda.gov/cber/

EMEA   European Agency for the evaluation of medicinal products: http://www.emea.eu.int/

ICH – International Conference on Harmonisation of Technical Requirements for Registration of Pharmaceuticals for Human Use: http://www.ich.org

Japanese Ministry of Health Labour and Welfare: http://www.mhlw.go.jp/english/

MCA – UK Medicines Control Agency: http://www.mca.gov.uk/

OECD – Organization for Economic Cooperation and Development:http://www.oecd.org

UK Pesticides Safety Directorate – accessed through http://www.defra.gov.uk/

UK Health and Safety Executive: http://www.hse.gov.uk/

Control of Substances Hazardous to Health regulations (COSHH): http://www.hse.gov.uk/hthdir/noframes/coshh/

Information links

US National Library of Medicine specialized information services:
TOXNET: http://toxnet.nlm.nih.gov/
PubMed: http://www.ncbi.nlm.nih.gov/entrez/query.fcgi

Toxicology societies

British Toxicology Society: www.thebts.org/
US Society of Toxicology: http://toxicology.org

European Society of Toxicolgy (Eurotox): http://www.eurotox.com
European Teratology Society: http://www.etsoc.com/
US Teratology Society: http://teratology.org/
British Society of Toxicological Pathologists: http://bstp.org.uk/
US Society of Toxicologic Pathologists: http://www.toxpath.org/

Organisations investigating and promoting alternatives to animals

USA: Johns Hopkins Center For Alternatives To Animal Testing (CAAT):
    http://caat.jhsph.edu/
Europe: European Centre for the Validation of Alternative Methods
    (ECVAM): Reports from ECVAM may be seen at:
    http://altweb.jhsph.edu/publications/ECVAM/ecvam.reports.htm
UK: Fund for the Replacement of Animals in Medical Experiments
    (FRAME):http://www.frame.org.uk

Select glossary

Acute toxicity study Single dose study in which administration is normally followed by 14 days observation and then macroscopic examination at necropsy.

ADI – acceptable daily intake The daily intake of a chemical that is expected to be without adverse effect when ingested over a lifetime.

ADME – absorption, distribution, metabolism and elimination The basic processes that influence pharmacokinetic behaviour and hence toxicity.

Angiogenesis The formation of new blood vessels, seen in embryos and tumours.

Apoptosis The process whereby cells are programmed to die. Reduced apoptosis can lead to tumour formation. It is an essential part of embryonic development, where effects may be associated with teratogenicity.

AUC – area under the concentration curve A measure of systemic exposure via plasma concentrations. Short half-life generally leads to a low AUC.

Biocoenosis An intergrated community of closely associated organisms.

Carcinogenicity bioassay A study to assess potential for carcinogenic action when the test substance is administered for up to 2.5 years in rodents. Study duration with transgenic animals may be 26 weeks.

Chromosomal mutation Any change in chromosome structure or number.

Chronic toxicity study Usually a toxicity study of 26 weeks or longer.

Clastogen or clastogenic Producing breakages in chromosomes.

Clearance Measure of the removal of a substance from blood or plasma, expressed in units such ml/min. Clearance may differ between organs and total clearance reflects all these values.

Dosage Synonymous with dose level (q.v.) – a rate at which a test system is dosed, e.g. milligrams per kilogram per day.

Dose An amount of compound administered on any one occasion, e.g. in milligrams per kilogram or, in clinical terms, milligrams per day.

Dose level The rate at which a compound is dosed, e.g. milligrams per kilogram per day.

Dose–response curve The curve resulting when response is plotted against dose. A large increase in response for a small increase in dose indicates a steep dose–response curve. Some chemicals, such as paracetamol, show an early slow increase in this curve with a steep increase when a threshold of toxicity is exceeded. The dose–response curve may also be significantly affected by relatively small changes in factors such as protein binding (see Therapeutic index).

Dose volume Usually used to define the volume rate for oral studies, e.g. millilitres per kilogram.

Gene mutation Change in the DNA at one or more bases: these may be insertion of a base (frameshift) or the substitution or misreading of one base for another.

Genotoxicity Modification or damage to genetic material.

α-2u Globulin Protein produced in large amounts in the liver of male rats and excreted in the urine. Chemicals such as d-limonene and trimethyl-pentanol form slowly degraded complexes with it, which accumulate in the kidney and lead to a male rat-specific nephropathy. The normal function of this protein may be to complex volatile pheromones and slow their release into the atmosphere.

Healthy worker effect The bias that can be introduced into epidemiological studies where a workforce is compared with the general population. The working population is expected to be healthier than the general population, which includes long-term sick and unemployed people as well as the healthy and other workers. This concept is now being questioned.

Hepatocytic hypertrophy Increased size of the hepatocytes, typically around the central vein of the liver lobule (centrilobular). It is characterised by greater distance between nuclei (increased cytoplasm) and is usually due to enzyme induction.

Hyperplasia An increase in a normal cell population, which can be seen in response to hormonal disturbances, to changes in the control of apoptosis or to increased cell turnover as a result of direct cellular toxicity.

LOAEL – lowest observed adverse effect level The lowest dose level or concentration at which adverse effects were seen.

Log P Octanol–water partition coefficient, a measure of lipophilicity which influences ADME. Skin permeability increases with log P over the mid-range: low and high log P values are associated with lower skin permeability.

α-2u (or μ) microglobulin See α-2u Globulin.

MRL – maximum residue limit The maximum acceptable concentration in foods for pesticides or veterinary drugs.

MTD – maximum tolerated dose The MTD for a chemical depends to a large extent on the type of test contemplated. Although it has been used extensively in relation to carcinogenicity bioassays to indicate a 10 per cent reduction in bodyweight gain, this is not appropriate in shorter studies where more severe toxicity is implied. Broadly the MTD in any test type is one that elicits toxicity but does not compromise the survival of the test system during the course of the experiment. The MTD for a short exposure or single administration is likely to be significantly higher than that for a long exposure or chronic toxicity study.

Mutation　A change in the DNA which may be transmitted by division and give rise to heritable changes, if the initial change is not lethal. A reverse mutation causes a reversion to the wild type, as in the Ames test; a forward mutation test detects mutants in wild-type bacteria.

NOAEL – no observed adverse effect level　The dose level or concentration that is associated with treatment-related change that is not considered to be adverse. This is a useful concept where there is no NOEL but where effects are transient or due to intended properties of the compound.

NOEL – no observed effect level　The dose level at which no treatment-related change was seen.

Octanol-water partition coefficient – see Log *P*.

OEL – occupational exposure limit　Average airborne concentrations of a chemical to which workers may be exposed over a defined period.

Peroxisome proliferation　Increase in the numbers of peroxisomes – cellular organelles having high levels of oxidative enzymes and probably involved in lipid metabolism. This increase is induced by several chemical classes including some hypolipodaemics and plasticisers such as diethylhexyl-phthalate and chlorinated compounds such as trichloroethylene. This proliferation, particularly in the liver of rodents, is associated with non-genotoxic carcinogenesis of little relevance to humans.

Pharmacokinetics　The study of the time course of the absorption, distribution and elimination of a compound from the body. This term usually refers to therapeutic doses, toxicokinetics being used for this in reference to toxicity studies.

Phase 1 metabolism　The process whereby molecules are made more polar to facilitate elimination, for instance by hydroxylation or hydrolysis. This process of detoxification may backfire when reactive metabolites are produced that result in direct toxicity on cellular macromolecules such as proteins or DNA.

Phase 2 metabolism　Conjugation of metabolites from phase 1 with polar endogenous molecules such as glucuronide, glycine, sulphate or glutathione to produce a more polar molecule that can be readily excreted in the urine or bile. Phase 2 metabolites are usually non-toxic although there are several exceptions to this general rule of thumb.

pK_a　The pH at which a molecule is 50 per cent ionized. This affects absorption, particularly across the intestinal mucosa. For example at low pH benzoic acid is mostly non-ionised: per cent ionisation increases as pH rises above 4, approaching 100 per cent ionised at pH 7. Thus, benzoic acid is best absorbed from low pH media such as those in the stomach.

STEL – short-term exposure limit　The upper airborne concentration that is acceptable for short-term exposure (e.g. not longer than 15 minutes experienced no more than four times in a day at intervals of not less than 1 hour) without prolonged or unacceptable adverse effect.

Subacute toxicity study   Usually a toxicity study of 28 days or less.

Subchronic toxicity study   Usually a toxicity study of 13 weeks.

TDI – tolerable daily intake   Used in similar contexts to ADI, for residues and food contaminants.

Therapeutic index   A measure of the difference between therapeutic levels or doses of a drug and those that are associated with toxicity. This is often related to the plasma concentration of unbound drug or chemical, as with phenytoin or warfarin (see dose–response curve).

TLV – threshold limit value   The upper permissible airborne concentration for occupational exposure.

TLV-C – threshold limit value-ceiling   An airborne concentration that should not be exceeded at any time.

Toxicodynamics   The study of the relationship between concentration at target tissues or plasma and toxic effect.

Toxicokinetics   The study of pharmacokinetics in toxicity studies. The knowledge of pharmacokinetics following single or repeated administration may be used to model or explain the effects expected in other species or in humans and may be related to toxicodynamics.

TWA – time weighted average   The average concentration to which nearly all workers may be exposed repeatedly without adverse effect, during a working day of 8 hours or a 40-hour week.

Notes

1 Introduction to toxicology: the necessity of measurement

1 Ellenhorn MJ. *Ellenhorn's Medical Toxicology*, 2nd edition. Philadelphia: Williams and Wilkins, 1997.
2 Harber VJ and Sutton JR. 'Endorphins and exercise'. *Sports Medicine* 1984; 1(2): 154–171.
3 Sforzo GA. 'Opioids and exercise. An update'. *Sports Medicine* 1989; 7(2): 109–124.
4 Shepherd RJ. 'Vehicle injuries to joggers. Case report and review'. *Journal of Sports Medicine and Physical Fitness* 1992; 32(3): 321–331.
5 Horton R. 'Genetically modified foods: absurd concern or welcome dialogue'. *The Lancet* 1999; 354(October 16): 1314–1315. Kuiper HA, Noteborn HPJM and Peijnenburg AACM. 'Adequacy of methods for testing the safety of genetically modified foods'. *The Lancet* 1999; 354 (October 16): 1315–1316. Ewen SWB and Pusztai A. 'Effect of diets containing genetically modified potatoes expressing *Galanthus nivalis* lectin on rat small intestine'. *The Lancet* 1999; 354(October 16): 1353–1354. Bateson PPG. 'Genetically modified potatoes (letter)'. *The Lancet* 1999; 354(October 16): 1382.
6 Toth B, Patil K, Taylor J et al. 'Cancer induction in mice by 4-hydroxy-benzenediazonium sulphate of the *Agaricus xanthodermus* mushroom'. *In vivo* 1989; 3(5): 301–305.
7 McManus BM, Toth B and Patil KD. 'Aortic rupture and aortic smooth muscle tumours in mice: induction by *p*-hydrazinobenzoic acid hydrochloride of the cultivated mushroom *Agaricus bisporus*'. *Laboratory Investigation* 1987; 57(1): 78–85.
8 Pilegaard K, Kristiansen E, Meyer OA et al. 'Failure of the cultivated mushroom (*Agaricus bisporus*) to induce tumors in the A/J mouse lung tumour model'. *Cancer Letters* 1997; 120(1): 79–85.
9 Toth B, Erickson J and Gannett P. 'Lack of carcinogenesis by the baked mushroom *Agaricus bisporus* in mice: different feeding regimen'. *In vivo* 1997; 11(3): 227–231.
10 Russell WMS and Burch RL. *The Principles of Humane Experimental Technique*. London: Methuen, 1959.

2 Normality: definition and maintenance

1 Nohynek GJ et al. 'Fat frail and dying young: survival, bodyweight and pathology of the Charles River Sprague–Dawley-derived rat prior to and since the introduction of the VAF variant in 1988'. *Human and Experimental Toxicology* 1993; 12: 87–98.
2 Giknis MLA and Clifford CB. 'Spontaneous neoplastic lesions in the Crl:CD-1® (ICR)BR mouse'. Charles River Laboratories, March 2000.

3   Charles River on-line literature. 'Spontaeous neoplastic lesions in the B6C3F₁/CrlBR mouse'. 1989. www.criver.com
4   Charles River on-line literature. 'Spontaeous neoplastic lesions in the CDF® (F-344)/CrlBR rat. 1990. www.criver.com

3   Determination of toxicity: basic principles

1   Festing MFW. 'Genetic variation in outbred rats and mice and its implication for toxicological screening'. *Journal of Experimental Animal Science* 1993; 35: 210–220.
2   Kacew S and Festing MFW. 'Role of rat strain in the differential sensitivty to pharmaceutical agents and naturally occurring substances'. *Journal of Toxicilogy and Environmental Health* 1996; 47(1): 1–30.
3   Bader A, Knop E, Fruhauf N *et al*. 'Reconstruction of liver tissue in vitro: geometry of characteristic flat bed, hollow fibre and spouted bed bioreactors with reference to the in vivo liver'. *Artificial Organs* 1995; 19(9): 941–950.
4   Bader A, Fruhauf N, Zech K *et al*. 'Development of a small-sclae bioreactor for drug metabolism studies maintaining heptospecific functions'. *Xenobiotica* 1998; 28(9): 815–825.
5   Belin V, Hodge T, Picaut P *et al*. 'The myocardial lesions produced by the potassium channel opener Aprikalim in monkeys and rats are prevented by blockage of cardiac b-adrenoreceptors'. *Fundamental and Applied Toxicology* 1996; 31(2): 259–267.
6   Cordier A, Amyes SJ and Woolley APAH. 'Correlation between fighting leasions and subcutaneous sarcoma in male B6C3F1 mice'. Proceedings of the 29th Annual Meeting of the Society of Toxicology. *The Toxicologist* 1990.

5   Determination: general and reproductive toxicology

1   Evans GO (ed.) *Animal Clinical Chemistry – A Primer for Toxicologists*. London: Taylor & Francis, 1996.
2   McCarver DG and Hines RN. 'The ontogeny of human drug-metabolizing enzymes: phase II conjugation enzymes and regulatory mechanisms'. *Journal of Pharmacology and Experimental Therapy* 2002; 300(2): 361–366.
3   Rasheed A, Hines RN and McCarver-May DG. 'Variation in induction of human placental CYP2E1: possible role in susceptibility to fetal alcohol syndrome'. *Toxicology and Applied Pharmacology* 1997; 144(2): 396–400.
4   Koukouritaki SB, Simpson P, Yeung CK *et al*. 'Human hepatic flavin-containing monooxygenase 1 (FMO1) and 3 (FMO3) developmental expression'. *Pediatric Research* 2002; 51(2): 236–243.
5   British Toxicology Society Working Party. 'Report on *in vitro* toxicology'. *Human and Experimental Toxicology* 1997; 16(suppl 1).
6   ICH Guideline on Reproductive Toxicity. ICH Guideline S5: Reprotox. http://www.ifpma.org/ich1.html
7   Creasy DM. 'Evaluation of testicular toxicity in safety evalutaion studies: the appropriate use of spermatic staging'. *Toxicology and Pathology* 1997; 25(2): 119–131.

6   Determination: genotoxicity and carcinogenicity

1   Festing MF. 'Use of a multistrain assay could improve the NTP carcinogenesis bioassay'. *Environmental Health Perspectives* 1995; 103(1): 44–52. Festing MFW. 'Properties of inbred strain and outbred stocks with special reference to toxicity testing'. *Journal of Toxicology and Environmental Health* 1979; 5(1): 53–68.

2 Data relevant to this study (presented by RW Tennant at a satellite symposium to Eurotox 2000) are at website http://dir.niehs.nih.gov/dirlecm/
3 Tennant RW. 'Application of transgenic models for toxicological characterization'. Crisp Data Base, National Institutes of Health, Bethesda, Maryland.
4 Tennant RW. 'Transgenic mouse models for identifying and charaterizing carcinogens'. Crisp Data Base, National Institutes of Health, Bethesda, Maryland.
5 Tennant RW. 'Evaluation and validation issues in the development of transgenic mouse carcinogeniticity bioassays'. *Environmental Health Perspectives* 1998; 106(suppl 2): 473–476.
6 Cohen SM, Robinson D and MacDonald J. 'Alternative models for carcinogenicity testing. *Toxicological Sciences* 2001; 64: 14–19.
7 Elcombe CR, Odum J, Foster JR *et al*. 'Prediction of rodent nongenotoxic carcinogenesis; evaluation of biochemical and tissue changes in rodents following exposure to nine nongenotoxic NTP carcinogens'. *Environmental Health Perspectives* 2002; 110(4): 363–375.

8 Determination: environmental toxicology and epidemiology

1 Wall R and Strong L. 'Environmental consequences of treating cattle with the antiparasitic drug ivermectin'. *Nature (London)* 1987; 327(6121): 418–421.
2 Madsen M *et al*. 'Treating cattle with ivermectin: effects on the fauna and decomposition of dung pats'. *Journal of Applied Ecology* 1990; 27(1): 1–15.
3 A Toxline search (http://www.toxnet.nlm.nih.gov) on 'caesium, Chernobyl and clay' brings up a selection of papers on the behaviour of caesium in soils.

9 Interpretation

1 Bell ML and Davis DL. 'Reassessment of the lethal London fog of 1952: novel indicators of acute and chronic consequences of acute exposure to air pollution'. *Environmental Health Perspectives* 2001; 109(suppl 3): 389–394.
2 Izzotti A, Parodi S, Quaglia A *et al*. 'The relationship between urban airborne pollution and short-term mortality: quantitative and qualitative aspects'. *European Journal of Epidemiology* 2000; 16(11): 1027–1034.
3 Bonner FW, Eason CT and Spencer AJ. 'Phenoxyisobutyrate derivatives: a review of animal toxicity'. *Research and Clinical Forums* 12(1): 23–45.
4 Rao MS, Dwivedi RS, Subbarao V *et al*. 'Induction of peroxisome proliferation and hepatic tumours in C57BL/6N mice by ciprofibrate, a hypolipidaemic compound'. *British Journal of Cancer* 1988; 58(1): 46–51.
5 Bonner FW, Deavy L, Astley N *et al*. 'Investigation of the mechanism of ciprofibrate induced thyroid hyperplasia in the rat'. Proceedings of the 30th Annual Meeting of the Society of Toxicology. *The Toxicologist* 1991; 11: 152.
6 Spencer A, Eason CT, Pattison A *et al*. 'Functional and morphological changes in the thyroid gland of Fischer 344 and Sprague-Dawley rats given bezafibrate and ciprofibrate'. *Human Toxicology* 1988; 8: 400.
7 Graham MJ, Wilson SA, Winham MA *et al*. 'Lack of peroxisome proliferation in marmoset liver following treatmnet with cirpofibrate for 3 years'. *Fundamental and Applied Toxicology* 1994; 22: 58–64.
8 Eason CT, Powles P, Henry G *et al*. 'The comparative pharmacokinetics and gastric toxicity of bezafibrate and ciprofibrate in the rat'. *Xenobiotica* 1989; 19(8): 913–925.
9 Christie AC 'Schizophrenia – is the potato the environmental culprit?' *Medical Hypotheses* 1999; 53(1): 80–86.

10 Friedman M, Rayburn JR and Bantle JA. 'Developmental toxicity of potato alkaloids in the frog embryop teratogenesis assay – Xenopus (FETAX)'. *Food and Chemical Toxicology* 1991; 29(8): 537–547.

11 Ewen SWB and Pusztai A. 'Effect of diets containing genetically modifed potatoes expressing *Galanthus nivalis* lectin on rat small intestine'. *The Lancet* 1999; 354: 1353–1354.

12 Horton R. 'Genetically modified foods: absurd concern or welcome dialogue?' *The Lancet* 1999; 354: 1314–1315.

13 Kuiper HA, Noteborn HPJM and Peijnenburg AACM. 'Adequacy of methods for testing the safety of genetically modified foods. *The Lancet* 1999; 354: 1315–1316.

10 Prediction of hazard

1 The development and validation of expert systems for predicting toxicity. Report and Rcommendations of ECVAM Workshop 24. http://altweb.jhsph.edu/publications/ECVAM/ecvam24.htm

2 Ellenhorn MJ. *Ellenhorn's Medical Toxicology*. Philadelphia: Williams and Wilkins, 1997.

11 Background to risk due to toxicity

1 Pilkington A, Buchanan D, Jamal GA *et al*. 'An epidemiological study of the relations between exposure to OP pesticides and neurological indices in sheep farmers'. *Occupational and Environmental Medicine* 2000; 58(11): 702–710.

2 Stephens R, Spurgeon A, Calvert IA *et al*. 'Neuropsychological effect of long-term exposure to OPs in sheep dip'. *Lancet* 1995; 345(8958): 1135–1139. Commentaries and authors' reply.

3 Mutch E, Blain PG and Williams FM. 'Interindividual variations in enzymes controlling OP toxicity in man'. *Human and Experimental Toxicology* 1992; 11(2): 109–116.

4 Geldmacher von Mallinckrodt M and Diepgen TL. 'The human serum paraoxonase polymorphism and specificity'. *Toxicological and Environmental Chemistry* 1988; 18: 79–196.

5 Mackness B, Durrington PN and Mackness MI. 'Low paraoxonase in Persian Gulf war veterans self-reporting Gulf War Syndrome'. *Biochemical and Biophysical Research Communications* 2000; 276(2): 729–733.

6 Virtue WA and Clayton JW. 'Sheep dip chemicals and water pollution'. *Science of the Total Environment* 1997; 194/195: 207–217.

7 Ames BN, Profet M and Swirsky Gold L. 'Nature's chemicals and synthetic chemicals: comparative toxicology'. *Proceedings of the National Academy of Sciences of the USA* revised 1990 and 'Dietary pesticides (99.99 per cent all natural)' at http://socrates.berkeley.edu/mutagen/ames.PNASII.html

8 Ballantyne B, Marrs T and Syversen T. *General and Applied Toxicology*, 2nd edition. London: Macmillan Reference, 2000.

9 Taylor SL and Hefle S. 'Will genetically modified foods be allergenic?' *Journal of Allergy and Clinical Immunology* 2000; 107(5).

10 *New Scientist* 11 September 2001.

11 *New Scientist* 21 October 2000.

12 *New Scientist* 19 February 2000.

13 *New Scientist* 18 December 1999.

14 Ames BN and Gold LS have published widely in this area, comparing natural with synthetic chemicals; see Ames BN, Profet M and Swirsky Gold L. 'Nature's

chemicals and synthetic chemicals: comparative toxicology'. *Proceedings of the National Academy of Sciences of the USA* revised 1990 and 'Dietary pesticides (99.99 per cent all natural)' at http://socrates.berkeley.edu/mutagen/ames.PNASII.html

15 Kellow A. *International Toxic Risk Management*. Cambridge: Cambridge University Press, 1999.

16 Illing P. *Toxicity and Risk – Context, Principles and Practice*. London: Taylor & Francis, 2001.

17 Kellow A. *International Toxic Risk Management – Ideals, Interests and Implementation*. Cambridge: Cambridge University Press, 1999.

18 ACSH website. http://www.acsh.org/publications/booklets/menu99.html

19 Friedman M, Rayburn JR and Bantle JA. 'Developmental toxicity of potato alkaloids in the frog embryop teratogenesis assay – Xenopus (FETAX)'. *Food and Chemical Toxicology* 1991; 29(8): 537–547.

20 Lappin G. 'Chemical toxins and body defences'. *Biologist* 2002; 49: 33–37.

21 Friedman M and McDonald GM. 'Postharvest changes in glycoalkaloid content of potatoes'. *Advances in Experimental Medicine and Biology* 1999; 459: 121–143.

22 Christie AC. 'Schizophrenia: is the potato the environmental culprit?' *Medical Hypotheses* 1999; 53(1): 80–86.

23 Scottish Executive. *Health in Scotland 2000*. http://www.scotland.gov.uk

12 Risk assessment in practice and setting exposure limits

1 Campbell DB. 'Extrapolation from animals to man. The integration of pharmaco-kinetics and pharmacodynamics'. *Annals of the New York Academy of Sciences* 1996; 801: 116–135.

2 Mahmood I and Balian JD. 'The pharmacokinetic principles behind scaling from preclinical results to phase 1 protocols'. *Clinical Pharmacokinetics* 1999; 36(1): 1–11.

3 Ritschel WA, Vachharajani NN, Johnson RD and Hussain AS. 'The allometrical approach for interspecies scaling of pharmacokinetic parameters'. *Comparative Biochemistry and Physiology* 1992; 103(2): 249–253.

4 Yates FE and Kugler PN. 'Similarity principles and intrinsic geometries: contrasting approaches to interspecies scaling'. *Journal of Pharmaceutical Sciences* 1986; 75(11): 1019–1027.

5 Gad SC. 'Trends in toxicology modelling for risk assessment'. In Salem H and Olajos EJ (eds) *Toxicology in Risk Assessment*. London: Taylor & Francis, 2000.

6 Witschi HR and Last JA. 'Toxic responses of the respiratory system'. In Curtis D Klassen (ed.) *Casarett and Doull's Toxicology*, 5th edition. New York: McGraw-Hill, 1996.

7 Biomarkers are discussed extensively in Ballantyne B, Marrs T and Syverssen T (eds) *General and Applied Toxicology*, 2nd edition (London: Macmillan Reference, 2000) and also in Curtis D Kalssen (ed.) *Casarett and Doull's Toxicology*, 5th edition (New York: McGraw-Hill, 1996) and in Salam H and Olajos EJ. *Toxicology in Risk Assessment* (London: Taylor & Francis, 2000).

8 Renwick AG. 'The use of an additional safety factor or uncertainty factor for nature of toxicity in the estimation of ADI and TDI values'. *Regulatory Toxicology and Pharmacology* 1995; 22(3): 250–261.

9 Renwick AG. ' Data derived safety factors for the evaluation of food additives and environmental contaminants'. *Food Additives and Contaminants* 1993; 10: 275–305.

10 WHO. 'Assessing human health risks of chemicals: derivation of guidance values for health-based exposure limits'. *Environmental Health Criteria* 170. Geneva: World Health Organization, 1994.

11 Essers A *et al*. 'Food plant toxicants and safety: risk assessment and regulation of inherent toxicants in plant foods'. *Environmental Toxicology and Pharmacology* 1998; 5(3): 155–172.

12 Illing P. Chapter 8 in *Toxicity and Risk – Context, Principles and Practice*. London: Taylor and Francis, 2001.

13 Ku RH. 'An overview of setting occupational exposure limits (OELs) for pharmaceuticals'. *Chemical Health and Safety* January/February 2000.

14 Chemical Industries Association. *Guidance on Allocating Occupational Exposure Bands*, Regulation 7. London: Chemical Industries Association, 1997. www.cia.org.uk

15 Association of the British Pharmaceutical Industry. *Guidance on Setting in-house Occupational Exposure Limits for Airborne Therapeutic Substances and their Intermediates*. London: ABPI, 1995. www.apbi.org.uk

13 Risk assessment and management in the workplace

1 Sunderman FW Jr, Aitio A, Morgan LG and Norseth T. 'Biological monitoring of nickel'. *Toxicology and Industrial Health* 1986; 2(1): 17–78.

14 Risk assessment: carcinogenicity; the environment; evolution and overview of risk assessment

1 Doll R, Morgan LG and Speizer FE. 'Cancers of the lung and nasal sinuses in nickel workers'. *British Journal of Cancer* 1970; 24(4): 623–632.

2 Morgan LG and Usher V. 'Health problems associated with nickel refining and use'. *Annals of Occupational Hygiene* 1994; 38(2): 189–198.

3 Kaldor J, Peto J, Easton D *et al*. 'Models of respiratory cancer in nickel refinery workers'. *Journal of the National Cancer Institute* 1986; 77(4): 841–848.

4 Burdon RH. *Genes and the Environment*. London: Taylor & Francis, 1999. See also numerous papers by BN Ames and L Swirsky Gold.

5 Dybing E. 'Genotoxic carcinogens – is there a threshold?' Notes from Eurotox Satallite Symposium, September 2000.

6 Williams GM, Iatropoulos MJ, Wang CX *et al*. 'Nonlinearities in 2-acetyl-aminofluorene exposure responses for genotoxic and epigenetic effects leading to initiation of carcinogenesis in rat liver'. *Toxicological Sciences* 1998; 45(2): 152–161.

7 Lutz WK. 'Dose-response relationships in chemical carcinogenesis: superposition of different mechanisms of action, resulting in linear–nonlinear curves, practical thresholds, J-shapes'. *Mutation Research* 1998; 405(2): 117–124.

8 Lutz WK and Kopp-Schneider A. 'Threshold dose response for tumour induction by genotoxic carcinogens modelled via cell-cycle delay'. *Toxicological Sciences* 1999; 49(1): 110–115.

9 Tomenson JA. 'Epidemiology in relation to toxicology'. In Ballantyne B, Marrs T and Syverssen T (eds) *General and Applied Toxicology*, 2nd edition. London: Macmillan Reference, 2000.

10 Ashby J, Brady A, Elcombe CR *et al*. 'Mechanistically-based human hazard assessment of peroxisome proliferator-induced hepatocarcinogenesis'. *Human and Experimental Toxicology* 1994; 13(suppl 2).

11 Riley DM and Fishbeck PS. 'History of methylene chloride in consumer products'. In Salem H and Olajos EJ (eds) *Toxicology in Risk Assessment*. London: Taylor and Francis, 2000.

12 Gibbs GW, Amsel J and Soden K. 'A cohort mortality study of cellulose triacetate-fiber workers exposed to methylene chloride'. *Journal of Occupational and Environmental Medicine* 1996; 38(7): 693–697.

13   Ojajarvi A, Partanen T, Ahlbom A *et al*. 'Risk of pancreative cancer in workers exposed to chlorinated hydrocarbon solvents and related compounds: a meta-analysis'. *American Journal of Epidemiology* 2001; 153(9): 841–850.

14   Hearne FT and Lifer JW. 'Mortality study of two overlapping cohorts of photographic film base manufacturing employees exposed to methylene chloride'. *Journal of Occupational and Environmental Medicine* 1999; 41(12): 1154–1169.

15   Green T. 'Methylene chloride induced mouse liver and lung tumours: an overview of the role of mechanistic studies in human safety assessment'. *Human and Experimental Toxicology* 1997; 16(1): 3–13.

16   Dell LD, Mundt KA, McDonald M *et al*. 'Critical review of the epidemiology literature on the potential cancer risks of methylene chloride'. *International Archives of Occupational and Environmental Health* 1999; 72(7): 429–442.

17   Ahlberg R *et al*. ECETOC/EFOA Task Force Report on Environmental Risk Assessment of MTBE, 2001. www.efoa.org/fr/mtbe_environment/EFOA-ECETOC per cent20report.pdf or through the EFOA website (www.efoa.org). See also: Abernathy CO. 'A drinking water advisory: consumer acceptability advice and health effects analysis on MTBE'. In Salem H and Olajos EJ (eds) *Toxicology in Risk Assessment*. London: Taylor & Francis, 2000. A search of the European Environment Agency website (www.eea.eu.int) for 'environmental risk assessment' showed 239 references.

18   Ames BN, Profet M and Swirsky Gold L. 'Nature's chemicals and synthetic chemicals: comparative toxicology'. *Proceedings of the National Academy of Sciences of the USA* revised 1990 and 'Dietary pesticides (99.99 per cent all natural)' at http://socrates.berkeley.edu/mutagen/ames.PNASII.html

19   Kellow A. *International Toxic Risk Management*. Cambridge: Cambridge University Press, 1999. See also Illing P. *Toxicity and Risk – Context, Principles and Practice*. London: Taylor & Francis, 2001.

20   Doull J. Chapter 1 in Salem H and Olajos EJ (eds) *Toxicology in Risk Assessment*. London: Taylor & Francis, 2000.

21   Riley DM and Fishbeck PS. 'History of methylene chloride in consumer products'. In Salem H and Olajos EJ (eds) *Toxicology in Risk Assessment*. London: Taylor & Francis, 2000.

Bibliography

General

Ballantyne, B, Marrs, T and Syversen, T. *General and Applied Toxicology*, 2nd edition. London: Macmillan Reference, 2000.

Ellenhorn, MJ. *Ellenhorn's Medical Toxicology*, 2nd edition. Philadelphia: Williams and Wilkins, 1997.

Heath, David. *An Introduction to Experimental Design and Statistics for Biology*. London: Taylor & Francis, 1995.

Hodgson, Ernest and Levi, Patricia E. *A Textbook of Modern Toxicology*, 2nd edition. New York: Appleton and Lange, 1997.

Hodgson, Ernest, Mailman, Richard B and Chambers, Janice E (eds) *Dictionary of Toxicology*, 2nd edition. London: Macmillan Reference, 1998.

Klassen, Curtis D (ed.) *Casarett and Doull's Toxicology*, 5th edition. New York: McGraw-Hill, 1996 (now available in a 6th edition).

Timbrell, John. *Principles of Biochemical Toxicology*, 3rd edition. London: Taylor & Francis, 2000.

Risk assessment and occupational toxicology

Illing, P. *Toxicity and Risk – Context, Principles and Practice*. London: Taylor & Francis, 2001.

Kellow, A. *International Toxic Risk Management*. Cambridge: Cambridge University Press, 1999.

Salem, H and Olajos, EJ (eds) *Toxicology in Risk Assessment*. London: Taylor & Francis, 2000.

Stacey, Neill H (ed.) *Occupational Toxicology*. London: Taylor & Francis, 1993.

Environmental toxicology

Shaw, Ian C and Chadwick, John. *Principles of Environmental Toxicology*. London: Taylor & Francis, 1998.

Walker, CH, Hopkins, SP, Silby, RM and Peakall, DB. *Principles of Ecotoxicology*, 2nd edition. London: Taylor & Francis, 2001.

Other texts

Burdon, Roy H. *Genes and the Environment*. London: Taylor & Francis, 1999.

Evans, GO (ed.) *Animal Clinical Chemistry – A Primer for Toxicologists*. London: Taylor & Francis, 1996.

Glaister, John. *Principles of Toxicological Pathology*. London: Taylor & Francis, 1986.

Kimber, Ian and Maurer, Thomas. *Toxicology of Contact Hypersensitivity*. London: Taylor & Francis, 1996.

Manser, Caroline E. *The Assessment of Stress in Laboratory Animals*. London: RSPCA, 1992.

Penreath, VW (ed.) *Neurotoxicology in Vitro*. London: Taylor & Francis, 1999.

Turton, J and Hooson, J. (eds) *Target Organ Pathology – a Basic Text*. London: Taylor & Francis, 1998.

Index

Note: *b* denotes a text box, *f* denotes a figure, *t* denotes a table

acceptable daily intake (ADI) 27, 153, 220, 253, 257, 300; *see also* exposure limits
accumulation 23, 26, 89, 97, 163, 164, 264–5; environmental 23, 146, 184, 282
acetaminophen: *see* paracetamol
2-acetylaminofluorene (AAF) 205, 276
absorption, distribution, metabolism and elimination (ADME) 21, 52, 65, 67, 80, 98, 163, 166, 171, 175, 181, 202, 205, 207, 221, 236, 242, 244, 251, 300; environmental 141; impact on toxicity 164 (*t*9.2); in pregnancy 96; in risk assessment 247, 273, 274, 277, 279
aflatoxin 2, 8, 179, 224, 228, 231, 253, 274
age: in comparison of historical controls 51–2, 156; in risk assessment 244, 248; in toxicity 15, 20–1, 37, 70, 164, 167, 171; related data analysis 130; test system 82
allergic sensitisation: *see* sensitisation
allometric scaling 236
American Conference of Governmental and Industrial Hygienists (ACGIH) 261, 287
American Council on Science and Health (ACSH) 8, 230 (*b*11.4), 308
Ames, Bruce (BN Ames) 8, 108, 284, 307
Ames test 38, 47, 61, 69, 108–13, 118, 177–8, 206, 210, 215
animal experiments, utility in risk assessment 292

animal husbandry 38–40, 44, 48, 51–2, 64, 68, 70, 156, 171, 194, 294
animals, legislation of use 57
apoptosis 17, 24, 120, 132, 133, 175, 274–6, 300

background data 45–53, 118, 121, 130, 155–6, 181, 290; in interpretation 166–7; *see also* historical control data
bacteria 38, 43, 69, 132; in environmental toxicology 143, 144, 163, 204; in genotoxicity 108–11, 113–14, 118; *see also individual species*
Balkan endemic nephropathy 7, 153, 231
baseline data: as normality 42, 45–53, 187, 243, 294
bees 32, 143, 145
benchmark dose (BMD) 255, 256
bioaccumulation 147, 282
bioavailability 22, 52, 61, 70, 165, 206; in risk assessment 228, 240–2, 244–6, 258, 280
biological markers (biomarkers) 186, 188, 241–2, 254, 266–8
birds, in environmental toxicology 142–5, 184
Biston betularia (peppered moth) 147
Buehler test 137–8

cadmium 23, 26, 165, 169
cancer: genetic association 107–8 (*t*6.1); *see also* carcinogenicity
carcinogen: classification (IARC) 179
carcinogenicity: factors in 134, 271; genotoxic 120–1, 275; non-genotoxic

9, 275, 296; markers of effect 132
(t6.5); mechanisms 8–9, 119–20, 123,
129, 131–2 (t6.5), 134, 182, 274, 275,
292, 295; risk assessment 270–9;
thresholds 274–6 (b14.2)
carcinogenicity assessment 119–31;
general principles 119–21;
interpretation 179–82 (t9.9); other
systems 120, 126 (b6.1), 131–4
carrying system: see formulation or
vehicles
cell culture: mammalian cells in
genotoxicity 109, 111, 114–16
chlorination of drinking water 228–9, 288
CHO assay 110, 113, 114, 177
cholinesterase inhibition 186, 188, 221
(b11.1), 230, 241–3, 254, 264
chorioallantoic membrane (CAM) test
137, 139
chromosomal damage (clastogenicity)
109–11, 114, 116–17
chromosome aberration tests 111–15,
118, 178, 206
ciprofibrate 189–91, 204
clastogenicity: see chromosomal damage
clinical chemistry 86–7; interpretation
172–3; liver function 86, 167; kidney
function 85, 86, 87, 167
clinical pathology 41, 50, 68, 84, 85–7,
93, 94, 102, 169, 172, 174; see also
clinical chemistry, haematology and
urinalysis
comet assay 110, 113, 116, 127, 131, 132,
207
compound categories 264; criteria for
classification 265 (t13.1)
computer models 201, 209–17; accuracy
of predictions 214–17; criteria for
success 210–13; endpoints predicted
210; strengths and weaknesses 213–14
confounding factors 155, 194; in
epidemiology 148, 185, 186, 187, 273;
in study design 67–8, 94
control groups, 110, 114–18, 130, 157,
273; as normality 41–4, 46, 48, 50;
size 67–8, 83 (t5.2), 101–2 (t5.4), 110,
123
controls 36, 40; and expectation 42, 46,
154–5; choice 68, validity of data 154
(b9.1)
corrositivity 78, 137, 210, 211, 213
Control of Substances Hazardous to

Health regulations (COSHH) 51, 58,
165, 254, 261, 266, 298
cytochrome P450 10, 15, 20, 109, 205, 247
cytotoxicity 74, 77, 111, 115, 178; studies
69

Daphnia magna 144–5, 283
data: handling in prediction of hazard
202–3, 235; quality 52, 69;
transformation 160 (f9.1), 161;
treatment 155, 161
DDT 4, 23, 26, 142, 147, 165, 179,
183–4, 285
Delaney amendment 197, 230, 286
dermal toxicity 82, 92–3, 263; factors in
136; test systems 81
dermatitis 10, 22; allergic contact 135–6;
contact 135–6
diet 3, 7–8, 22, 231, 241, 280; as test
article carrier 62–3; as a risk factor
185–6, 222, 230 (b11.4), 270; in
animal studies 44–5, 64, 121, 123–5,
129, 193
di-ethyl-hexylphthalate (DEHP) 128,
249
diethyl stilboestrol (diethylstilbestrol) 16,
17, 34, 97, 106, 175, 197, 274
digitalis 11, 13
DNA: damage 8, 18, 31, 64, 113, 116,
127, 132, 176, 177, 207, 272, 275,
278; repair 23, 27, 109, 114, 115, 132,
134, 136, 271; vulnerability 271–2
(b14.1)
dog (beagle): in general toxicology 40,
81, 83, 92, 204
dog whelk 146–7
dominant lethal test 117
dose levels 54, 84, 110, 234, 238, 242,
247, 251, 274–7, 300; choice 58, 63,
69–71, 124, 125, 129, 130, 174, 192,
208; computer prediction 210, 215,
241; selection for exposure limit
calculation 254–9; test concentration
62–3, 69–70, 110, 118
dose range-finding (sighting study)
69–70, 94, 100, 110, 129, 155;
troubleshooting 70
dose–response (curve) 8, 13, 21, 27, 90,
94, 166; in genotoxicology 111, 177–8
(t9.6, 9.7); in risk assessment 30, 220,
244, 246, 255, 257, 259, 262, 265,
275, 294, 300; U-shaped 8, 167, 180

Drosophila melanogaster (fruit fly) 204, 297; in genotoxicity 112; in reproductive toxicology 99

earthworms 143, 145
ecotoxicology: *see* environmental toxicology
electrocardiogram (ECG) 78, 93, 171; confounding factors 68; timing 93
embryotoxicity 73, 265; studies 98, 100, 102, 202
endogenous chemicals 11–12, 19, 23, 26, 76, 109, 142; in calculation of exposure limits 256; in risk assessment 223, 225, 228, 230–1(*b*11.4), 279
environmental toxicology 140–7; interpretation 182–4 (*t*9.10); predicted environmental no effect concentration (PNEC) 282, 283; predicted environmental exposure (PEC) 282, 283
epidemiology 148–50; and background incidence 149, 185; carcinogenicity 273; interpretation 185, 186 (*t*9.11)
Escherichia coli 51, 110, 112, 113, 114
ethics of toxicological assessment 28–31, 84
ethinyl oestradiol 255, 256
European Centre for the Validation of Alternative Methods (ECVAM) 73, 79, 209, 210, 295, 299, 307
expert systems 108, 208; *see also* computer models
exposure: assessment 161–6 (*b*9.2), 219, 239–43 (*b*12.1); integration of exposure information 161–6; markers of 184, 188; measurement 241–2; monitoring 267, 268; prediction 240–1
exposure limits 136, 234, 248, 252–8, 261; dose level selection for calculation 254–9; occupational 253, 266, 267, 268, 279; setting 256, 257 (*b* 12.4)

ferret 82
fertility 97, 100, 102, 105, 106, 175, 176, 202, 265; studies 98, 100, 101, 103
fibrates 15, 182; *see also* ciprofibrate
field tests and studies 145–7
first dose in man 196, 249

fish 32, 99, 184, 293; in environmental toxicology 143, 145
formulation 30, 52, 61, 70, 71, 73, 92, 94, 164, 165, 171, 198, 228, 242–5, 258, 266; dermal 61–2
Fund for the Replacement of Animals in Medical Experiments (FRAME) 295, 299
fruit fly: *see Drosophila melanogaster*

Gaian concept 140
general toxicology 80–94; examinations 84–9 (*b*5.2); interpretation 169–74 (*t*9.3 9.4); study duration 84
genetically modified: crops or foods 3, 37, 63, 143; risk 224–5 (*b*11.2), 288; *see also* potatoes
genomics 20, 74, 75, 132, 133, 134, 279, 296
genotoxicity 107–18, 180, 181, 198, 202, 204, 206–7, 271, 274, 275, 301; interpretation 175–9 (*t*9.6, 9.7); positive controls 110 (*t*6.2); test system characterisation 112, 118
α-2u globulin 8–9, 89, 123, 180, 199, 203, 205, 274, 301
Good Laboratory Practice (GLP) 57, 69, 201, 292
guinea pig 3, 4, 31, 43, 58–9, 137–8, 139, 203, 205

haematology 51, 86; interpretation 172
hamster 4, 21, 121; in general toxicology 39, 81 (*b*5.1)
hazard 8–9, 54–5; human-relevant 195–6, 202 (*b*10.1), 218, 262; versus risk 196
Health and Safety at Work Act 261
Health and Safety Executive (UK) 58, 235, 261, 266, 298
hepatocyte 20, 25, 51, 65, 77, 109, 172, 199, 278; couplets 77; cultures 29, 66, 75, 78, 113–15; hypertrophy 90, 247, 301
hepatotoxicity 24, 198, 218, 254; markers 87
histological processing (histopathology) 87, 92, 102, 103, 125–6, 133; as confounding factor 130
historical control data 41, 50, 67–8, 86, 98–9, 122, 174, 176, 180, 194, 294; criteria for comparison 51–3; drift 48–9; number of data points 49–50;

ranges 40, 42, 45, 47–9; *see also*
    background data
4-hydrazinobenzoic acid 30, 198, 208;
    structure 209 (*f*10.1); *see also*
    mushrooms

immunotoxicity 106, 168, 172, 297; and
    stress 39, 91, 171
individual data sets, interpretation 169
inhalation toxicology: *see* respiratory
    toxicology
intercellular gap junctions 18, 132, 133,
    292
intermediates (in synthetic pathways) 6,
    207, 260, 263, 268
International Conference on
    Harmonisation (ICH) 54, 56, 101,
    102, 298
invertebrates 293; in environmental
    toxicology 144–5
4-ipomeanol 19; mechanism of toxicity
    20; structure 20
irritation: dermal 135, 137, 138–9; ocular
    75, 136, 137, 138–9; *see also*
    sensitisation
isoniazid 14, 21, 28, 197
ivermectin 141, 148

LC$_{50}$ (test) 144, 145, 210
LD$_{50}$ (test) 4, 58, 82–3, 210, 214, 221, 231
lead 23, 26, 201, 228, 244, 269
limulus amoebocyte lysate (LAL) test 31,
    58, 78
local lymph node assay (LLNA) 31, 58–9,
    65, 137, 139
log P (partition coefficient) 134, 136,
    143, 163, 208, 211, 214, 236, 301
low dose extrapolation 272, 276

Magnusson and Kligmann test: *see*
    maximisation test
margin of exposure 256
margin of safety 13, 27, 105, 204, 229,
    230, 234, 244, 246, 248, 249, 250–2
markers: *see* biological markers
Material Safety Data Sheet (MSDS) 135,
    263
maximisation test 58, 137–8
maximum residue limit (MRL) 253, 287,
    302; *see also* exposure limits
maximum tolerated dose (MTD) 69–70,
    124, 129, 181, 210, 214–15, 302

mesocosms 143, 145–6, 183, 281; *see also*
    field tests and studies
metabolism 5, 10, 14–15, 17–18, 21–6,
    28, 37–8, 44, 50, 64–7, 70, 80–1, 89,
    116–17, 124, 133, 164–5, 171, 174–5,
    178, 180–1, 189, 193, 196, 200, 205,
    211–12, 216, 236, 244, 247, 277, 298;
    first pass 179, 206; phase 1 21, 109,
    302; phase 2 65, 109, 302
methyl tertiary butyl ether (MTBE)
    282–4 (*b*14.4)
methylene chloride 228, 275;
    carcinogenicity case study 277–9
    (*b*14.3); evolution in risk assessment
    286–7 (*b*14.6)
micronucleus test 110, 111, 113, 119,
    206; interpretation 177, 178
minipig: in general toxicology 81, 92; in
    reproductive toxicology 97–8, 100,
    102, 105
models 219, 233, 234, 235, 284, 288; in
    carcinogenicity 238–9, 274, 277, 280;
    physiologically based pharmacokinetic
    (PBPK) 134, 217, 235–8, 287; *see also*
    computer models
monkey: *see* non-human primate
mouse: in genotoxicity 112, 113, 117,
    119; *see also* rodents
mouse coat colour spot test 112
mouse ear swelling test (MEST) 43, 138
mouse lymphoma L5178Y TK± assay
    110–14, 206; interpretation 178
MTD: *see* maximum tolerated dose
mushrooms 2, 8, 208; carcinogenicity 3,
    7, 29–30 (*b*1.2), 197–8, 230
mutagenicity: *see* genotoxicity

National Toxicology Programme (NTP)
    121
natural chemicals 6, 230 (*b*11.4);
    medicines and remedies 9–10 (*b*1.1);
    versus synthetic 11–13
necrosis 9, 14, 15, 17, 20, 24, 90, 138,
    170, 172, 218
neurotoxicity 91, 210
nickel 261; monitoring 268; refining,
    workforce precautions 271
no observed adverse effect level
    (NOAEL) 166–7, 264, 302; in
    calculation of exposure limits 247–8,
    251, 254–9
no observed effect level (NOEL) 166–7,

302; in calculation of exposure limits
247–9, 251, 254–9
non-human primate 42, 57, 68, 204, 292;
in general toxicology 81–2, 87, 92, 94,
173; in reproductive toxicology 97–8,
105
normal distribution 6, 35–6 (f2.1), 159,
238
normal range 42, 166, 169; defining 47–8

occupation and risk 220–5, 232, 266
occupational disease 260–1, 266, 271
occupational exposure bands 253, 258
occupational exposure limits: see exposure
limits
Occupational Safety and Health
Administration (OSHA) 253, 261, 287
occupational toxicology 22, 58;
interpretation 185–9 (t9.11)
octanol–water partition coefficient: see
log P
OECD guidelines 144, 146, 283, 298
organ weights 83, 87–8, 99
organic foods 231
organophosphate 92, 188, 206, 213, 242,
264; and enzyme aging 18, 206;
insecticides 4, 18, 221; see also
cholinesterase inhibition

paracetamol (acetaminophen) 3, 4, 6,
15–16, 21, 22, 24, 177, 198, 301;
prediction of toxicity 218 (b10.3)
paraquat 23–6, 92; mechanism of toxicity
19
pathology: morphological 47, 130, 172,
173–4, 181, 182
peregrine falcon 142, 147
peri- and post-natal development:
generally 95, 100, 202; studies 82,
101–3, 104–5
permissible exposure limits 253; see also
exposure limits
peroxisome proliferation 131, 171, 181,
196, 302; specificity in rodents 9, 189,
204, 275
peroxisome proliferators 87, 127–8, 180,
199, 277
personal protection equipment (PPE)
261, 264, 266, 267 (b13.1), 268, 269
pharmacogenomics 217
pharmacokinetics 64, 65, 67, 80, 82, 119,
124, 180, 181, 190, 199, 205, 302; and

risk 236, 252, 263, 265, 274, 277;
prediction 134
phenytoin 4, 13, 21, 23, 303
photocarcinogenicity studies 123–4, 180
phototoxicity 8, 22, 136
physicochemical properties: see test
substance
physiologically based pharmacokinetic
models (PBPK) see models
pollution 3, 141–2, 147, 183, 184, 223,
280–1, 284; see also environmental
toxicology
polymorphism (genetic or metabolic) 21,
171, 199, 217, 221, 242, 243, 266
post-mortem examinations 84, 87–8, 101,
172
potatoes 192, 230, 286; genetically
modified 12, 45, 191–4, 225; sweet 20
PPE: see personal protection equipment
predicted environmental exposure (PEC):
see environmental toxicology
predicted no effect concentration
(PNEC): see environmental
toxicology
proteomics 20, 74, 75, 132, 133, 279, 296

Quantitative Structure Activity
Relationship (QSAR) 126, 210, 216
QT interval 56, 78, 168, 171

3 Rs: see reduction, refinement,
replacement
rabbit 4, 31, 52, 58, 62, 78; in general
toxicology 81–2, 92; in irritation
studies 137–9; in reproductive
toxicology 48, 97–8, 100–2, 104, 105,
176
rat: see rodents
receptors in toxicity 5, 11, 14, 17–18, 60,
131, 165, 193, 214; interspecies
differences 171, 247
recovery: see reversibility
reduction, refinement, replacement (3Rs)
31, 58, 67, 292, 294
renal toxicity 21, 56, 73, 153, 169, 170,
199; markers 173
reproductive toxicology 95–106;
alternative test systems 99;
interpetation (t9.6); parameters
measured 103 (t5.5), 174–5
respiratory toxicology 92
reversibility (irreversibility), 17–18, 23,

24–5, 191, 193, 280; in general
    toxicology 83, 84, 89–90, 94, 103; in
    hazard prediction 202, 204, 218; in
    interpretation 157, 174; in risk
    assessment 226, 244, 247–8, 250, 254,
    262, 265
ricin 18
risk: acceptability 226–7, 228, 233, 243,
    248, 251, 256, 257, 259, 279, 281,
    285, 289; and natural chemicals
    229–31; versus hazard 196
risk management 219, 220, 222, 233, 250,
    290; international 284–5 (b 14.5);
    workplace 264–7 (b13.1), 268
rodents: fertility 105; in carcinogenicity
    121–3; in general toxicology 81, 83,
    84; in genotoxicity 112, 113, 117,
    119; in reproductive toxicology 97–8,
    100–1, 102, 104
route of administration (dosing or
    exposure) 4–5, 61–4, 92, 111, 117, 123,
    156, 171; in risk assessment 245, 262
route of exposure: see route of
    administration

S-9 mix 109–10, 111, 114, 115, 166, 178,
    207
safety factors 243–51; and hazard
    weighting 251; choosing 250–1
    (b12.3); rationale 251–2
safety margins: see margin of safety
Salmonella typhimurium 38, 51, 108;
    strains 110, 113–14
sensitisation: allergic 136; allergic, in
    guinea pigs 137, 138; allergic, in mice
    137; see also irritation
sighting study: see dose range-finding
significance (biological, statistical,
    toxicological) 157–8, 167, 168, 186
single cell gel electrophoresis assay: see
    comet assay
sister chromatid exchange (SCE) 116,
    117, 168
statistics 156–61; statistical process
    158–61 (f9.1)
stress 22, 52, 91, 129, 174, 292; effects on
    test system 38–40, 45, 68, 93–4, 119,
    176; in interpretation 154, 171, 178
structure activity relationship 208; see
    also QSAR
Syrian hamster embryo (SHE) cell
    transformation assay 133

target organ toxicity 18, 170, 172, 173,
    248, 262; expression of toxicity 22–3;
    determinants 23–7; factors 23 (t1.3)
TCDD see tetrachlorodibenzo-p-dioxin
telemetry 38, 40, 51, 68, 85, 93, 171
test concentrations: see dose levels
test substance 60–1; form 70–1, 94, 201,
    204, 234, 242, 243–5, 258; impurities
    60; physicochemical characteristics
    61, 140, 143, 228, 246; solvents
    (residual) 60
tetrachlorodibenzo-p-dioxin (TCDD) 3,
    23, 26, 60, 179, 198, 203, 281, 284,
    286; acute toxicity 4
tetrodotoxin 5, 18
thalidomide 16, 34, 35, 56–7, 96, 148,
    197, 290, 292; influence on test
    system choice 97; occupational
    exposure limit 255–6
threshold limit value 253
thresholds 75, 158, 168, 255, 264; of
    toxicity 163, 165, 176, 178, 182, 188,
    204, 206–7, 236, 244, 246–7, 265; in
    carcinogenicity 271, 274–6; storage
    169; response 177
thyroid 127, 132, 133, 170; change and
    ciprofibrate 189–90; hormones 23, 26;
    thyroid stimulating hormone (TSH) 26
time weighted average (TWA) 253, 278,
    287, 303; see also exposure limits
tolerable daily intake 253, 303; see also
    exposure limits
toxic change: cellular basis and
    consequences 16–20
toxicokinetics 67, 68, 93–4, 180, 182,
    202, 250, 252, 303; see also
    pharmacokinetics
toxicology in silico 74–7; see also computer
    models
transgenic 12; animals 38, 64, 117, 127
    (b6.2), 179, 204, 291, 293, 294;
    studies in transgenic animals 122,
    127–8 (t6.4)
troubleshooting: dose range-finding 70
    (b3.2); general toxicology 171(t9.4);
    genotoxicity 178 (t9.7); reproductive
    toxicity 176 (t9.5)
tryptophan 60, 162; in genotoxicity
    112–14

unscheduled DNA synthesis (UDS) 66,
    109, 110, 113, 115, 116, 118, 177, 178

urinalysis 87, 172

validation 59, 117, 295; computer models
    215; methods *in vitro* 73–4, 78, 112,
    292; test system 65
vehicles (as test substance carriers) 52,
    67–8, 93, 94, 156, 162, 165, 206;

choice 61–4, 92; inappropriate 98,
    105, 176; *see also* formulation
vinyl chloride 22, 35, 148, 149, 185, 222,
    273
vitamin A 7, 8, 97, 167

workforce diversity 266–7